GENE EXPRESSION IN MUSCLE

ADVANCES IN EXPERIMENTAL MEDICINE AND BIOLOGY

Recent Volumes in this Series

Volume 175
NEUROTRANSMITTER RECEPTORS: Mechanisms of Action and Regulation
Edited by Shozo Kito, Tomio Segawa, Kinya Kuriyama, Henry I. Yamamura, and Richard W. Olsen

Volume 176
HUMAN TROPHOBLAST NEOPLASMS
Edited by Roland A. Pattillo and Robert O. Hussa

Volume 177
NUTRITIONAL AND TOXICOLOGICAL ASPECTS OF FOOD SAFETY
Edited by Mendel Friedman

Volume 178
PHOSPHATE AND MINERAL METABOLISM
Edited by Shaul G. Massry, Giuseppe Maschio, and Eberhard Ritz

Volume 179
PROTEINS INVOLVED IN DNA REPLICATION
Edited by Ulrich Hübscher and Silvio Spadari

Volume 180
OXYGEN TRANSPORT TO TISSUE – VI
Edited by Duane Bruley, Haim I. Bicher, and Daniel Reneau

Volume 181
GENE EXPRESSION AND CELL-CELL INTERACTIONS IN THE DEVELOPING NERVOUS SYSTEM
Edited by Jean M. Lauder and Phillip G. Nelson

Volume 182
GENE EXPRESSION IN MUSCLE
Edited by Richard C. Strohman and Stewart Wolf

A Continuation Order Plan is available for this series. A continuation order will bring delivery of each new volume immediately upon publication. Volumes are billed only upon actual shipment. For further information please contact the publisher.

GENE EXPRESSION IN MUSCLE

Edited by

Richard C. Strohman

University of California
Berkeley, California

and

Stewart Wolf

Totts Gap Medical Research Laboratories
Bangor, Pennsylvania, and
Temple University
Philadelphia, Pennsylvania

PLENUM PRESS • NEW YORK AND LONDON

Library of Congress Cataloging in Publication Data

Totts Gap Colloquium on Gene Expression in Muscle (1983: Bangor, Pa.)
Gene expression in muscle.

(Advances in experimental medicine and biology; v. 182)
"Proceedings of the Totts Gap Colloquium on Gene Expression in Muscle, held October 12–14, 1983, in Bangor, Pennsylvania, under the sponsorship of the Muscular Dystrophy Association"—T.p. verso.
Bibliography: p.
Includes index.
1. Muscular dystrophy in children—Genetic aspects—Congresses. 2. Gene expression—Congresses. 3. X chromosome—Abnormalities—Congresses. I. Strohman, Richard C. II. Wolf, Stewart, 1914- . III. Muscular Dystrophy Association. IV. Title. V. Series. [DNLM: 1. Gene Expression Regulation—congresses. 2. Genetic Marker—congresses. 3. Muscles—embryology—congresses. 4. Muscular Dystrophy—familial & genetic—congresses. W1 AD559 v.182/WE 559 T7212g 1983]
RJ482.D9T68 1983 618.92′74 84-26468

DOI 10.1007/978-1-4684-4907-5

Proceedings of the Totts Gap Colloquium on Gene Expression in Muscle,
held October 12–14, 1983, in Bangor, Pennsylvania,
under the sponsorship of the Muscular Dystrophy Association

MyCopy version of the original edition 1985

A Division of Plenum Publishing Corporation
233 Spring Street, New York, N.Y. 10013

PREFACE

This volume contains the edited transcript of an interdisciplinary colloquium held at Totts Gap Medical Research Laboratories, Bangor, Pennsylvania on October 12-14, 1983 under the sponsorship of the Muscular Dystrophy Association.

The aim was to illuminate the pathogenic mechanism of Duchenne Muscular Dystrophy through a synthesis of available data on gene expression in muscle. In the informal give and take of the colloquium, the participants found themselves engaged in mutual education and enlightenment as they attempted to put together what is known and to highlight what is not known about the subject.

Significant research into muscle as a tissue and muscle disease began only about 50 years ago although the description of muscular dystrophy by Guillaume Benjamin Amand Duchenne de Boulogne had been published in 1862. By 1943 it was clear that Duchenne muscular dystrophy was an X-linked genetic disorder. Up to the present, however, the offending gene has not been identified although its location on the short arm of the X chromosome has been approximately determined. The gene product associated with the initial disturbance in skeletal muscle has also remained elusive up to now. Moreover, investigations into the mechanisms of the muscle degeneration have been hampered by ignorance of the fundamental phenotypic expression of the genetic disorder. The pathological picture of muscle degeneration with fat and collagen replacement of muscle cells is familiar, but as yet there has been no clear identification of the initial lesion. It has not even been established whether the basic disturbance is impaired control of muscle growth, accelerated catabolism in muscle cells, or defective structural or contractile protein synthesis. Most investigators believe that the flagrant morphologic changes seen in muscle biopsies of even early cases of dystrophy are secondary to a more unitary and fundamental disorder of gene expression. It is known that approximately 1/3 of cases of Duchenne Muscular Dystrophy are the result of a new mutation, presumably in the grandparents, that is passed along to the patient's mother. This high rate of mutation encourages the speculation that the disorder involves a single gene. Although the clearest phenotypic marker, increased serum concentration of creatine kinase, is usually detectable at birth and often in the amniotic fluid of the fetus, morphologic changes in muscle have not been detected prior to the onset of symptoms at age 2-4.

The elusiveness of the initial lesion in vivo has led investigators to seek it in cultures of developing muscle cells. Work with these cultures has uncovered much knowledge of myoblast differentiation and muscle cell maturation but has shown the process to be unexpectedly complex. Although gene expression in muscle proteins has been observed to vary from the embryonic state to the neonatal and to the adult form, the morphological characteristics of embryonic fibers are indistinguishable from their neonatal and adult counterparts. Nevertheless, the different muscle protein isoforms must represent the expression of different genes or at least different gene transcript processing for some proteins.

The pertinent data and interpretations from a variety of approaches to these problems have been arranged in the following chapters in what we hope is a logical sequence.

The editors acknowledge with thanks the invaluable assistance of Joy Colarusso Lowe, who with skill, patience and precision, produced the manuscript for publication.

Richard Strohman
Stewart Wolf

CONTENTS

PART I

BACKGROUND

CHAPTER 1: CLINICAL PERSPECTIVE: PHENOTYPIC EXPRESSION IN MUSCULAR DYSTROPHY

Lewis P. Rowland

Department of Neurology
Columbia University, College of Physicians and Surgeons
New York, NY

My assignment is to introduce molecular biologists and developmental biologists to the clinical concept of muscular dystrophy, and to provide a brief summary of previous studies of possibly significant primary gene expression in these inherited diseases of muscle.

The failure thus far to discover an abnormal gene produce in these diseases stems from the difficulty of identifying the initial disturbance in a cascade of effects leading to almost total degeneration of muscle. Nevertheless, there is some information and I shall try to review the essentials. There have been several reviews and conferences on related topics in the past decade (1-6).

Muscle weakness can arise from a disturbance in the motor nerve, the peripheral nerve, or from muscle itself. The idea that separate diseases can affect primarily one of these three anatomic structures was first suggested by neuropathologists of the 19th century. Assignment of the source of the trouble is accomplished through clinical neurologic examination; electromyography and measurement of nerve conduction velocity; morphologic study of muscle biopsy; and biochemical study of blood and muscle. When it is determined that the patient's symptoms are due to dysfunction of muscle in the absence of clinical or laboratory evidence of altered neural function, the disorder is classified as a myopathy.

A muscular dystrophy is a myopathy with four special characteristics: (1) It is inherited. (2) Symptoms consist solely or primarily of weakness. (3) The weakness is progressive. (4)

The morphologic changes imply degeneration and regeneration of muscle, with no evidence of abnormal storage of a metabolic product within muscle fibers (although fat and connective tissue accumulate to replace the degenerated muscle).

Not all inherited myopathies are classified as muscular dystrophies. For instance, some heritable myopathies are manifest by myoglobinuria (appearance of the muscle pigment in the urine) and there may not be any muscle weakness between attacks of myoglobinuria. Other disorders are manifest by myotonia, without weakness, and some by symptoms similar to cramps. Although inherited, these conditions are not called dystrophies. In other conditions, there is weakness but, unlike the dystrophies, the weakness does not become progressively more severe; instead the weakness may be episodic and occur in attacks, as in familial periodic paralysis, or the weakness may be fixed, never getting worse, as in some congenital myopathies. Finally, there are conditions that may resemble muscular dystrophies clinically but differ because there is abnormal storage of lipid or glycogen within the muscle fibers. These and other closely related metabolic myopathies will be reviewed later in this volume by Miranda.

Within the category of muscular dystrophy there are many different diseases that can be differentiated on clinical and genetic grounds. To take just two examples (Table 1), the Duchenne and facioscapulohumeral (FSH) types differ in pattern of inheritance (expression in boys alone or both sexes); age at onset; first symptoms in pelvic girdle or shoulder girdle muscles; whether the face is affected; presence of pseudohypertrophy; rate of progression and ultimate effect on life expectancy; serum content of sarcoplasmic enzymes; and severity of necrosis and regeneration in muscle. Limb-girdle dystrophy, probably heterogeneous, differs from both Duchenne and FSH. These clinical and biologic differences all imply different abnormalities of different genes and different gene products. Duchenne dystrophy itself provides little evidence of heterogeneity; within limits of the rate of progression, the clinical picture is homogeneous. Attempts to identify subtypes by the association with mental retardation have not, to my mind, been successful because there is no uniform association with retardation within families and because the retardation, unlike the myopathy, is not progressive.

On the other hand, Becker dystrophy has always seemed to clinicians as though it ought to be allelic with Duchenne dystrophy because it is similar in all respects except for the age at onset and rate of progression. In contrast to Duchenne dystrophy, almost all boys with Becker dystrophy are still walking by age 12 and they may live long after age 30. Evidence from molecular genetics suggests that the two disorders are, in fact, allelic (7).

TABLE 1

Classification of Muscular Dystrophies

Genetics	Duchenne X-Linked	FSH Autosomal Dominant	Limb-Girdle Autosomal Recessive
Girls Affected	No	Yes	Yes
Onset of Symptoms	Before age 5	Adolescence	Adolescence
Initial Symptoms	Legs	Arms, Face	Either
Face Affected	No	Yes	Maybe
Hypertrophy	Yes	No	Rare
Disability	Adolescence	Variable, May be Asymptomatic	Either
Age at Death	20-30	After 60	Either
CK (Normal, 1-50)	5,000	75-500	75-5,000

Any theory of Duchenne dystrophy must explain three fundamental characteristics: progressively more severe weakness; progressive degeneration and disappearance of skeletal muscle; and increased serum activity of sarcoplasmic enzymes.

Affected boys can be recognized clinically as soon as they begin to walk. At first they can walk, with increasing difficulty. Usually between the ages of 9 and 12, they stop walking. By age 21, they are virtually paralyzed from the neck down; breathing becomes restricted and they become susceptible to pulmonary infections. These clinical changes parallel progressive loss of muscle because regeneration cannot keep pace with degeneration; at the end, skeletal muscle has virtually disappeared and there is only fat and connective tissue where there should be muscle fibers.

DR. STROHMAN: Are there any hints we could get about the early stages? Are some muscles particularly affected in the early stages? Is there a sequence?

Distribution of Cellular Changes & Theories of Pathogenesis

DR. ROWLAND: There is no distinction on the basis of muscle fiber-types. Human muscles are almost all mixed with respect to histologic fiber-type and all fiber-types are affected by the dystrophic process. Muscles of the pelvic girdle are affected first in Duchenne dystrophy, and other muscles are affected first in FSH dystrophy. Similarly, the face is always affected in FSH but never (except slightly and terminally) in Duchenne dystrophy. These differences are unexplained. Also, proximal limb muscles are affected first and more severely than distal muscles. In almost all muscular dystrophies the patients may have trouble running or climbing stairs because they cannot lift the legs adequately but movements about the ankles are not limited, or they may have trouble raising their arms when the hands are still strong. However, there are exceptions because there are also some "distal myopathies." Duchenne himself blamed the predilection for proximal muscles on some kind of embryonal distinction between proximal and distal muscles but no one has been able to advance a coherent molecular explanation for these differences. Ultimately, all limb and trunk muscles are affected.

Histologically, the dystrophic process is characterized by evidence of degeneration and regeneration of muscle fibers in apparently random fashion. Sometimes fibers are affected in groups suggesting that the pattern might imply micro-infarcts but several studies of the micro-circulation of Duchenne muscle have failed to unveil any consistent abnormality. More characteristic are so-called "opaque" fibers that are the site of shortened sarcomeres, which may be important in necrosis as discussed later. The appearance of fat and connective tissue is thought to be a reaction to the degeneration but some investigators believe that the entire disorder could be due to an abnormality of connective tissue that is literally out of control, proliferating and choking muscle fibers. Hypertrophy of some muscle fibers is another Duchenne characteristic that has to be explained. Again, there is no accepted theory for these changes.

The third characteristic, high serum concentrations of creatine kinase and other sarcoplasmic enzymes has given rise to the "membrane theory" of Duchenne dystrophy, which can be stated as follows (4).

"The genetic fault of Duchenne dystrophy affects an enzyme or structural protein that is absent, decreased in amount or rendered functionally abnormal because of an altered amino acid sequence. The nature of the presumed abnormality of composition is not known, it could affect a structural protein or an enzyme of the membrane, or an abnormal enzyme function may lead to abnormal placement of lipids, proteins or glycoconjugates in the membrane. Whatever its nature, the membrane abnormality in turn, causes the symptomatic weakness and progressive degeneration of muscle cells."

The serum enzyme abnormality was the first evidence of altered membrane function and it is still the most persuasive evidence that the primary fault affects surface membranes. But high serum enzyme activity found is so consistent that it can now be considered a defining characteristic of the disease. If a young boy had symptoms and signs that suggested Duchenne dystrophy but the serum enzyme levels were normal, it would not be possible to make the diagnosis of Duchenne dystrophy; some other disease would have to be identified.

The Membrane Theory

Therefore, any theory of the disease must explain the serum enzyme abnormality. For reasons that have been discussed elsewhere (4-6), the circulating enzyme molecules are thought to have originated in muscle; it is believed that the enzymes leak from muscle, that there is abnormally increased efflux from muscle. Two theories have been advanced to explain the abnormal efflux:

1) There are holes or physical interruptions of the surface membrane and the enzyme molecules escape through these holes. At the Mayo Clinic, B. Mokri and A.G. Engel (8) provided evidence of these lesions, which they called "delta lesions." The holes could be part of the dystrophic process itself or could be due to an abnormal composition of the membrane that makes it more fragile.

2) In the other theory, physical holes that can be seen with the electron microscope are not necessarily the source of enzyme leakage. There could be an alteration of the basic functions of a cell membrane that maintain the differences in composition of intra- and extra-cellular fluids. If this function fails, soluble intracellular enzymes could escape to extracellular spaces.

These two theories are not mutually exclusive; an altered membrane might function abnormally at first and might be expressed by increased propensity to physical interruptions.

Physical evidence of altered surface membranes in Duchenne dystrophy has been provided by the freeze-fracture studies of Schotland, Bonilla and their colleagues at the University of Pennsylvania (9). They have found abnormal patterns of intramembranous particles, orthogonal arrays, caveolae, cholesterol and concanavalin A binding sites. These ultrastructural abnormalities are of great interest and are consistent with the membrane theory but they do not provide a clue to the genetic fault and there have been few studies of the biochemistry of isolated membranes.

Two integral proteins of muscle surface membranes - $(Na^+ + K^+)$-ATPase and adenylate cyclase - have shown abnormal responses to biochemical controls. That is, the ATPase is not inhibited by ouabain (as the normal enzyme is) and the cyclase is not stimulated by catecholamines as the normal enzyme is. However, these reported abnormalities both require confirmation and, in any case, they are thought to be secondary abnormalities, due to some other alteration of the membrane that should provide the normal environment of enzymatic activity. Studies of the structure and function of cell membranes with special reference to muscular dystrophy have been reviewed in the published proceedings of another colloquium (10) other theories of the pathogenesis of Duchenne muscular dystrophy, none of which have obtained strong support from experimental studies, stem from indications of abnormalities in structural or contractile proteins (11-19).

Electrophoretic studies of contractile proteins seem to have started in our laboratory (17), very few studies followed until the introduction of two-dimensional gels (18-19).

In 1981 Fitzsimons and Hoh (20) reported electrophoretic evidence of fetal forms of myosin light chains in Duchenne dystrophy (which they attributed to immature regenerating fibers). They found similar patterns in an entirely different disorder, a neurogenic disease of motor neurons called Werdnig-Hoffmann disease or infantile spinal muscular atrophy. In that condition they attributed the persistence of fetal forms of myosin light chains to the lack of innervation, which might be necessary for the maturation of developing muscle.

In another study, at the University of Tokyo, Takagi and ɔnaka (21) found a peculiar population of fibers in Duchenne ıscle. In normal muscle, they could define fast and slow fibers ı the basis of physiologic responses to strontium. In Duchenne ıscle, some fibers gave intermediate values that were not seen in ɔrmal muscle. They thought these intermediate fibers might be ɜtal-type fibers which could have persisted because a state of rrested development or because of the abundance of regenerating ibers.

One other physiologic study is worth mentioning although it was not carried out directly on human muscle. As we shall discuss shortly, one of the major theories to account for the necrosis of Duchenne muscle is that calcium enters the muscle cell in abnormal amounts (another measure of the abnormality of cell permeability). High intracellular concentrations of calcium might also affect the contractility of muscle. Therefore it was of interest when Takamori et al (22) reported that the physiologic properties of mammalian muscle treated with the calcium ionophore (A23187) differed from those of human dystrophic muscle.

In summary, while there is still no convincing evidence that a mutant form of contractile protein is the altered gene product in Duchenne dystrophy or any other form of muscular dystrophy, human or veterinary, continued study is warranted with newer techniques including in vitro culture of muscle cells.

Sarcoplasmic Reticulum

Another major area of study has been the sarcoplasmic reticulum (SR). Unlike many of the other laboratory studies in Duchenne dystrophy that have tended to give discordant results, there has been consistency of the results in five different studies of SR (13, 23-26). Both the initial rate of calcium-uptake and the total calcium-uptake are less than controls. There has been inconsistency, however, about the magnesium-ATPase, which was high in one study, low in another and normal in two. Samaha and Congedo (27) thought they could subdivide Duchenne cases on the basis of SR abnormality.

Despite this implication of biologic abnormality of SR, there is nothing in the clinical manifestations of Duchenne dystrophy that might suggest a primary (or secondary) disorder of relaxation of muscle. Other explanations were therefore sought by Takagi et al (25) who found that the lipid composition of SR membranes from Duchenne muscle differed from normal. They then analyzed the lipid composition of a membrane preparation that started with normal fat and connective tissue (but not muscle) and followed the same method they had used to prepare SR membranes. Making reasonable assumptions about the amount of contamination of the Duchenne muscle by fat and connective tissue, the apparent abnormality of lipid composition of Duchenne SR could be attributed to the membranes from contaminating non-muscle tissues. If so, the abnormal Ca-uptake of Duchenne SR could have been due to contamination by membranes from fat and connective tissue that lacked ability to bind calcium and thereby lowered the activity of the SR preparation.

That interpretation was later reinforced by Dux and Martonosi (28) who measured a "crystallization index," the proportion of SR vesicles that contained crystalline regions in electronmicroscopic examination. That index was lower in Duchenne SR than in adult controls but on vesicles that contained Ca^{2+}-ATPase crystals, there was no significant difference in the distribution or dimensions of the crystals in normal and dystrophic muscle. They therefore attributed the lower crystallization index to contamination by fat and connective tissue membranes.

Physiologic studies of SR have been few and inconsistent. Wood et al (29) found evidence of abnormal calcium regulation in single skinned fibers but that was not confirmed by Takagi et al (30).

Several features of Duchenne muscle have immature or fetal characteristics including myosin light chain patterns (31) and contractile properties of skinned fibers (29). Others include freeze-fracture changes (9) and isozyme patterns of soluble enzymes and other biochemical changes (31). These abnormalities have suggested to some investigators that the disease might be due to an "arrest of maturation." However, Duchenne muscle is replete with regenerating fibers until the disease is advanced; the number of these regenerating fibers may be sufficient to account for the biochemical evidence of immaturity. Indeed, Miike (32) found that human fetal fibers do not stain with acridine orange, but regenerating fibers do. In Duchenne muscle, he found there was no histochemical evidence that the fibers are fetal. Therefore, it is difficult to attribute the disease to an arrest of maturation.

Maturation of Dystrophic Muscle

When the membrane theory of Duchenne dystrophy was articulated in 1976 (33), it was not clear how an abnormality of surface membranes could account for either the progressive necrosis and degeneration, or the clinical weakness. Theories to explain the necrosis have evolved in the past seven years. The dominant theory assumes that the cellular barrier to the high external concentration of calcium is impaired and more than the normal amount of calcium ion enters the cell, either because of impaired permeability functions or because of the physical holes in the delta lesions, or both. Increased amounts of calcium have been detected histochemically and by direct measurement (34). As a result of the focally increased intracellular concentration of calcium, there is focal hypercontraction of the filaments in the area (seen in cross-section as an opaque fiber). The local hypercontraction stretches and disrupts filaments at remote sites, and that disruption could be the start of necrosis, which may be repaired at first, but ultimately, degeneration exceeds the reparative capacity of the muscle.

Necrosis

Alternative theories attribute the noxious effects of increased calcium content to increased energy-dependent uptake of calcium by mitochondria (an "energy seal"), activation of proteases, or depolymerization of microtubules. This is all still theoretical but studies of the effects of calcium ionophores or injected calcium have supported the theory that high intracellular content of calcium can be noxious.

Still another factor in Duchenne necrosis could be an immunologic mechanism because Engel and Biesecker (35) found that complement activation in necrotic muscle leads to formation of the membrane attack complex.

Use of Cells other than Muscle to Study Duchenne Dystrophy

Direct biochemical study of Duchenne muscle faces two major handicaps. First, the amount of muscle that can be obtained from a child is limited (1.0 gram would be generous). Second, the muscle is contaminated by fat and connective tissue; any membrane preparation cannot be assumed to arise only from muscle because of these contaminating cells. To circumvent these problems, investigators of the past decade have used other cells, especially the erythrocyte, even though there has never been the slightest suggestion of hematologic abnormality in the disease. The results of red blood cell studies have been almost entirely inconsistent; although numerous physical and biochemical properties have been analyzed, there is not a single piece of evidence that would implicate a particular erythrocyte membrane protein as the important gene product (4,6).

Cultured muscle has also been used, but faces different problems. First, the cells are not immortal so the amount is limited. Second, cultured muscle (without innervation) does not mature, as Dr. Miranda will discuss. Third, fibroblasts are also seen in cultured muscle and it remains uncertain whether unfused cells are myoblasts or fibroblasts. So far, except for Dr. Blau's observations that will follow, no consistent abnormalities have been identified in cultured Duchenne muscle.

Dr. Miranda will discuss the possibility that failure to demonstrate abnormality in cultured muscle may be due to the persistent immaturity of these cells, and he will discuss possible solutions to that problem, because the abnormality of Duchenne dystrophy may be expressed only in mature muscle. Immortalization of Duchenne cells, or use of human-rodent hybrids to study X-linked gene products may alter the presently uncertain picture (36).

Other cells that have been used are the lymphocyte (for studies of capping as a measure of membrane fluidity) or the fibroblast. In general, these cells have also given rise to conflicting results (4,6). Within the past few months, there have been reports of increased membrane permeability of fibroblasts (37), greater susceptibility to detachment by trypsin (38), or decreased intracellular adhesiveness (39).

DR. EPSTEIN: What evidence is there of consistency among neurologists in the diagnosis of Duchenne dystrophy?

DR. ROWLAND: The agreement is very close in the case of Duchenne much more so than say, limb girdle dystrophy because there is very little heterogeneity in Duchenne dystrophy. If you take a child who has the right physical appearance and you add the serum enzyme and then you add again a pattern of X-linked recessive inheritance, you get a very stereotyped picture. It may be difficult to sort out Duchenne from Becker but the difference, essentially one of timing and severity, shows up when you are dealing with families. If you take a kid at age 5, you can not say to the parents, the kid will be off his feet by age 12 and be in a wheelchair because he may have a Becker form and he may go on longer. Becker's make up a small percentage of dystrophies.

DR. EPSTEIN: What about the boy with a high CPK and muscle weakness that comes into a rehabilitation medicine department.

DR. ROWLAND: Except for Becker which would account for 10% of the cases, 90% will be Duchenne. The only other evidence of heterogeneity is Alan Emery's attempt to segregate patients and families on the basis of associated mental retardation and I don't think that is strong evidence.

DR. EPSTEIN: What about control?

DR. ROWLAND: The control is probably aged matched controlled and that is a problem in the same muscle. It is a problem because the conventional muscle biopsy for Duchenne dystrophy for most dystrophies is quadroceps. The reason we take that is it is a nice big muscle and it is convenient. But then you have a hard time getting normal controls. We get normal controls from adults who have muscle symptoms but psychiatric disorders. We have to do a muscle biopsy to prove they don't have a muscle disease. There are not many studies of normal muscle from paid volunteers and there certainly are not many from children.

DR. BLAU: What is the source of normal control muscle samples?

DR. ROWLAND: There are two popular places to get controls of children. One is from orthopedic procedures and the other is the rectus abdominus from normal kids having appendectomies. In orthopedic operations you rarely get the belly of the quadraceps, the muscle most typically biopsied in dystrophic patients.

DR. FISCHMAN: Does Duchenne dystrophy involve muscles of the face?

DR. ROWLAND: Only terminally.

DR. WOOD: We studied sternocleidomastoid muscles where both fiber types are represented and found very little involvement in a 12 year old patient with Duchenne dystrophy. On the other hand his deltoid and biceps muscles were clearly affected.

DR. KEDES: Could the distribution of involvement be related in part to growth and hence the need to elongate? The head size certainly doesn't change much following infancy. Do head muscles grow less than limb muscles?

DR. STROHMAN: It seems to me that we really ought to know about that. Do we have any single fiber studies in the human where within the same muscle you could begin to look at whether or not one fiber is early affected and perhaps another fiber is not and you could begin to make a judgment about whether the fiber that isn't affected becomes involved later only secondarily. Would that be a good strategy to use?

DR. WOOD: The earliest age of patients contributing to fiber studies is 6 months. Histologically, Type I and Type II fast and slow fibers do not differ at that age. Both fiber types are affected in humans. Although in animal muscles with pure muscle types the fast, white glycolytic muscles are selectively involved and there is little if any degeneration in slow, red oxidative muscle groups. Most human muscles are of mixed fiber types and both are involved in the dystrophic process.

DR. HOLTZER: What about hypertrophy? Is there a systematic sequence and disappearance of hypertrophy?

DR. ROWLAND: The appearance of hypertrophy ultimately goes when everything goes. Pseudohypertrophy rather than hypertrophy is the word that has been used since the turn of the century because although the muscles look large, there is massive infiltration with fat and connective tissue. Nevertheless, one of the histologic characteristics of Duchenne muscle is that abnormally large as well as abnormally small fibers are seen under the microscope. Is it some fundamental control abnormality or is the fiber hypertrophy compensatory for adjacent fibers that are degenerating?

DR. HOLTZER: Does this fiber hypertrophy appear before degeneration, with degeneration or after degeneration?

DR. ROWLAND: The variability in muscle fiber size is found in biopsies taken in the earliest stage of the disease but there is already clinical weakness.

DR. HOLTZER: Are there any signs of degeneration in a hypertrophied fiber or is it pure hypertrophy and the next one will be clearly degenerated?

DR. WOOD: We studied single fibers from dystrophic patients and were able to distinguish functional differences between thick and thin fibers. In Duchenne dystrophy there is segmental development of morphological abnormalities as well as physiological and possibly biochemical abnormalities.

DR. FISCHMAN: In the case of cardiac hypertrophy from aortic stenosis, for example, a fiber undergoing hypertrophy can reach a certain diameter and no more before beginning to degenerate.

DR. KEDES: Does the nuclear cytoplasmic ratio stay the same when a fiber is hypertrophied, or is there a recruitment of a more nucleid rather than the same number of nuclei making a more massive protein?

DR. EASTWOOD: It is my impression that the nuclear cytoplasmic ratio is changed in hypertrophied fibers.

DR. SCHULTZ: In the compensatory hypertrophy model, the hypertrophy induced by removing one of the synergistic muscles causes an increase in satellite cell proliferation. There is an increase in nuclei.

CHAPTER 2: ONTOLOGIC PERSPECTIVE: TERMINAL DIFFERENTIATION AND MATURATION AS DIFFERENTLY REGULATED STAGES IN MUSCLE DEVELOPMENT

Richard C. Strohman* and Stewart Wolf**

*Department of Zoology, University of California
Berkeley, CA: **Totts Gap Medical Research Laboratories
Bangor, PA

Dr. Rowland has described the well defined and rather uniform phenotypic expression of Duchenne muscular dystrophy. Efforts to identify a trigger for the ineluctable sequence of degenerative changes in muscle associated with that disease have thus far been frustrated. Nevertheless, because the characteristic weakness appears only late in infancy, and for other reasons as well, a defect in the genetic regulation of muscle cell development seems likely. Recently acquired knowledge of protein synthesis and recently developed tools for the study of cellular development have opened the door to new efforts to monitor the developmental sequence from satellite cell to myotube-building myoblast and ultimately to adult mature myocyte. The presentations that follow will examine the requirements for muscle cell differentiation and maturation, the gene regulated stages of development and their possible involvement in the mechanisms of Duchenne dystrophy. The proteins of the myofibrils, myosins, actins and troponin have been and still are primary targets for study as they reflect the two distinct stages of muscle cell development, differentiation and maturation.

Gene Expression During Terminal Differentiation

During skeletal muscle terminal differentiation there is a profound shift in gene expression. After presumptive myoblasts withdraw from the cell cycle and fuse to form the embryonic muscle fiber there are large increases in, and in most cases *de novo* synthesis of, all the proteins of the myofibril (40-41). While there may be a few exceptions, there is general agreement that this shift in expression is regulated at the level of gene transcription and that the many genes involved may be coordinated in their activation (42-45).

Moreover, since terminal differentiation will occur in vitro in completely defined medium and without nerve (46) the coordination of muscle gene expression at this stage of development is assumed to reside in a program already determined earlier in the cell lineage (47). Of course, cell environments may be established that extend presumptive myoblast cell proliferation and delay and even reverse the terminal shift in gene expression (48-49), but the event itself appears to be inevitable once the myoblast has withdrawn from the cell cycle. The questions here are complex and include the following:

1. What constitutes the determination event through which the early cell becomes committed to muscle?

2. How is this commitment maintained without expression through the many divisions of the stem cell population?

3. What is the mechanism of terminal expression and its presumed coordination involving many genes that results in the formation of the embryonic muscle fiber?

Much of our workshop is concerned with this last question. As we will see, the embryonic skeletal muscle fiber is quite complex in terms not only of its presumed coordination of muscle specific genes but complex also in terms of the heterogeneity of protein isoforms expressed.

While the mechanisms of terminal myogenesis remain to be worked out, later events of fiber growth and maturation are providing still other dimensions to the question of regulated gene expression.

Gene Expression During Muscle Maturation In Vivo

For example, in the case of fast muscle, although terminal myogenesis clearly establishes functional muscle fibers, these fibers may contain both fast and slow myosin light chains (50-52) fast and slow forms of C-protein (53) embryonic or fetal and cardiac isoforms of myosin heavy chains (53-59), and cardiac forms of alpha actin (60). So the embryonic fast muscle fiber is a cell of complex gene expression in which we find fast and slow and cardiac specific gene sequences expressed along with their specified protein isoforms and together with embryonic rather than adult gene sequences for entities such as the myosin heavy chain. Clearly a great deal of regulation needs to occur as the embryonic fiber sorts itself out so that it finally expresses the genes characteristic of the stable adult state.

This transition from embryonic to adult fiber type we call maturation. The attendent regulation of gene expression from embryonic to adult isoforms is evidently without coordination.

That is, there is evidence, some of which will be discussed at this meeting, favoring a lack of temporal correlation in the appearance of the different isoforms and of their respective transcripts. Thus the embryonic isoform for one protein may persist during neonatal development much longer than the embryonic isoform for another muscle-specific protein (61). The impact of nerves and innervation on the maturational process is also in need of further definition. Nerve appears to be unnecessary for the expression of some adult isoforms (62) but appears to be critical for the expression of others (63-64). The nerve-muscle interaction is further complicated by the fact that nerve is nevertheless a powerful determinant of muscle type in the adult. Cross-innervated adult muscle will, for example, switch to the muscle type characteristic of the innervating motor neuron (65-67). The genes for fast versus slow muscle isoforms may therefore be under different controls than those genes coding for embryonic versus neonatal or adult isoforms.

Fiber Maturation *in vitro*

From the work cited above it seems that while terminal differentiation is coordinated and determined early in embryonic life, fiber maturation appears to be more stochastic and a process more open to environmental signals. Experimental evidence from *in vitro* myogenesis confirms this apparent difference. For example, as we have mentioned, terminal myogenesis will occur *in vitro* in defined medium without nerve cells. Maturation, however, as defined by the orderly replacement of embryonic by first neonatal and then by adult isoforms, is difficult to achieve in cell culture and at this time, while there has been some progress (68) the expression of a *complete* adult muscle phenotype *in vitro* has not been accomplished. Dr. Whalen as well as others here will address this issue more completely.

Instead of maturing, muscle fibers in culture appear to be stuck in an embryonic pattern of gene expression. For example, cultured rat and chicken muscle fibers express an embryonic myosin heavy chain together with embryonic patterns of tropomyosin and myosin light chains. But in addition, they also express cardiac alpha actin in the mouse as well as in the chicken (69). The appearance of cardiac alpha actin in skeletal muscle is part of an embryonic pattern of gene expression. In human muscle culture there is a coexpression of fetal together with adult myosin light chains but the nature of the overall pattern of human muscle genes expressed in culture has yet to be defined (70).

The conclusion, therefore, is that without the proper signals muscle fiber maturation does not occur in culture. Obvious signs of the dystrophic process also do not occur in culture when muscle cells from dystrophic patients are used (71). The relationship between these two observations will be discussed more fully in the next paragraphs. A large part of this meeting will dwell upon the possibility of inducing adult gene patterns in culture using nerve co-cultures, hormones, trophic factors, and electrical stimulation. A second conclusion that may be drawn now is that the mechanisms regulating gene expression during terminal differentiation may be quite different from the mechanisms regulating gene expression during fiber maturation.

Given the background cited above, we will not attempt to summarize the various contributions of the workshop from the point of view of their relationship to muscle diseases. One question squarely put to this meeting is, "What is the relationship between studies of regulated gene expression in muscle and a possible cure for muscle wasting disease?" The various contributors made it clear that there are many areas in which researchers are finding possible linkages to muscle diseases.

Relationship of Basic Research in Muscle Fiber Differentiation and Maturation to Muscle Diseases

The muscle satellite cell is a source of new muscle not only during regeneration following injury but in normal growth and maturation as well (72). It is possible that a deficiency in the satellite cell population may be involved as the primary defect in Duchenne dystrophy. This is the very provocative notion advanced by Dr. Blau and it is discussed thoroughly in her paper. Dr. Schultz provides us with some recent insights into satellite cell number in different skeletal muscles of the rat and some work from our own laboratory and Dr. Whalen will discuss the differences in gene expression of satellite cells from different muscles as they differentiate in culture.

Satellite Cells

A second area of emerging importance to muscle disease is emphasized in Dr. Hauschka's session. The role of mitogens in terminal differentiation is presumably critical in maintaining the stem line and in regulating muscle cell fusion. At the same time, we are made aware of the critical role such factors might play in muscle injury and in abnormal or deficient muscle growth. The presence of growth factors in the muscle would presumably be required to promote division of the satellite cell under appropriate conditions (injury, disease, etc.). Yet there is very little that we now know about the presence of these factors in normal or abnormal muscles. The work of Dr. Ozawa has been extremely important here and we have an extension of his findings discussed by Dr. Oh and by Dr. Matsuda.

Growth Factors

Thus, the early work on the cellular biology of the satellite cell, so elegantly announced by the studies of Dr. Mauro and the publication of the Symposium on Muscle Regeneration is continuing and is being merged with molecular studies that will hopefully produce another level of understanding of the way in which the source of new muscle is regulated both in the normal and in the diseased state.

Protein Isoform Expression

We have already mentioned the extensive work showing that many muscle proteins exist as families with the different isoforms within each family being expressed at different times during development. That is, there are isoforms that are expressed in the fetal stages, in the neonatal stages and during the adult stages of development and growth. It is possible that the gene for Duchenne or Beckers dystrophy is a member of the adult set of genes rather than of the fetal or neonatal sets. We do not yet know what the gene product is. We do however have the example from the early work of the Columbia group that relates a muscle deficiency disease to the presence of an adult rather than an embryonic protein isoform. In this disease, McArdle disease, the deficient enzyme is expressed as an adult isoform. The embryonic isoform of the same enzyme is normal. Dr. Miranda gives a thorough discussion of isoenzymes in diseased muscle in his paper.

Dr. Fischman's session discussed several key issues, the first has to do with a linkage between expression of myofibrillar protein isoforms on the one hand, and on the other, the assembly of muscle filaments. The second area has to do with the expression of the different isoforms in muscle culture and how this expression might be related to dystrophy.

A further opportunity may be present here in that the weight of the evidence from cell culture studies indicates that muscle cultured from Duchenne patients is normal (71). We also know that cultured muscle in general expresses an embryonic pattern of muscle genes. If we can identify the conditions necessary for the expression of a complete adult phenotype in culture then it is possible that we will also have identified the conditions necessary for the expression of the gene for Duchenne or Beckers dystrophy. This cell culture approach represents an attempt to identify directly the defective gene product and is complimentary to studies utilizing recombinant DNA approaches to identify the specific gene sequences involved.

Related to this problem of isoform expression and its control is the role played by hormones and stimulation by motor neurons. Drs. Hoh and Bandman provide us with a basic description of the kinds of myosin isoforms being expressed in a normal and dystrophic muscle. They present the clear suggestion that in dystrophic muscle there is at least a partial failure for the muscle to mature since there is a persistent expression of embryonic or neonatal markers.

Against this background of isoform expression in normal and diseased muscle Drs. Rubinstein and Kelly present their findings on the effects of hormones on muscle isoform expression and Dr. Pette gives us his recent information on the role of electrical stimulation in the control of muscle gene expression and isoform appearance.

A question that has been asked for years has been, "What is the function of the different protein isoforms?" Until recently there has been little if any effort made to provide an answer. In her paper, Dr. Lowey develops an analysis of the sequence alterations that appear in the different myosin heavy chain isoforms and, in addition, informs us about the enzymatic differences that are present or absent when one compares the different myosin isoenzymes. These results may have a large impact on the question of filament and myofibrillar assembly and are therefore extremely relevant to the question of structural abnormalities in diseased muscle.

Assembly of Muscle Filaments & Fibrils

Assembly was not a major topic of this workshop but it is clear that the work on isform expression is going to play an important role in future discussion on assembly. Susan Lowey's work has already been mentioned in this context. Dr. Garrels, in his paper, has identified some new actin-associated proteins using quantitative two-dimensional electrophoresis and many questions can be raised concerning their role both in assembly and in regulation of muscle activity.

Dr. Holtzer describes the effects of the tumor promoter (TPA) on fibrillar disassembly and reassembly and has begun the task of examining the mode of action of this drug in causing the disassembly of muscle fibrillar structure. These studies appear to be leading the way in understanding the relationship between cytoplasmic filament organization and myofibrillar assembly.

Dr. Epstein shows us how different myosin heavy chains are used to construct the same thick filament (hybrid filaments) in the nematode and studies like his will be critical in examining the fate of the different myosin heavy chain isoforms as the earlier fetal and neonatal types are replaced by the adult types.

Are hybrid thick filaments also formed during transitions of muscle development in vertebrates? Another question that comes up in this context is related to the sequence of synthetic events during satellite cell recruitment into growing muscle fibers.

Fibers formed from satellite cells during regeneration *in vivo* or *in vitro* recapitulate embryological development in that they synthesize embryonic and adult myosins sequentially. Do satellite cell nuclei that enter adult muscle also program the synthesis of embryonic myosin heavy chains? If so, do these embryonic heavy chains form hybrid thick filaments with existing adult heavy chains? What is the consequence for assembly in having, as has been suggested by Drs. Ho and Bandman, for dystrophic muscle a persistent expression of embryonic or neonatal myosins in a fiber surrounded by an adult environment? The answers to these questions could have an important bearing on our understanding of muscle disease.

The last session of this workshop focused on gene expression as analyzed by recombinant DNA studies. As a bridge to these studies, Dr. Blau presented her work on gene expression in muscle cell hybrids and heterokaryons. In a heterokaryon produced from the fusion of a mouse muscle cell (line) with a human amniotic cell she has demonstrated the activation of human genes for CPK and myosin light chains in the mouse muscle formed in culture. These experiments have great potential in identification of cytoplasmic factors that are required for gene activation.

Recombinant DNA Approaches

Drs. Kedes, Buckingham, Yaffe and Strehler have developed a number of cDNA probes for myosin heavy and light chains, for alpha skeletal and cardiac actin. They are able to follow changes in mRNA transcripts of these genes during development and find an amazing amount of coexpression of fetal, cardiac and adult genes during early development. In addition, Dr. Yaffe reports on the expression and regulation of cloned genes in myogenic cells and discusses possibilities for analyzing those DNA sequences that code for the regulated expression of specific structural genes during development. Both Dr. Buckingham and Dr. Yaffe and his collaborators have continued to develop chromosomal assignments for the genes coding for myofibrillar proteins. Dr. Strehler reviews the myosin heavy chain gene family and provides structural details that may also lead to the identification of DNA sequences that carry information for the regulation of tissue and stage specific expression of the different myosin heavy chain isoforms.

Finally, Dr. Kunkel reviews the work analyzing the human X chromosome and the attempts to develop useful restriction fragment length polymorphisms for the human X-linked muscular dystrophies.

In conclusion, this meeting is one which attempts to focus results of basic research on the problem of a particular set of muscle diseases. We are extremely gratified that more and more investigators are taking the opportunity to work with the interesting system that developing and maturing skeletal muscle in fact has become. And we are extremely grateful to this small but critical group of people who have come together to share and compare results.

PART II

PHENOTYPIC EXPRESSION & MOLECULAR MARKERS FOR MUSCLE DISEASES

CHAPTER 3: HEREDITARY METABOLIC MYOPATHIES

Armand F. Miranda,* Tiziana Mongini* and
Salvatore DiMauro*

*H. Houston Merritt Clinical Research Center for
Muscular Dystrophy and Related Diseases
Columbia University, New York, NY

There are nine known hereditary enzyme defects of glycogen metabolism and glycolysis affecting skeletal muscle. "Metabolic myopathie" can be classified into two main groups: 1. Deficiencies of enzymes that occur in single molecular forms which are already present in fetal tissues and continue to be synthesized throughout life. Defects of these "household enzymes" usually cause functional impairment of muscle, as well as other organs and tissues. 2. Deficiencies of enzymes that occur in multi-molecular forms in different tissues (isozymes) which normally undergo transitions during myogenesis and muscle maturation. This developmentally-regulated process involves a gradual shift from one or more isozymes present in fetal muscle, to a muscle-specific form, which persists throughout post-natal life.

Muscle-isozymes may also be present in non-muscle tissues (e.g. brain, heart) where they constitute a fraction of the total enzyme activity, the rest being due to other "non-muscle" isozymes. Deficiencies of muscle-specific isozymes may, therefore, also cause functional impairment of other tissues as well, although this is not common, because the genetic lack of muscle isozyme in non-muscle tissues is usually compensated by normal catalytic activity of the non-muscle isozymes, which are coded on different gene loci.

* Supported by Grants NS-1176 and NS-18446 from the National Institute of Neurological and Communicative Disorders and Stroke and by the Muscular Dystrophy Association, Inc.
Dr. Mongini was supported by a post-doctoral fellowship from Odine Mauriziano and U.I.L.D.M., Section of Turin, Italy.

Studies of differentiating muscle cultures from afflicted patients have led to a more complete understanding of muscle-isozyme regulation, because mutations that affect these muscle-specific isozymes are not phenotypically expressed in immature muscle. As a consequence, the full phenotypic expression of the "muscle isozyme" myopathies occurs only at more advanced stages of muscle differentiation, probably when nerve-muscle associations become established. A few genetic disorders affecting mitochondrial enzymes of lipid oxidation have also been recognized recently (73-74).

In this chapter we shall review most of the well-characterized hereditary myopathies caused by defects of enzymes of glycogen-breakdown and glycolysis (Figure 1), discuss one disorder (Mucolipidosis type II) which, unlike other known muscle enzyme deficiencies, appears to affect _immature_ rather than _mature_ muscle (75-76), and consider the potential use of nerve-muscle co-cultures as a model for studying the muscle isozyme myopathies _in vitro_.

I. Myopathies Caused by "Household" Enzyme Deficiencies

Several hereditary metabolic glycogenoses have been reproduced in muscle culture, showing reduced or absent activity of the affected enzymes and accumulation of glycogen as seen in intact muscle from patients (77-82). These were due to defects of enzymes that do not occur in multimolecular forms in different tissues, and are normally present in both immature and mature muscle.

Acid Maltase (AM: alpha glucosidase) Deficiency: AM is a lysosomal acid hydrolase that catalyzes the degradation of glycogen, acting on both alpha 1-4 and 1-6 glucosyl linkages (Figure 1) (74,83,84). AM is present in all tissues and at all stages of muscle development as a single molecular form. The gene locus for AM is on the human chromosome 17 (85-87).

Although lysosomal glycogen breakdown by AM is not directly involved in energy metabolism, this enzyme must play a crucial role in muscle since hereditary AM deficiency (AMD) causes profound generalized weakness in infants (Pompe disease) and a less severe myopathy in children and adults (88-91). Since AM occurs as a single molecular form in all tissues, AMD is a generalized disorder (74,83,84). The morphologic hallmark of the disease is the presence of numerous membrane-bounded glycogen deposits _in vivo_ and in culture (74,77,83,92). Extralysosomal glycogen, is also increased, but it may derive from the "bursting" of glycogen-laden lysosomes (74,77,83). Biochemical studies with radioactive precursors suggest that there is no detectable AM

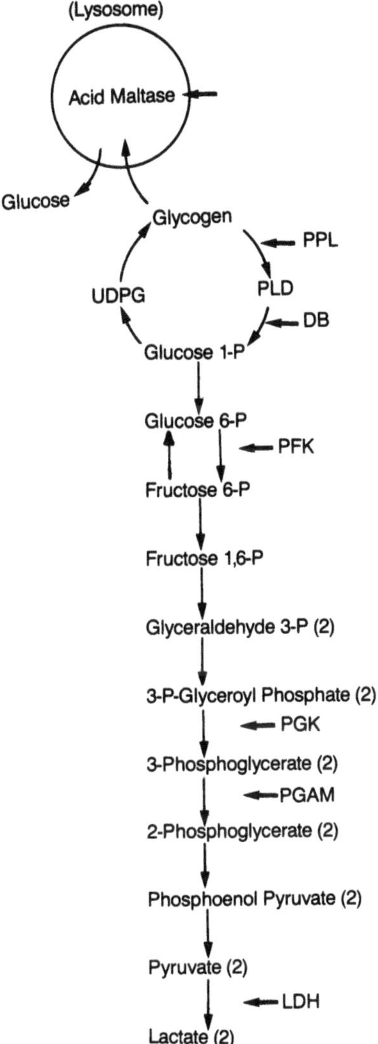

FIGURE 1: Scheme of glycogen metabolism and glycolysis. Horizontal arrows indicate the metabolic block caused by deficiencies of: Acid maltase (alpha-glucosidase), phosphorylase (PPL), glycogen debrancher enzyme (DB), phosphofructokinase (PFK), phosphoglycerate kinase (PGK), phosphoglycerate mutase (PGAM) and lactate dehydrogenase (LDH).

synthesis in cultured fibroblasts from patients with infantile AMD (92). Immunologic analysis also fails to show detectable cross-reacting AM protein in most patients (82,83,88,93,94). However, in the later-onset variants (juvenile and adult-AMD) there is some residual AM activity and presence of immunologically cross-reacting protein (82,83,88,93,95). In these forms of AMD, myopathy is the predominant clinical feature, and the disease is more benign than infantile AMD (74,91,92). This residual AM activity which can be as much as 20% of normal, probably explains the milder clinical presentation in late-onset AMD (95). These AMD variants are probably due to different mutations of the same gene locus since somatic cell hybridization of cells from patients with infantile and late-onset AMD patients does not restore AM activity (92,96). It is puzzling why the lack of lysosomal AM activity cannot be compensated by extralysosomal glycogenolytic enzymes, which do not appear to be affected in AMD.

Debrancher Enzyme (DB) Deficiency: DB catalyzes the breakdown of limit-dextrin, produced by the action of glycogen phosphorylase. DB has a dual catalytic action, involving first the transfer of maltotriosyl units from donor glycogen to acceptor glycogen, followed by the hydrolysis of alpha-1,6-glucosidic linkages (Figure 1). The "transferase" and "1,6-glucosidase" reactions can be measured separately with appropriate substrates. There is no evidence that DB exists in more than one molecular form in mammalian tissues.

DB deficiency (Cori-Forbes disease) is usually identified in childhood and causes liver symptoms, sometimes with mild cirrhosis and growth retardation. Curiously, clinical symptoms usually disappear after puberty, and some affected adults are found to be clinically "normal." The enzyme deficiency can be demonstrated in most tissues including muscle, but clinical muscle disease is relatively uncommon, usually manifesting in adult life (74,83,97, 98). The most important features in DB myopathy are weakness and wasting without myglobinuria. Some patients also have slowing of motor nerve conduction velocity. Cardiac symptoms were reported in some patients (96,97).

Since DB appears to exist as a single molecular form in all tissues, DB deficiency can be identified in cultured skin fibroblasts and in cultured muscle cells at all stages of differentiation (81,99). Enzyme activity is virtually absent in these cultured cells and there is excessive amount of glycogen which is mostly free in the cytoplasm, although some of it is contained within membrane-bounded "sacs." In the cells from patients studied *in vitro* the deficiency involved both transferase and 1,6-glucosidase functions of DB, although in a few patients only one of the two catalytic functions may be affected (91,92). DB deficiency is autosomally inherited, but the structural enzyme locus has not yet been assigned.

Phosphoglycerate Kinase (PGK) Deficiency: PGK catalyzes the formation of 3-phosphoglycerate from 3-phosphoglyceroyl phosphate (Figure 1). Two molecular forms have been described in human tissues. PGK-1, coded on the X-chromosome is present in all tissues except spermatogenic cells in which another isozyme (PGK II) is expressed (chromosomal localization is still unknown) (100). Additional molecular forms may be present, but it is not yet clear whether these are due to post-translational modifications (78-80).

Several human PGK mutations have been described some of which are clinically silent. In others, hemoloytic anemia and variable brain dysfunction are the characteristic features. In two mutant enzymes, single amino acid substitutions have been identified (78,79,100,101). A new clinical variant, characterized by exercise-induced myoglobinuria without hemolytic anemia has recently been found in a 15-year-old boy. Kinetic and electrophoretic studies indicate that this variant is different from other mutations that were described previously but amino acid sequence analysis has not yet been done (78,79).

PGK deficiency was studied in skin fibroblasts and skeletal muscle in vitro and the enzyme defect can be demonstrated in both types of cultures. However, there is no abnormal glycogen in cultured muscle, just as no glycogen storage was seen in the patient's muscle biopsy (80). This may be attributed to the presence of some residual activity that may be sufficient for normal or near normal glycogen breakdown. SV40-transformed fibroblasts from the patient showed surprisingly normal or near normal PGK activity as compared with the non-transformed skin fibroblasts. In addition, acrylamide gel electrophoresis showed the appearance of a second band of PGK, that was not seen in electropherograms from intact muscle or untransformed fibroblasts. It is not yet known whether this "new" PGK represents a post-transational modification. However, it seems unlikely that this novel PGK band is a product of a mutant gene, because its appearance accompanied the normalization or near-normalization of enzyme levels in SV40 transformed fibroblasts from the patient (78).

Cellulose acetate electropherograms of human fetal muscle analyzed at different gestational stages (16-24 weeks), showed no distinct fetal and adult isozymes of PGK. However, this observation should be confirmed, using more sensitive techniques and should include analysis of earlier fetal stages (89).

Of the nine known hereditary metabolic myopathies affecting enzymes of glycogen degradation and glycolysis, at least four are due to deficiencies of muscle-specific isozymes. The affected enzymes are: phosphorylase, phosphofructokinase, phosphoglycerate mutase and lactate dehydrogenase (Figure 1). The converse situation, myopathies caused by deficiencies of isozymes that are abundant in fetal muscle and low or absent in adult muscle, has not yet been discovered. LDH-H deficiency has been reported, but there was no evidence of myopathy (102). There is, however, one type of mucolipidosis (type II; I-cell disease) that appears to affect muscle, only at early stages of differentiation (75,76).

II. Myopathies Caused by Muscle-Specific Enzyme Deficiencies

Phosphorylase (PPL) Deficiency: PPL catalyzes the first step in glycogen breakdown by removing alpha-1-4-glycosyl residues from the peripheral branches of glycogen: the products of this reaction are glucose-1-phosphate and limit-dextrin (Figure 1). In mammalian tissues, including humans, PPL occurs in at least three tissue-specific forms (liver type; brain type; muscle type) that are under separate genetic control (103). During myogenesis, a non-muscle ("brain"-type PPL) isozyme is gradually replaced by the muscle-specific form. At intermediate stages of muscle differentiation, three PPL isozymes can be demonstrated by histochemical staining or autoradiography of electropherograms: a slow-migrating band is muscle PPL, made up of four identical subunits, a faster "brain type" homotetramer and an intermediate hybrid isozyme consisting of two subunits each of muscle and "brain" isozyme (104-107). While in normal mature skeletal muscle, only the muscle specific isozyme is expressed, in cardiac muscle all three PPL forms are present throughout adult life, and the electrophoretic pattern is similar to that of fetal skeletal muscle at an intermediate stage of differentiation (Figure 2) (105,107,108,109). Muscle PPL isozyme is also present in brain (about 25% of total activity), the remaining PPL activity being due to "brain PPL" (110).

Myophosphorylase deficiency (McArdle disease), was the first genetic defect of glycogen metabolism to be described in 1961 (111) and the enzyme defect was documented several years later (112,113). In its "typical" form, myophosphorylase deficiency presents in adolescence or early adulthood with muscle pain, cramps and sometimes myoglobinuria, ususally following brief intense exercise, when glycogen is the main source of muscle energy (74-83). A severe, rapidly fatal form of McArdle disease has been described and other clinical variants characterized by weakness of early onset (114) or, more commonly, late onset have also been described (92,96). The molecular basis for this clinical heterogeneity has not yet been explained.

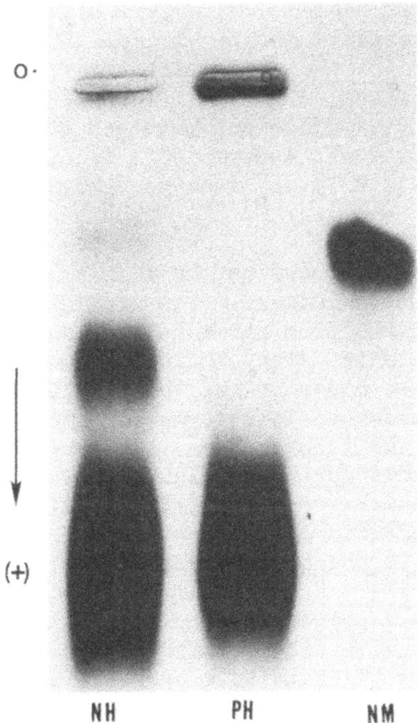

FIGURE 2: Native acrylamide slab gel electrophoresis of homogenates of normal heart (NH), heart from a patient with fetal, infantile myophosphorylase deficiency (PH)and normal muscle (NM). The gel was overloaded to reveal minor bands, and stained to reveal phosphorylase isozyme activities. (Reproduced with publisher's permission: Neurology 29:1539, 1979. Harcourt Brace Javanovich, Inc.)

In heart muscle, about 40% of the total PPL activity can be inhibited by anti-muscle isozyme antibody, the rest being represented by a different isozyme which is unaffected in McArdle disease (104,109,110). Direct evidence for this came from studies of cardiac muscle obtained at autopsy from a baby with the severe fatal variant of McArdle disease (115). Immunological and electrophoretic analysis of the patient's heart muscle showed the presence of a single, more anodic PPL isozyme, while both the muscle isozyme and the hybrid form were absent (Figure 2) (116). Dissociation and reassociation studies of the subunits from normal adult skeletal muscle PPL and PPL from the patient's heart showed that the intermediate PPL band is, indeed a hybrid of the two isozymes, as previously demonstrated in studies of PPL purified from rabbit tissues (109,116). Although muscle-PPL was absent in the patient's heart, there was no clinical evidence of cardiac dysfunction in this baby or in other patients with typical McArdle disease. This suggests that the residual cardiac isozyme is functionally adequate in patients with myophosphorylase deficiency.

In liver tissue, a different glycogen PPL isozyme is present. In patients with liver PPL isozyme deficiency, muscle is unaffected suggesting that it is a "true" isozyme, coded on a separate gene locus.

PPL deficiency was the first hereditary metabolic myopathy to be studied in muscle culture. The findings were quite surprising since cultured myotubes from patients showed a normal histochemical reaction and regenerating areas in intact muscle from the same patients also stained normally for PPL (117). Reappearance of PPL activity was confirmed in more recent biochemical studies (104,106,118). In two laboratories, the PPL activity in cultured myotubes (104,106) did not react with anti-muscle-PPL antibody and, by electrophresis, did not co-migrate with adult muscle PPL: instead, it migrated with one of the bands found in fetal muscle, probably identical to the brain isozyme (92,104,119).

Since there is no glycogen accumulation in McArdle muscle cultures, the non-muscle PPL isozyme in cultured myotubes from patients is probably adequate to support normal glycogen degradation.

Although only "brain" PPL can be demonstrated in electropherograms of normal muscle cultures stained by conventional histochemical technique, more sensitive methods, such as immunocytochemistry and autoradiography of the acrylamide gels show small amounts of muscle PPL isozyme (120). In fact, initiation of muscle PPL activity in muscle cultures is not nerve-dependent, since trace amounts of muscle-PPL antigen are present in cultured myotubes grown in complete absence of nervous tissue or whole embryo extract (120). This suggests that nerve influences are not required for initiation of muscle PPL synthesis, but further maturation of the muscle PPL isozyme pattern cannot occur in the absence of nerve.

Several studies remain to be done. First, long-term nerve-muscle co-cultures might establish conclusively whether nerve factors are required for muscle PPL isozyme maturation. Secondly, although McArdle disease is attributed to a mutation of the structural gene of the muscle-PPL isozyme subunit, this has not yet been proven. Supportive evidence for this hypothesis may come from the demonstration that muscle PPL fails to appear in innervated muscle cultures from affected patients. Conclusive evidence of a structural gene mutation in McArdle disease can be obtained by molecular analysis of the M-PPL subunit isozyme gene.

Phosphofructokinase (PFK) Deficiency: PFK catalyzes the formation of fructose-1,6-diphosphate from fructose-6-phosphate, a major rate-limiting reaction of glycolysis (Figure 1). Like PPL, PFK occurs in multimolecular forms in mammalian tissues. In humans, three distinct PFK subunits were identified: muscle (M); liver (L) and platelet (P), also labeled F for fibroblast by some investigators (121-125). These subunits can hybridize to yield as many as fifteen homo- and hetero-tetramers (122). The genes coding for PFK-M, L and P have recently been assigned to chromosomes 1, 21 and 10, respectively (125,126-128). Developmental changes in PFK isozyme patterns have been studied in detail in several human fetal tissues from 8 to 40 weeks gestation and in muscle culture (129-131). In all fetal tissues studied, including skeletal muscle, isozymes containing all three PFK subunits are synthesized at 8 to 12 weeks of gestation (129,130). In skeletal muscle, PFK isozymes containing subunits M and P predominate but L-containing isozymes are also present. At mid-gestation, PFK-L subunits are no longer detectable, but small amounts of PFK P are still found. A significant rise in total PFK activity at 25 weeks of gestation coincides with an increase of PFK-M-containing isozymes (130), and shortly before birth only PFK-M_4 is present in skeletal muscle. In heart muscle at early stages of gestation P and M subunit-containing isozymes predominate (130). Unlike skeletal muscle, however, the major proportion of total PFK activity is due to PFK-P_4 and PFK-M_4 at 36-40 weeks of gestation, but some PFK-L isozymes persist throughout adult life. In brain, all three subunits are already expressed prenatally, as early as at 10 weeks of gestation. In postnatal brain, the major proportion of PFK activity is due to PFK-M isozymes. PFK-L isozymes decline somewhat, but persist throughout adult life. Major alterations in isozyme patterns are also observed in developing liver, but there is a persistent predominance of PFK-L (130).

Muscle PFK deficiency (Tarui disease) is due to genetic lack of PFK-M activity probably due to genetic mutation of the gene structure (123,131-133). Tarui disease usually causes exercise intolerance, cramps and myoglobinuria and a mild hemolytic trait. In most patients the myopathic changes predominate, while in a few individuals hemolysis is the more prominent clinical feature (133). In adult heart, most PFK activity is due to PFK-M and P isozymes (130). The resulting partial deficiency of PFK activity in heart of patients does not appear to affect cardiac function. The most prominent pathologic expression of PFK-M deficiency in non-muscle cells affects erythrocytes, and consists of hemolysis, thus indicating that PFK-M is crucial for normal erythrocyte functions (133).

In normal mature skeletal muscle only PFK-M subunits are expressed (123,124). PFK-M-containing isozymes, although present in small amounts, can be demonstrated in cultured skin fibroblasts, myoblasts and myotubes by ion exchange chromatography and by immunological studies with monoclonal antibodies against PFK-M (134). Biochemical studies of myotube cultures from patients with PFK-M deficiency indicate that total enzyme activity is normal and there is no glycogen accumulation (92,134). This can be attributed to the predominance of functional non-muscle PFK isozymes (PFK-L and P). Chromatographic and immunological studies of muscle cultures from PFK-M-deficient patients and unaffected controls show that all the PFK activity in patients is due to PFK-L and P containing isozymes. In the control cultures, at least 15% of total PFK activity is due to PFK-M isozymes. Although PFK-M activity is absent in the patient's cultures, immunocytochemical analysis consistently shows the presence of immunologically cross-reacting PFK-M-containing protein in cultured cells, including undifferentiated myoblasts and fibroblasts (130). Based on these data, the following conclusions can be drawn:

1. Unlike other muscle-specific isozyme proteins, PFK-M is already synthesized in small amounts in unfused, mononuclear cells, including mitotic cells, as demonstrated by staining with monoclonal antibodies.

2. Cultures from PFK-M deficient patients contain abundant PFK-L and PFK-P isozymes, characteristic of fetal muscle.

3. At early stages of myogenesis in cultures, PFK-L and P isozymes can maintain normal glycogen metabolism in PFK-M deficient muscle cells, since cultures from patients are morphologically normal and there is no glycogen accumulation in cultured myotubes.

4. In muscle cultures from five unrelated patients, PFK-M deficiency is due to _inactive_ PFK-M protein, not to lack of PFK-M _synthesis_, since there is immunocytochemical evidence of PFK-M cross-reacting protein.

Studies of more mature muscle cultures co-cultivated with neuronal tissues may show predominance or exclusive presence of PFK-M_4 isozyme. In such cultures from patients it may be possible to demonstrate characteristic glycogen accumulation, thus allowing an analysis of the developmental pathobiology of PFK-M deficiency _in vitro_.

Phosphoglycerate Mutase (PGAM) Deficiency: PGAM is a dimer molecule that catalyzes the formation of 2-phosphoglycerate from 3-phosphoglycerate (Figure 1) (135). Two different subunits are present in human tissues, designated PGAM-B ("brain") and PGAM-M ("muscle"). A hybrid dimer MB is also present in tissues that synthesize both M and B subunits (135). During myogenesis there is a gradual transition from PGAM-B to PGAM-M (135-137). In normal mature skeletal muscle PGAM-MM is the predominant isozyme (about 95% or more of the total). Comparison of the developmentally-regulated conversion of PGAM with that of creatine kinase (CK), an oxidative dimer enzyme abundant in muscle, shows that CK matures earlier than PGAM (92). PGAM isozyme transition is, therefore, a useful marker to evaluate more advanced muscle maturation, *in vivo* and *in vitro*.

In cardiac muscle, both PGAM-M and PGAM-B subunits are produced throughout adult life. The M-subunit containing enzymes make up about 70% or more of total activity, resembling the isozyme pattern of fetal skeletal muscle (Figure 3). In other organs such as the brain, connective tissue, erythrocytes and liver, total enzyme activity is totally due to PGAM-BB (Figure 3) (135-137). There is sufficient indirect evidence that the B and M subunits are coded on different genes.

The first patient with PGAM-M subunit deficiency was recognized recently by DiMauro et al (136,137) and two more patients have since been identified (83). All patients developed myoglobinuria after intense exercise, but analysis of the muscle biopsies showed only mild or no increase of glycogen. Areas of regeneration were the only abnormal feature in two of the three patients, but this was probably a consequence of recent necrosis.

Because PGAM-BB is the only isozyme found in connective tissue, deficiency of PGAM-M subunits cannot be diagnosed in amniocytes or cultured skin fibroblasts. Even in non-innervated cultured myotubes from patients total PGAM activity was normal due to predominance of PGAM-BB (136,137). Some PGAM-MB and MM isozyme activity was demonstrated electrophoretically in normal human muscle cultures after more prolonged cultivation (up to 8 weeks) (120), but complete conversion from PGAM-BB to PGAM-MM was only observed in normal human muscle cultures that were co-cultivated with fetal mouse spinal cord complex (117). The phenotypic expression of PGAM-M deficiency *in vitro* can probably be demonstrated in such nerve-muscle cultures, but this has not yet been done.

Lactate Dehydrogenase (LDH), Deficiency: LDH catalyzes the formation of lactate from pyruvate, the final step of anaerobic glycolysis (Figure 1). LDH exists as a tetrameric molecule. Two isozyme subunits LDH-1 (H or A) and LDH-5 (M or B) hybridize randomly under physiologic conditions yielding five homo and heterotetramers (M_4, M_3, H_1, M_2H_2, M, H_3, H_4) (119). LDH-M and LDH-H subunits are coded on chromosomes 11 and 12, respectively (138,139). During myogenesis or muscle regeneration there is a conversion from anodic (LDH-H) to cathodic LDH-M isozymes, but the

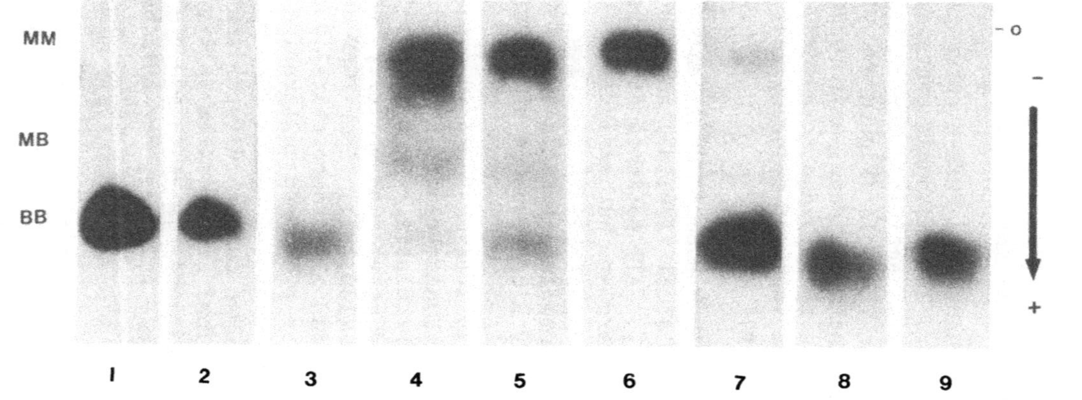

FIGURE 3: Cellulose acetate electrophoresis of phosphoglycerate mutase isozyme activities in various human tissue extracts and muscle culture from controls and a patient with M-subunit PGAM deficiency: Lane 1, normal brain; lane 2, normal liver; lane 3, erthyrocytes; lane 4, heart; lane 5, fetal skeletal muscle (22 wks gestation); lane 6, normal skeletal muscle; lane 7, patient's skeletal muscle (overloaded sample); lane 8, patient's myotube culture; lane 9, control myotube culture.

conversion is never complete. LDH-H subunits are generally produced in small but detectable amounts even in normal mature skeletal muscle. In cardiac muscle LDH-H and LDH-M isozymes also continue to co-exist during muscle development but LDH-H isozymes predominate in mature heart (119).

Both LDH-H and LDH-M subunit deficiencies have been demonstrated in Japanese kindreds (102,140,141). LDH-H deficiency does not appear to cause clinical problems but LDH-M deficiency was shown to cause myoglobinuria, following brief intense exercise. Like PGAM-M deficiency, however, there was no obvious accumulation of glycogen, the pathologic hallmark of other enzyme deficiencies of glycogen metabolism (e.g. PPL, DB and PFK deficiencies). Lack of glycogen accumulation in muscle from patients with PGAM-M and LDH-M subunit deficiencies is probably due to residual activity of non-muscle isozymes (PGAM-BB; LDH-H_4) which appear to be sufficient for normal or near normal glycogen metabolism in muscle at rest.

Because both LDH subunits are synthesized in different proportions in all tissues, LDH-M deficiency can be demonstrated in aminocytes and cultured skin fibroblasts. In electropherograms from cultured fibroblasts of a patient with LDH-M subunit deficiency only a single band of LDH enzyme activity is present, which co-migrated with LDH-H_4 isozyme of normal cells (141). Muscle culture studies have not yet been done in these patients, but the isozyme profile ought to show a single LDH-H_4 band, as demonstrated in cultured fibroblasts, since both subunits are synthesized in normal cultured myotubes (119).

Inclusion Body or I-cell Disease (Mucolipidosis type 11): All the known hereditary isozyme myopathies are due to deficiencies of subunits of muscle-specific isozymes that are low or absent at early stages of myogenesis, while they are present in large amounts in normal mature muscle. There is one lysosomal disorder, however, that can be classified as a metabolic myopathy of immature muscle and is no longer expressed as the muscle attains maturity: I-cell disease is a rapidly fatal genetic disorder in which normal processing of many, but not all lysosomal acid hydrolases is defective, due to deficiency of an acetylglucosamine transferase needed for proper packaging of enzymes into lysosomes (142). Cells from patients, including cultured skin fibroblasts, show large numbers of lysosomal structures (hence the name "inclusion" body disease) and abnormal leakage of lysosomal enzymes in the extracellular medium (76,143).

I-cell disease is not considered a metabolic myopathy because muscle biopsies, unlike other tissues, do not show any decrease of intracellular lysosomal enzymes and there is no abnormal increase of lysosomes in muscle fibers. However, when muscle from these patients is grown in culture, both mononuclear cells and myotubes show abundant lysosomal inclusions (76). In more mature, partially cross-striated myotubes obtained through more prolonged cultivation, abnormal lysosomal inclusions are no longer present (76). The disappearance of inclusions with maturation is not confined to <u>cultured</u> muscle because in muscle biopsies satellite cells, the dormant <u>myogenic precursors</u> of regenerating muscle fibers (144), also show abundant lysosomes, whereas <u>mature</u> muscle fibers do not (75). Based on these findings, I-cell disease can be considered a metabolic myopathy causing pathologic changes in muscle only at early stages of differentiation.

Because not all lysosomal enzymes are affected in I-cell disease, cells from these patients may serve as a model to study the metabolism of lysosomal enzymes in muscle: I-cell studies suggest that there are at least two types of regulation of lysosomal enzyme metabolism and one of these is under developmental control in muscle, conceivably involving multimolecular isozyme forms.

III. Muscle Maturation in Culture

Human muscle cultures grown in the absence of nerve do not mature beyond the fetal stage, even after several weeks <u>in vitro</u> (92,119,120,145). This explains why muscle cultures from patients with hereditary muscle-specific isozyme deficiencies do not exhibit characteristic pathologic alterations since the non-muscle ("fetal") isozymes that are still abundant in such myotube cultures are sufficient to allow normal metabolism. Lack of complete muscle maturation is not unique to human cultures derived from <u>mature</u> muscle, but has also been noted in cultures obtained from human <u>fetal</u> muscle, which showed only fetal-specific myosin light chain (145). Therefore, to study the developmental pathobiology of "muscle isozyme myopathies" <u>in vitro</u> it is essential to optimize the conditions that promote advanced maturation. Morphologic studies of long-term organotypic nerve-muscle co-cultures, in which human muscle fibers are innervated with motor neurons from fetal mouse spinal cord complex, showed well-developed regenerated muscle straps with well-aligned sarcomeres, subsarcolemmal nuclei, and prominent triads (146-148). In such co-cultures, virtually complete isozyme maturation of an oxidative enzyme (CK) and glycolytic enzyme (PGAM) were noted after 3 months <u>in vitro</u> (146). Electronmicroscopic analysis of these cultures also showed well-developed motor endplates (146). Complete isozyme transition of CK and PGAM has not been observed in nerve-muscle co-cultures that lack nerve muscle contacts; this suggests that innervation is required for muscle maturation and maintenance of the differential state. In these uninnervated organotypic nerve-muscle co-cultures, transition of CK-BB to CK-MM was more advanced after

2 1/2 months *in vitro*, than had been attained in similar long-term cultures, grown aneurally. In two cultures, CK-M containing isozymes represented as much as 80% of the total CK activity, while in the same cultures the PGAM-MM activity was less than 50% of total. These findings not only confirm that developmentally-regulated isozyme transitions in muscle are not synchronous, but also suggest and that functional innervation may be more important for the maturation of some multimolecular isozyme systems (e.g. PGAM) than for others (e.g. CK).

Studies of organotypically-grown nerve-muscle co-cultures from mouse, showed the presence of adult fast myosin isozyme in some of the regenerating fibers (149). The possible mechanisms by which the nerve may promote muscle maturation were considered (135).

There is evidence that contractile activity of the developing muscle straps may contribute toward regulation of myosin synthesis (150). However, inhibition of contractility with tetrodotoxin in fetal rat myotube cultures did not cause a great change in total CK activity, while, unexpectedly, it caused a significant *rise* in total phosphorylase activity (151). It was not specified which phosphorylase isozyme increased. While contractility may play a role in isozyme maturation, other factors must be involved, because in the heart, an organ that contracts continuously, full conversion of isozymes such as, CK, PPL, PGAM, PFK does not occur. More detailed biochemical analysis of nerve-muscle co-cultures are needed to determine the role of contractility and trophic nerve influences on maturation of structural isoproteins and multimolecular isozymes of the major metabolic pathways.

DR. WOOD: Considering the lack of transition from fetal to adult development in muscle cultures, we seem to observe two kinds of events: in one situation the "adult" enzyme appears but the "fetal" enzyme doesn't go away. In another situation the "fetal" enzyme remains and the adult enzyme never appears. In other words, in some instances the genes that code for adult enzyme are turned on while the genes coding for "fetal" enzymes are turned off. In other cases, the genes coding for adult enzyme are not turned on.

DR. MIRANDA: For some glycoltyic enzymes (e.g. lactate dehydrogenase, LDH) both isozyme subunits continue to be synthesized in muscle culture (and *in vivo* throughout adult life). But even in this situation, there is a shift during muscle development, from anodic to cathodic isozyme. Creatine kinase (CK) isozyme transition occurs quite early during myogenesis: both *in vivo* and *in vitro*, there is detectable muscle-isozyme activity at the time of myoblast fusion. The glycolytic enzyme, phosphoglycerate mutase (PGAM), on the other hand, appears to differentiate more slowly: the complete shift from fetal to mature isozyme pattern cannot be demonstrated in immature aneural cultures, but does occur in nerve-muscle co-cultures. The isozyme transitions that we observe in aneural culture, therefore, reflect the immaturity of the myotubes. The adult isozymes, at least in normal muscle, should appear, provided we can "push" the maturation process by optimizing the conditions.

DR. YAFFE: Maybe the differences observed in culture are due to the presence of unfused myoblasts in the myotube cultures. One control would be to remove the myoblasts from the cultures.

DR. MIRANDA: That is an important point, we must realize, however, that it is very difficult to eliminate <u>all</u> unfused muscle cells, even in cultures derived from clones. To circumvent this problem, we removed the mononuclear cells (and small myotubes) mechanically, by filtration of trypsinized uninnervated myotube cultures through a fine mesh stainless steel sieve. Even in such pure myotube preparations, both CK-B and CK-M-containing isozymes are detectable by electrophoresis. Moreover, immunocytochemical staining with anti CK-B and anti CK-M antibodies show the presence of B and M subunit-containing isozymes in all myotubes that we looked at.

DR. BLAU: CK isozyme transition occurs relatively early in development; have you also studied changes of heavy chain myosin?

DR. MIRANDA: No, I have not studied myosin.

DR. RUBINSTEIN: Is it possible that the satellite cells from adult muscle fibers are different from primary embryonic myoblasts? Have you studied innervated cultures derived from embryonic muscle cells?

DR. MIRANDA: No I haven't. But this is definitely something worth looking into. Drs. Shimada, Fischman and Moscona (152) have demonstrated several years ago that myotubes derived from dissociated embryonic avain muscle and neurons can form nerve-muscle connections in culture, but to my knowledge isozyme transitions have not yet been studied in such cultures.

DR. FISCHMAN: Using the "organotypic" approach of nerve-muscle culture has a lot of advantages despite its complexity of interactions within the spinal cord. At present we don't know what they are. It might be feasible to overlay established primary muscle cultures with sections of spinal cord.

DR. MIRANDA: We have tried some of these, using cultures derived from mature human muscle but, have so far have not been able to attain the high degree of differentiation that we saw in the organotypic muscle cultures of Peterson (145).

DR. WHALEN: Perhaps we should comment on the use of the word "innervation" in nerve-muscle co-cultures. There have been studies over the years demonstrating innervation electrophysiologically. In our experiments we found cultures maturing between 2-4 weeks. There are large and small diameter fibers in these cultures. If one takes that as some evidence of innervation then only some myotubes are innervated. I think that one would be hard put to demonstrate synapses on more than a few fibers in a given number of cultures. In the Maximov system, one does not see the pretzel-shape organization of synaptic membrane. Although one sees regions of concentrated acetylcholine receptors and by silver staining one can demonstrate nerve fibers coming close to synaptic structures, but it is not clear whether they actually terminate there. Therefore, one should be careful about assuming that the cells are innervated. The steps of maturation, cross-striation and contractility require the presence of spinal cord in this system. Thus, although the process is nerve-dependent in a certain sense, that doesn't necessarily mean that the cells are innervated. Ventral horn cells will produce maturation, but so will the dorsal side of the spinal cord.

DR. FISCHMAN: Dr. Miranda, have you observed that both ventral and dorsal halves of the spinal cord are equally effective in maturation promotion?

DR. MIRANDA: From the morphologic studies of Peterson and Crain it would appear that innervation is essential for muscle maturation and long-term maintenance of the differentiated state. Our preliminary isozyme studies with Peterson and Masurovsky show virtually complete isozyme maturation of CK and PGAM in 3-month-old nerve-muscle culture. With regard to synapse function, we noted electronmicroscopically, very well-developed motor-end plates after 3 months, showing secondary clefts and numerous clear vesicles in the presynaptic region. We have not yet done isozyme analysis of individual fibers, but that may be possible as well. If this were done, we might witness fully mature isozyme patterns in less than 3 months. From the earlier studies of Peterson and co-workers it would appear that non-innervated muscle fibers might exist in early co-cultures, but these are not likely to survive after several months _in vitro_. In our system we are unable to keep uninnervated myotubes in a healthy state for more than 2 months, not even when fibroblast overgrowth does not pose a problem. In two co-cultures that showed no evidence of nerve-muscle contacts we did not get complete maturation of CK and PGAM, but in all the cultures we looked at, both ventral _and_ dorsal aspects of the spinal cord were present.

DR. BLAU: Have you looked at the effect of nerve extracts?

DR. MIRANDA: No we did not, but we did examine the effects of high concentration chick embryo extract, which should contain extractable nerve components, but we never got the high degree of isozyme maturation that we saw in innervated organotypic muscle culture.

CHAPTER 4: MYOSIN ISOFORMS IN NORMAL AND DYSTROPHIC HUMAN AND MURINE MUSCLES

Joseph F.Y. Hoh* and R.B. Fitzsimons*

*Department of Physiology
University of Sydney
NSW, 2006, Australia

Introduction

Myosin is the contractile protein in muscle which forms the cross-bridge with actin to transduce the free energy of hydrolysis of ATP into mechanical work and heat. The rate of energy transduction is a function of the kinetics of myosin as a mechano-enzyme. Myosin exists as a large family of isoenzymic forms differing from each other in subunit composition, ATPase activity and consequently the rate of energy transduction. The functional significance of myosin polymorphism lies in the fact that each type of muscle fiber has its unique type of isomyosin which determines its intrinsic contractile dynamics. This diversity of isomyosin types is matched by the wide range of muscle fiber types. Muscle fibers associated with a specific isomyosin type may also have different isoforms of other myofibrillar proteins as well as varying proportions of glycoltyic and oxidative enzymes. These differences allow muscle fibers with different contractile properties to be classified histochemically into a number of types.

Myosin is a multi-subunit protein consisting of a pair of heavy chains and two pairs of light chains. The structure of each isomyosin is coded by a distinct set of genes. The expression of these genes changes during development as well as during post-natal life in response to appropriate physiological stimuli. Thus, the contractile characteristic of a striated muscle fiber can be exquisitely matched to the requirement of a particular function or to the changing functional demands made upon it during life.

In this presentation, the types of isomyosins found in normal murine and human muscles will be described, and changes in isomyosins occurring in murine and human muscular dystrophy and in human infantile spinal muscular atrophy (153-154) will be reviewed. The significance of these changes are discussed in relation to changes in contractile properties of diseases muscles and mechanisms which regulate isomyosin gene expression during development and post-natal life.

Isomyosins in Normal and Dystrophic Mouse Muscles

The normal fast-twitch extensor digitorum longus (EDL) and the slow-twitch soleus muscles contain between them 5 isomyosins which can be resolved by pyrophosphate gel electrophoresis. Normal soleus contains two isomyosins, a dominant slow-migrating component (slow isomyosin: SM), together with a smaller amount of a distinctly faster migrating component (intermediate isomyosin: IM). These isomyosins are distinct in electrophoretic mobility compared with the three isomyosins (FM1, FM2 and FM3) in the EDL. Traces of SM are found in some of the EDL muscles. Normal gastrocnemius muscle contains the three fast isomyosins together with trace amounts of IM and SM. The relative amounts of isomyosins in these mouse muscles are summarized in Figure 4

Isomyosins from dystrophic (ReJ 129 dy/dy) mouse muscles reveal no components not already present in the normal muscles. However, there is a general shift of isomyosin distribution towards the slower migrating form in all the muscles studied. Dystrophic soleus muscles contain 78-100% SM. Dystrophic EDL muscles contain 34% of IM, an isomyosin not normally present in mouse EDL. Furthermore, the distribution of the fast isomyosins are skewed in favor of FM3. The increase in the amounts of SM and IM, as well as skewing in the distribution of the fast isomyosins, is also seen in the dystrophic gastrocnemius muscles (Figure 4).

Although dystrophic muscle fibers are more difficult to classify histochemically (probably because of the presence of multiple types of myosins in the same fiber), the observed isomyosin shifts were shown to be accompanied with changes in fiber type distribution. The soleus, which normally contains type 1 and type 2A fibers, showed an increase in the slow type 1 fibers with dystrophy, while the gastrocnemius muscle, which normally has a predominance of type 2B fibers, showed an increase in the proportion of both type 1 and type 2A fibers (154).

Newborn mouse muscles contain three fetal isomyosin components which can be distinguished electrophoretically from adult isomyosins. As shown in Figure 5, the slowest of the

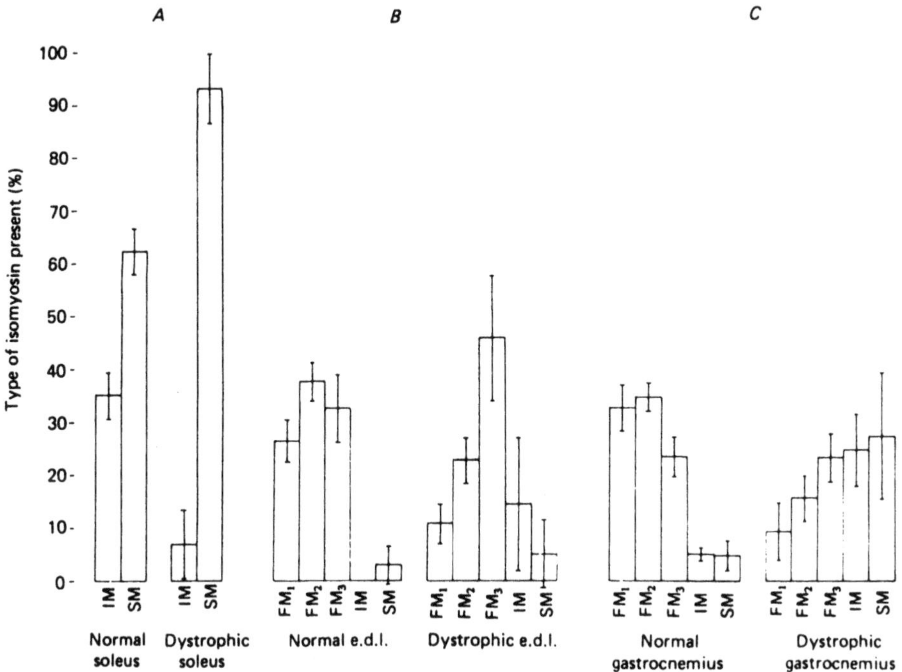

FIGURE 4: Histogram illustrating the mean percentage of each isomyosin in: A, normal (n=12) and dystrophic (n=12) soleus muscles. There is a relative increase in the percentage of SM, and decrease in the percentage of IM in dystrophic soleus, when compared with normal soleus. B, normal (n=9) and dystrophic (n=9) EDL (e.d.l.) muscles. Significant amounts of IM are present in dystrophic EDL, which thus contains an abnormally low percentage of fast (FM1-FM3) isomyosins. FM3 constitutes a greater proportion, and FM1 a lesser proportion of this fast myosin complement in dystrophic EDL, than of fast myosin in normal EDL. C, normal (n=10) and dystrophic (n=10) gastrocnemius muscles. Dystrophic gastrocnemius muscles contain higher than normal percentages of SM and IM. FM3 is clearly present in greatest amounts, and FM1 in least amount of the fast isomyosins in dystrophic gastrocnemius, although these three fast isomyosins are present in approximately equal proportions in normal gastrocnemius. Error bar = +/- S.D. Reproduced from Fitzsimons and Hoh (1981a) by courtesy of the editors of The Journal of Physiology.

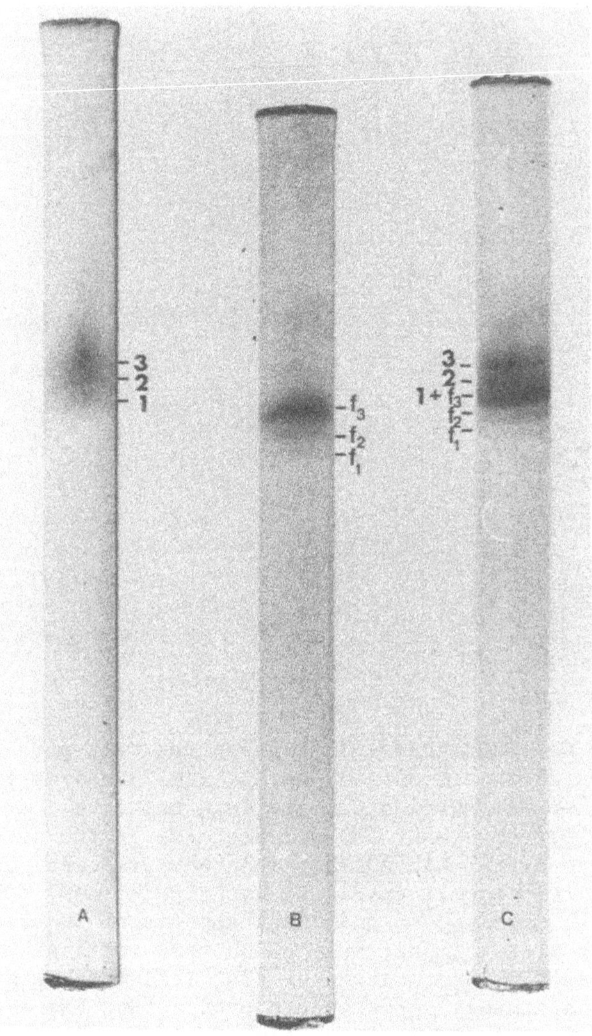

FIGURE 5: Pyrophosphate gel electrophoresis of intact murine isomyosins in 4.5% polyacrylamide. A, normal fast isomyosins of EDL, bands numbered 1-3 corresponding to FM1-FM3. B, isomyosins from newborn mouse skeletal muscle. Three components (f1, f2, and f3) are detected. C, coelectrophoresis of A and B, f3 comigrates with FM1, while f2 and f3 are electrophoretically distinct from mature isomyosins. These fetal components have never been detected in muscles of matured dystrophic mice.

fetal components co-migrate with the fastest of the EDL fast isomyosins. In none of the dystrophic muscles studied could fetal myosin components be detected. This is in great contrast with human dystrophic muscles in which fetal isomyosins were always found (see below).

Normal mouse EDL and SOl muscles differ in force:velocity properties, the Vmax for the former being two-fold higher than the Vmax for the latter (155-157). Such a difference implies that the contractile machinery of the EDL is capable of transducing energy at twice the rate of the SOL. The difference in energetics resides in the difference in kinetic properties of their cross-bridges, i.e., in the different isomyosins they contain: the FM in the EDL and the IM and SM of the soleus. The mouse diaphragm has been shown to have a force:velocity curve intermediate between the force:velocity curves of the EDL and soleus muscles (157). Myosin extracted from this muscle has been shown to contain 84% of an isomyosin which can be established as IM on the basis of electrophoretic co-migration with the IM from mouse soleus (Hoh and Chow, unpublished observations). Thus IM is associated with muscle fibers with a speed of contraction intermediate between the fast-twitch and slow-twitch fibers. In the rat, the presence of IM (isomyosin 4) (158) is associated with motor units which have isometric contraction time intermediate between those of fast-twitch of slow-twitch muscle fibers (159-160). Motor unit studies on the mouse soleus are consistent with, but have not established the presence of, a similar population of intermediate motor units (161).

Douglas and Baskin (1971) reported that the maximal velocities of dystrophic (ReJ 129 dy/dy) mouse EDL and SOl muscles were unaltered, but the force:velocity curves of both muscles fell below the curve for the respective normal muscles. The observed shifts in isomyosin and fiber type distributions can adequately explain these changes. To see this clearly it is necessary to consider the effect of isomyosin heterogeneity of a muscle on its force:velocity curve. If a muscle contains both fast-twitch and slow-twitch muscle fibers, during an isotonic contraction the two types of fibers will each contract independently in parallel in such a way that their respective force:velocity properties are obeyed. Thus, the Vmax of the whole muscle will be determined by the fast fibers. At velocities between the maximal velocities of the fast-twitch and slow-twitch fibers, only the fast-twitch fibers will bear the load. Below the Vmax of the slow-twitch fibers, both fast and slow components will bear the load. The fast-twitch fibers will, however, bear proportionally the greater load, in accordance with the force: velocity characteristics of these muscles. Since the Vmax of a muscle containing fibers of different speed would be that of the fastest fiber, the unaltered maximal velocities for the dystrophic muscles can be accounted for by the fact that the fast isomyosins are still present in dystrophic EDL, and IM is still present in dystrophic SOL. The fact that the force:velocity curves for both dystrophic EDL and SOL muscles fall below the curves for the respective normal muscles can therefore be explained by the reduction in the proportion of the faster fiber component, as evidenced by the shift in their isomyosin distributions toward the slower form.

Endo et al (1983) have compared the Vmax of chemically skinned single dystrophic EDL fibers with normal EDL fibers using the slack test. Their results confirm that Vmax of dystrophic EDL fibers remained unaltered. However, if isomyosins IM and SM reported here for dystrophic EDL are present in different fibers, a small fraction of fibers from the dystrophic EDL would be expected to show a reduced Vmax. Such fibers were not found by these authors. The absence of such fibers in this study may be due to a sampling problem (162).

Douglas and Baskin (1971) also showed that whereas the contraction times of both dystrophic EDL and SOL muscles and the half-relaxation time of the dystrophic SOL muscle showed only minor differences from those of corresponding normal muscles, the half-relaxation time of the dystrophic EDL was considerably longer than the value of normal EDL muscle. Similar increase in half-relaxation times have also been observed for the principally fast-twitch gastrocnemius muscle (163-164) and the tibialis anterior (165), but not the soleus (164). Increases in half-relaxation times have also been reported in the EDL (166) and the fast-twitch extensor carpi radialis longus (167) muscles of the C57BL/6J dy-2J/dy-2J strain of dystrophic mouse. A similar increase in half-relaxation time is also seen in human dystrophic muscles (see below). Thus, this change appears to be well established in both murine and human dystrophic muscles.

The reduced half-relaxation time of dystrophic mouse fast-twitch muscles has led some investigators to suggest that an abnormality in the properties of the sarcoplasmic reticulum may exist in these muscles (163,164,168). A recent investigation suggests that this is not the case (169). The occurrence of shifts in isomyosin and fiber-type distributions offer an entirely different perspective on this problem. The time course of the isometric twitch of a muscle is necessarily a function of its fiber-type composition. During the isometric contraction of a muscle with different types of fibers, each type of fiber will contract and relax independently with a characteristic time-course, so that the isometric myogram of the whole muscle would be given by the algebraic summation of the twitch tension-time curves of the fiber type components. The increase in SM and IM observed in the dystrophic EDL and gastrocnemius muscles increases the number of slow and intermediate motor units which contribute tension to the isometric twitch of the whole muscle in the region of the relaxation time of the fast-twitch muscle fibers. This leads to an apparent increase in half-relaxation time of fast-twitch muscles. In the case of the slow-twitch soleus muscle, a decrease in the amount of IM relative to SM will lead to a marginal increase in contraction-time of the whole muscle without significantly affecting the time-course of the half-relaxation. Thus, the time-course of the isometric twitch of dystrophic muscles can be satisfactorily explained in terms of shifts in isomyosin and fiber type distributions.

Isomyosins in Normal Adult, Developing and Dystrophic Human Muscles

Myosin from normal human subjects consists of two distinct forms of slow myosin (SM1 and SM2) and three fast-migrating components (FM1, FM2 and FM3). These slow and fast isomyosins are found in type 1 and type 2 fibers respectively (170). Although human type 2 fibers can be further subdivided into 2A and 2B fibers on the basis of acid sensitivities of their myosin ATPases (171) and immunohistochemistry (172), no further heterogeneity could be resolved by pyrophosphate gel electrophoresis in 4%, 2.4% and 5% gels. In view of the biochemical (173) and immunochemical (174) evidences for two structurally distinct types of fast muscle myosins corresponding to the type 2A (fast-red) and type 2B (fast-white) fibers in experimental animals, it is probable that the human fast isomyosins separated by pyrophosphate gels contain both types of isomyosin which failed to be resolved by gel electrophoresis.

During normal human fetal development, two distinct groups of early myosin components, f5 (possibly f4-f5) and f1-f4 (possibly f1-f3), appear and disappear in succession before being finally replaced by adult isomyosins. Myosin from fetuses (16-20 gestation) contains a dominent isomyosin component (f5) which co-migrates with FM1 in 4% gels, being clearly distinct from FM2 (Figure 6). Traces of other isomyosins (f3, f3, f4 and SM) are also present in these embryos. At birth, adult isomyosins already predominate; in addition, four fetal components, f1-f4 are also present (Figure 7). The fetal isoforms persist normally until the 4th week of neonatal life. These changes in isomyosins during development are similar to changes in the rat (175) and rabbit (176), except that the relaxation to the time of birth the adult isoforms appear earliest in human muscle, then in rabbit, and lastly rat.

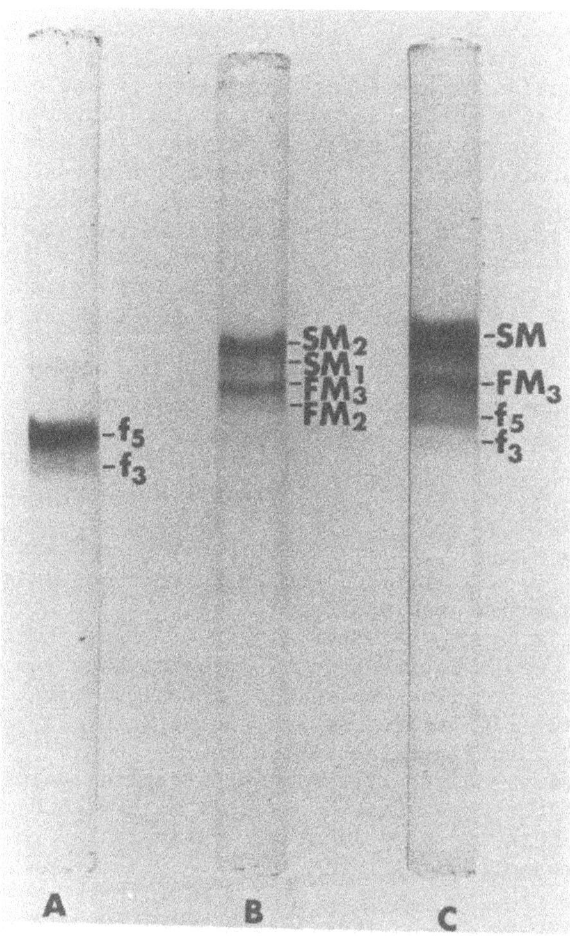

FIGURE 6: Isomyosins from human fetuses analyzed in 4% pyrophosphate gels. A, early fetal (16-20 week) myosin containing the dominant f5 (embryonic) component and faster-migrating f3 (fetal). Any f4 present would co-migrate with f5 in this 4% gel. There is a trace of slow myosin present. B, normal mature human skeletal myosin, containing 2 slow components (SM1 and SM2) and 2 fast components (FM3 and FM2). This particular sample contains hardly any FM1. C, mixture of A and B. f5 migrates ahead of FM2, in the position of FM1. Gel B contains less mature myosin than does gel C, permitting clear resolution of slow myosins SM1 and SM2.

Reproduced from Fitzsimons and Hoh (1981a) by courtesy of the editors of the Journal of Neurological Sciences.

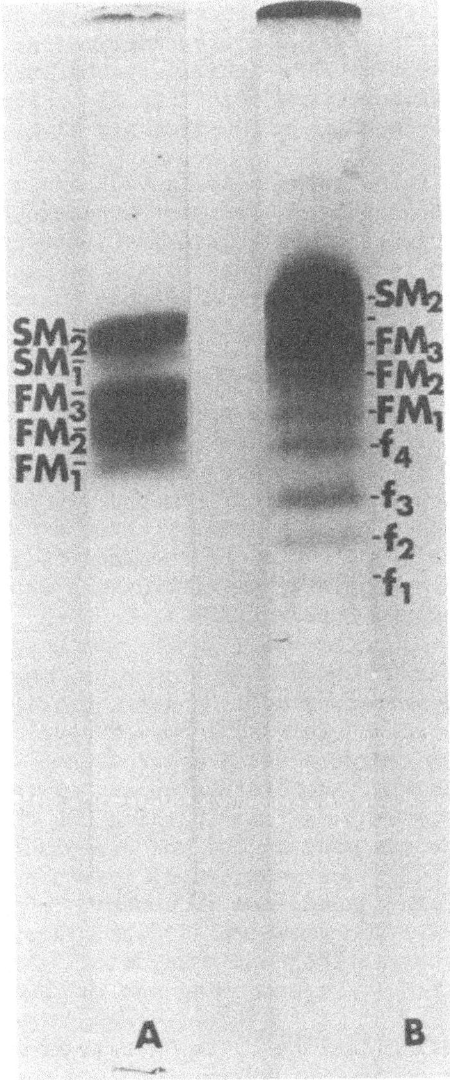

FIGURE 7: Human isomyosins in 4.5% polyacrylamide gels from (A) normal mature skeletal muscle, containing a mixture of histochemical fiber types. There are 2 slow (SM1, SM2) and 3 fast (FM1-FM3) isomyosins. (B) Normal neonatal skeletal muscle. In addition to the mature isomyosins there are 4 fetal isomyosins, f1-f4.

Reproduced from Fitzsimons and Hoh (1981a) by courtesy of the editors of the Journal of the Neurological Sciences.

Muscles from patients with Duchenne muscular dystrophy who, in addition to the normal fast and slow isomyosins, the presence of fetal components f1-f4. This is illustrated in Figure 8. These components constitute from less than 1% to about 12% of the total myosin, and are found in all patients analyzed.

The presence of fetal isomyosins in Duchenne muscles is correlated with the presence of variable proportions of type 2C fibers (177). This histochemical class of fibers is heterogeneous. It is associated with fetal isomyosin, since neonatal rat (178) and human fetal muscle fibers (179) show this histochemical characteristic. However, type 2C fibers are also occasionally present in adult human muscle fibers, especially in athletes undergoing training (180-181). In this context, it has been shown to be due to the coexistence of FM and SM (182) in fibers undergoing fiber-type transformation. Since the type 2C fibers in Duchenne muscle have characteristics of regenerating fibers, they presumably contain fetal isomyosin. However, it is not possible to rule out the possibility that some of these fibers may contain both SM and FM, especially in view of the fact that they tend to occur in segments of a single fiber alternating with segments which stain normally type 1 and type 2 (177).

Duchenne muscle contains a large number of regenerating cells (183-184). Since regenerating cells undergo proliferation, fusion and maturation as myoblasts do during normal development, it is reasonable to propose that the fetal myosins seen in Duchenne muscle are synthesized in regeneration cells. This view finds support in experiments done in rats in which EDL and tibialis anterior muscles were removed, minced and reimplanted back into the original muscle bed. One week later, myosin extracted from the regenerating muscle can be seen to contain fetal myosin components (Figure 9). The presence of fetal isomyosins (185), fetal myosin heavy chains (186) and embryonic light chains (187) has been reported in regenerating rat muscles.

Another interesting feature of the myosin from dystrophic patients is that the content of SM is increased compared with normal subjects, as shown in Table 2. These differences in the distribution of isomyosins are highly significant ($P<0.001$), and adequately account for the marked reduction of the half-relaxation time and the moderate increase in the contraction time of isometric twitches of human dystrophic muscles (188-191) along the same principles referred to above for dystrophic mouse muscles. Thus, a shift in isomyosin distribution towards the slow form occurs in both human

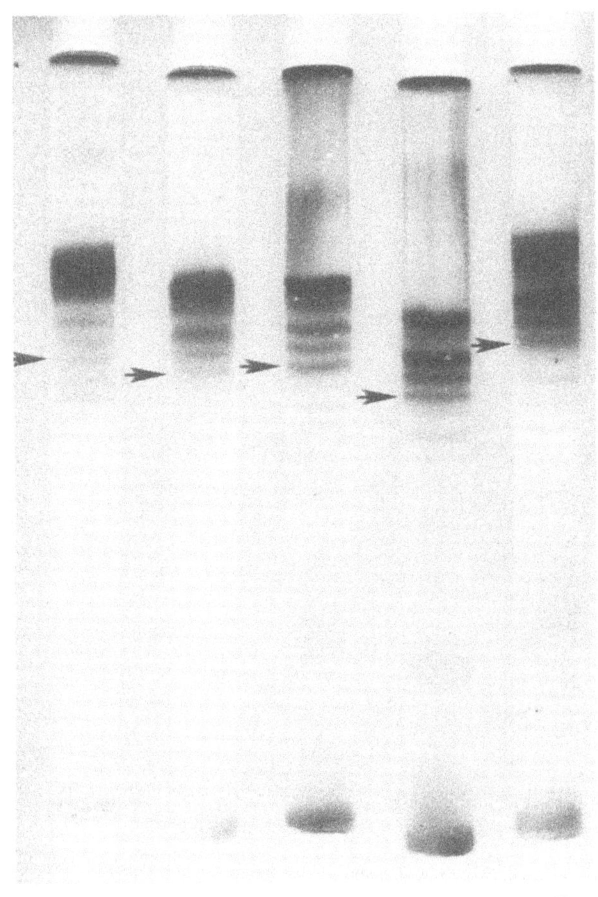

FIGURE 8: Myosins from 5 different skeletal muscle samples from patients with Duchenne muscular dystrophy. Four fast-migrating "fetal" myosin bands were seen in each case, and are most clearly demonstrated photographically in gels C and D. FM1 is arrowed in each gel. Some myosin samples contain a marked excess of slow myosin, in particular, SM2. In these cases the distinction between SM1 and SM2 was often blurred, but it is most clearly illustrated in gel C. These 4.5% gels are from different electrophoretic runs. Reproduced from Fitzsimons and Hoh (1981a) by courtesy of the editors of the Journal of the Neurological Sciences.

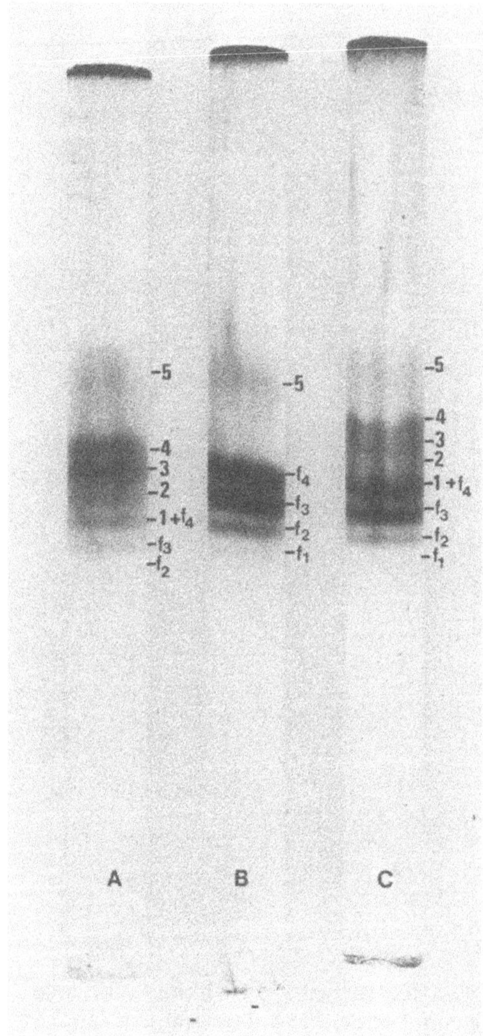

FIGURE 9: Fetal isomyosins in regenerating rat muscles. A, myosin from regenerating rat leg muscle, 1 week after injury. There are 2 isomyosins migrating ahead of isomyosins 1-4 which are found in normal rat fast-twitch muscles. B, rat fetal myosins (from back muscles of 4-day-old rat), showing 4 fetal/embryonic components f1-f4. C, combination of A and B. The 2 additional isomyosins in rat regenerate co-migrate with fetal isomyosins f2 and f3.

TABLE 2

Content of slow isomyosins in normal and dystrophic human muscles expressed as percentage of total myosin. The differences between normal and dystrophic muscles are highly significant ($p<0.001$, Student's t test).

Muscle	Normal	Dystrophic
Deltoid	54.2 + 13.7% (n = 6)	78.4 + 7.1% (n = 17)
Vastus lateralis	48.4 + 10.4% (n = 12)	64.2 + 8.7% (n = 17)

and murine muscular dystrophy, suggesting that a common mechanism may be responsible.

It is now well established that the different types of muscle fibers in mammals are susceptible to interconversions from one fiber-type into another in response to various stimuli (192-193). For example, sustained stimulation at 10 Hz of a fast-twitch muscle in the rabbit leads to a switch in the synthesis of both the light chains and heavy chains characteristic of fast isomyosin to those of slow isomyosin (194-195), while intermittant stimulation increases the proportion of type 2A fibers (196). The fact that human muscle fibers can indeed undergo fiber type transformations have been documented in athletes undergoing training (180, 181, 197).

In the light of the dynamic nature of mammalian muscle fibers, we postulate that shifts in isomyosin distribution towards the slow and intermediate forms in dystrophic muscles represent a nonspecific adaptive response to increases usage, especially in response to increased gravitational load on postural muscles weakened by disease. It has been proposed that the normal impulse activity associated with postural reflexes provides the necessary stimulus for maintaining the synthesis of slow isomyosin in type 1 muscle fibers (198). Consistent with this view, increases in the proportion of type 1 fibers in the rat soleus have been reported to occur in response to increased gravitational load associated with increase in body weight during normal growth (199), with chronic exposure to elevated g force by centrifugation (193,200) and with synergist denervation (201). In contrast, when postural activity of the rat soleus is prevented by cordotomy (158) or by suspending the hind-quarters (198), a shift away from slow isomyosin towards the intermediate isomyosin becomes evident.

Atrophy of muscle tissue due to whatever cause would lead to a situation where the surviving muscle fibers would tend to be more intensively used than normal for postural maintenance and as well as phasic functions. This tendency to overuse would, through the mechanisms discussed above, lead to a shift in isomyosin and the fiber-type distributions towards the slow and intermediate types. Such a mechanism would be quite non-specific and would be expected to occur in other diseases in which muscular atrophy and weakness are prominent features. Consistent with this view, an increase in the proportion of slow isomyosin or type 1 muscle fibers is indeed quite commonly observed in neuromuscular diseases (170), being observed in spheroid body myopathy, central core disease, multicore disease and congenital type 1 fiber predominance. Similar findings have been reported by others (202-203). An increase in the proportion of type 1 muscle fibers is observed in anorexia nervosa (204). In this condition, nutritional atrophy of muscle fibers are usually associated with a high level of physical activity, and there is a complete absence of type 2B fibers. Reversing the argument that increased gravitational load would shift the distribution of isomyosins and muscle fiber types in the direction of the slow forms, it may be postulated that the reverse change, namely, slow to fast fiber type transformation, should occur in antigravity muscles of patients confined to the wheelchair, immobilized in plaster cast or after prolonged bed rest. Slow to fast fiber type transformation is also expected to occur in muscles of astronauts living in a micro-gravity environment for a protracted period of time.

An alternative hypothesis has been proposed (167) for the slowing of dystrophic (C57Bl/6J dy-2J/dy/2J) mouse fast-twitch muscles. According to this view, slow isomyosin is synthesized in response to spontaneous twitching of hindlimb muscles (205) which occurs in this strain of mice, possibly related to the presence of amyelination of lumbar spinal roots. While the spontaneous activity may indeed increase the level of total activity of these muscles, and so contribute to the observed isomyosin changes, it is not an essential feature of the dystrophic process leading to the slowing of the affected fast-twitch muscles. Spontaneous activity was not observed in the hindlimb muscles of the ReJ 129 dystrophic mice. The dystrophic EDL in which Parry and Desypris showed spontaneous electromyographic activity, did not contain type 1 fibers at all, whereas slowing of fast-twitch fibers occurred in the extensor carpi longus in this strain of mice even though no spontaneous activity was recorded (206). It is likely that slowing in all these muscles is due to the presence of IM in all these muscles in addition to the possible presence of SM. These changes probably arise as a result of increased activity in response to increase load on the weakened dystrophic muscles, irrespective of the presence or absence of spontaneous activity.

Isomyosins in Infantile Spinal Muscular Atrophy

Skeletal muscles from patients with infantile spinal muscular atrophy (Wernig-Hoffmann disease) have been shown to contain fetal isomyosins (153). Figure 10 shows examples from 4 different patients. The relative proportions of the various fetal components to each other are very similar to the fetal isomyosins in neonatal muscles. The percentage of fetal isomyosins present in infantile muscular atrophy varied up to a maximum of 55% of the total myosin, and frequently exceeded the amounts in Duchenne muscles.

The presence of fetal isomyosins in infantile spinal muscular atrophy is correlated with the appearance of myoblasts and myotubes (207,208), which are typical of fetal muscle tissue. This disease is associated with a drastic reduction (to 1/3 - 1/11 of controls) in the number of motoneurons in the spinal cord (209,210). These observations suggest that ultrastructual and isomyosin changes associated with the normal process of muscle cell differentiation are dependent on the availability of an adequate nerve supply.

The concept that the nerve is important for the induction of adult isomyosins during normal development is consistent with experimental findings. During normal development, 3 types of isomyosins appear and disappear in succession: embryonic, fetal (neonatal) and adult isoforms (153,175). In primary rat muscle cell cultures, only embryonic and fetal forms are expressed (211) (Hoh and Hughes, unpublished observations). However, when adult muscle fibers regenerating _in vitro_ are allowed to be innervated by neural explants, fast isomyosins are expressed (212).

The view that the nerve is required for the expression of adult myosin is apparently contradicted by certain clinical and experimental observations. A large amount of fetal isomyosin was found in a muscle biopsy from an adult patient with non-specific myalgia and fatigue (213). Three fetal components were present (f1, f2 and f3) and these form 1/3 of the total myosin. Light and electron microscopic analyses of the muscle tissue from this patient failed to reveal any abnormality. In particular, evidence of muscle atrophy, degeneration or regeneration was absent. Routine EMG analysis was also normal, suggesting the absence of abnormalities in innervation. The absence of atrophy suggests that trophic function of the nerve may be distinct from the mechanism regulating fetal isomyosin gene expression. The fact that apparently normal innervation could not suppress fetal isomyosin gene expression suggests that this process may involve something independent of, or in addition to, functional innervation of muscle fibers.

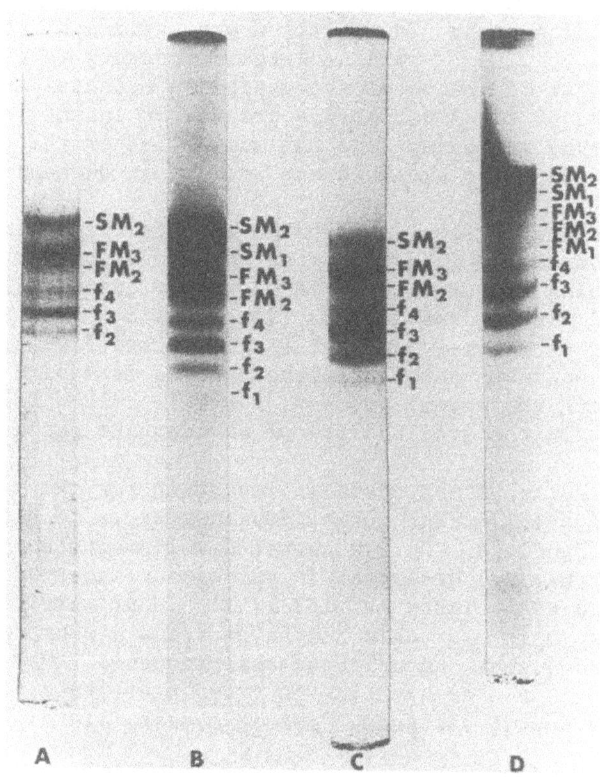

FIGURE 10: Gels containing myosins from muscles of 4 different patients affected by infantile spinal muscular atrophy. A and B, 4.5% gels. FM3 is the prominent fast myosin. There is no FM1 or f5. Fetal myosins f2-f4 are clearly, and f1, faintly seen. C, 4.5% gel. Approximately 55% of the myosin is present as fetal (f1-f4) components. The muscle specimen used was from a histochemical "bloch," which appeared to consist virtually entirely of hypotrophic fibers. D, 5% gel. In this example of myosin from spinal muscular atrophy there is an excess of slow myosin, and trace amounts of fast isomyosins, FM1-FM3, which are separated from the more widely spaced fetal isomyosins, f1-f4. All gels are from different electrophoretic runs. Reproduced from Fitzsimons and Hoh (1981a) by courtesy of the editors of the Journal of Neurological Sciences.

There is also experimental evidence that innervation may not be necessary for isomyosin differentiation. In a developing rat, fast isomyosins are not normally detected before the 10th day of post-natal life (175). Denervation of a fast muscle at 7 days of age did not prevent the subsequent appearance of fast myosin heavy chain (214). During regeneration of denervated adult soleus muscle, isomyosins which are similar in heavy chain structure to adult fast and fetal isomyosins but distinct from them appear 15 days after injuring the muscle by ischaemia and bupivacaine injection (187).

A possible explanation for these apparently contradictory findings on the role of the nerve in muscle differentiation may be that differentiating muscle cells require a factor or factors from the nerve. Muscles are already innervated before birth. Innervation may, without causing immediate adult myosin gene expression, commit the innervated cells to differentiate along a specific pathway. Furthermore, denervation *in vivo* may lead to the release of the postulated factors from the nerve stump into the general circulation. An abnormality in the structure and function of the postulated factors in the patient with non-specific myalgia may account for the fact that apparently normal innervation may not be sufficient for normal development. Clearly, more *in vitro* studies on muscle cell differentiation are called for to unravel the problem of how the normal process of muscle differentiation comes about and how these mechanisms may go wrong in neuromuscular diseases.

DR. RUBINSTEIN: We produced a monoclonal antibody which reacts with embryonic myosin and shows the same specificity in rat and human. Donald Schotland supplied a number of muscle biopsy samples to section and stain with this antibody. In specimens from normal muscles there was no binding, but in those that appeared under the light microscope to be dystrophic there was binding in the very small, apparently regenerating fibers. As Dr. Hoh said, embryonic myosin is clearly expressed in these regenerating fibers. We also found a small amount of embryonic myosin antibody in denervated fibers. We don't know whether that represents additional incorporation of satellite cells into these fibers or whether the nuclei pre-existing in the fibers were reexpressing it. Thus embryonic myosin may be expressed in diseased human muscle, probably in regenerating fibers, and perhaps in denervated muscle.

DR. BANDMAN: In diseased muscles do you see a shift toward an increased amount of slow myosin with an increased proportion of slow fibers?

DR. HOH: All we can say is that the distribution correlates. In the disease you do find more than Type 1 fibers.

DR. STROHMAN: Earlier we asked Dr. Rowland whether in Duchenne patients you could see some differential expression of the dystrophic process in the two different fiber types. It seems to me from your data that the slow fibers are accentuated in this case, suggesting that they were less affected in the disease than the fast.

DR. HOH: It is simply the way muscle reacts to the disease.

DR. EPSTEIN: When you see the fetal myosin increase in these situations, is the fetal myosin restricted to special fibers that do not contain the other myosins or does more than one isozyme exist in the same fiber?

DR. HOH: We have no data yet. It is important to resolve that question.

DR. FISCHMAN: In the 5 electrophoretic variants of isoforms, are these heavy chains? Can you elaborate on what the 5 electrophoretic variants may be?

DR. HOH: We haven't specifically examined the nature of light or heavy chains.

DR. ROWLAND: I want to ask Dr. Hoh about the exercise tolerance. In a patient with good exercise tolerance and normal muscle biopsy, you might assume that is nothing wrong with his muscles although he is shown to have fetal myosins. Aren't there normal people going around who are going to turn out to have fetal myosins?

DR. HOH: No. We have studied a variety of normal volunteers as well as patients whose muscle specimens were obtained during abdominal and orthopedic surgery.

DR. WHALEN: For a long time I was confused about the 5 bands referred to as embryonic and fetal but as you showed here and point out in your earlier papers, the F1 is always very minor and migrates in a fashion indistinguishable from the fibroblastic type myosin. If one discounts that, one is left with 4 bands, and as you said the data suggest that F2, F3 and F4 are fetal cum neonatal. I have no idea about the light chain content except the embryonic light chain is always very minor.

DR. HOH: Even in the early fetuses?

DR. WHALEN: In the early human fetus, I don't know, but certainly in the rat one can never go back far enough to have as much as 30 percent of embryonic light chain. In response to Henry Epstein's question, the conclusion would be that the small fibers have both adult fast myosin and fetal myosin.

DR. STROHMAN: Are you saying that the slow type fibers are showing less regeneration or fetal expression than fast type fibers?

DR. WHALEN: You have to see these biopsies to believe it. You have very small fibers which stain histochemically as Type 2 and very large type grouped fibers staining as class Type 1 and they are probably innervated and look healthy. It is in the very small fiber that one has both fast and fetal myosin.

DR. KEDES: Relating to the issue of not only getting to the isoforms existing in the single fiber, we are trying to decide which nucleus in that fiber is responsible for producing which isoform. Is it the newly recruited nucleus coming in from a satellite cell that is producing fetal type isoforms or are the nuclei already within the fiber capable of undergoing gene switching and revert to making fetal myosin? In the long run we are going to have to answer that question.

DR. FISCHMAN: I was going to ask if Dr. Umeda could comment on that. The cardiac system with the thyroxin stimulation. Can a single ventricular myonucleus transcribe to myosin heavy chains?

DR. UMEDA: I assume that the nuclei in the myocytes are capable of transcribing the genes.

DR. STROHMAN: That question has got to be answered and it cannot be necessarily predicted from what one knows about the expression of new satellite cells in completely regenerating fibers. In that case all of the fibers are gone and you have satellite cells dividing and making brand new fibers. Thus, in regenerating fibers, the first mode of expression is an embryonic one, embryonic myosin heavy chain and embryonic patterns of tropomyosin. Then within a week or so the process goes completely over to the adult patterns. The question is whether or not as new satellite cells move into pre-existing fibers does expression in those pre-existing fibers revert to fetal or embryonic patterns.

DR. WOOD: I would like to suggest that single fiber analysis is extremely important in answering these questions. By studying the entire fiber length one must determine whether or not the entire fiber undergoes a transformation from fast to slow, or slow to fast at the same time as certain nuclei are turned on to produce genes from one form throughout the cell. Alternatively genes might be causing sarcomeres to act differently from one another, displaying fast type, slow type and possible fetal type in the same fiber. If you have different isoforms in different regions of the same fiber, that itself could create a pathological condition.

DR. STREHLER: I think we can learn something from training athletes. It has been shown that there is a shift from fast myosin during training but there is no increase in cell number.

DR. PETTE: It is known from training studies we can also transform fast into slow fibers not only with regard to the enzymes but in regard to the sarcoplasmic reticulum and the myosin, but this is shown even better in the electrostimulation experiment where you can transform pre-existing fibers into fast and slow fibers. There is not loss of fibers no increase in fibers.

DR. WHALEN: In agreement with the studies of enzyme analysis we have found that the heavy chain transition is very complete when it goes from fast to slow. The first heavy chain transition seems to take place from Type 2B myosin heavy chain to Type 2A and then to slow myosin.

DR. BLAU: If I understood Dr. Pette correctly, one could get the switch from fast to slow in the absence of additional nuclei to the fiber. Can one get the switch from fetal to adult myosin isozyme expression?

DR. PETTE: I have no experience with that. We only looked for light chains. There the stimulation showed an increase in the synthesis of slow fiber myosin.

DR. BLAU: Developmental transition may require something else?

DR. PETTE: Yes.

CHAPTER 5: DISTRIBUTION OF SLOW MYOSIN IN DYSTROPHIC CHICKEN MUSCLE

Everett Bandman

Department of Food Science and Technology
University of California
Davis, CA

Introduction

Avian muscular dystrophy is a disorder that preferentially affects the development of fast twitch muscles (215,218). Previous research using anatomical, histochemical, and biochemical methods have demonstrated clear dystrophic abnormalities in the posterior latissimus dorsi (PLD) while the anterior latissimus dorsi (ALD), a slow tonic muscle, is unaffected by the disease (216,219). Most of this research has been performed on normal and dystrophic chickens of different genetic backgrounds. While avian muscular dystrophy is caused by a single autosomal recessive gene, the dystrophic gene causes relatively rapid fiber atrophy when placed on a New Hampshire background (217,220). These effects are most likely due to differences in the rate of muscle growth in the two breeds. Since inbred lines of normal and dystrophic chickens now exist that contain greater than 90% of their genes in common, these strains (normal line 03 and dystrophic line 433) were used for the current study to ensure that the differences observed between normal and dystrophic muscles were due to the disease.

The adult PLD contains focally innervated fast twitch fibers that are histochemically Type 2 (or α_W in the chicken) (221). The PLD is histochemically distinct from the ALD by 8 days of embryonic development (222). While the PLD is histochemically Type 2 at 8 days of embryonic development, previous studies have demonstrated

* I would like to acknowledge the expert technical assistance of Mr. Sam Matoba and Ms. Penelope Means and the helpful advice of Dr. George Cardinet. This research was supported by a grant from MDA to E. Bandman and by NIH Grant 1 R01 AM31731-01.

slow myosin light chains and slow myosin isozyme during development of the PLD (223). These slow myosin components appear during normal development so that by 90 days ex ovo the PLD contains only fast myosin components (223).

We have previously shown that the PLD in dystrophic chickens continues to contain slow myosin components even in fully mature one year old birds (223). The purpose of the present study was to determine the cytodistribution of these slow myosin components. This was accomplished through immunocytochemistry using an antibody specific for slow myosin heavy chain and the histochemical ATPase reaction following acid pretreatment.

The interpretation of the immunocytochemical results in this study are based on the specificity of the antisera used. Antisera were raised in rabbits immunized with either adult fast or adult slow myosin heavy chains. The antigen used was homogenized SDS polyacrylamide gel containing the myosin heavy chain from the pectoralis major (fast) or anterior latissimus dorsi (slow). The specificity of the antisera was tested using "Western blot analysis." It was found that these antisera reacted predominantly against the antigen used for immunization. However, these antisera did cross react with the reciprocal antigens. These cross reacting antibodies were removed by absorbing antislow myosin heavy chain antisera with fast myosin coupled to Sepharose and by absorbing antifast myosin heavy chain antisera with slow myosin coupled to Sepharose. The resulting antibodies did not cross react as judged by "Western blot analysis" (Figure 11).

Immunocytochemical Analysis

In order to demonstrate the immunocytochemical specificity of the antibodies, a mixed fiber type muscle (Medial Gastrocnemius) was reacted with the both antifast and antislow myosin heavy chain antibody. Bound antibody was localized using horseradish peroxidase coupled to Staph Protein A. As shown in Figure 12, a reciprocal staining pattern is observed. In addition, those fibers that react with the antislow antibody are identical to those that demonstrate acid-stable ATPase activity indicating they are Type 1 or slow fibers. Thus, Western blot analysis demonstrates that the antislow myosin heavy chain reacts only with slow heavy chain and immunocytochemistry indicates that the antibody reacts only with histochemically Type I fibers.

The PLD was dissected from normal and dystrophic chickens at -4d, 0d, 10d, 20d, 40d, 60d, 90d, 120d and 1 year. The muscles were placed side by side and frozen in liquid freon. Transverse sections were cut at 9-14μ and serial sections were reacted with either antifast or antislow myosin heavy chain antibody. Serial sections were also reacted for myosin ATPase after acid or alkaline

FIGURE 11: Specificity of antislow and antifast MHC antibodies by "Western Blot" analysis. Embryonic pectoralis, adult pectoralis and neonatal ALD myosin heavy chains were electrophoretically transferred to nitrocellulose and cut into replicate strips. One strip was stained with amido black (Strip B) to identify the position of the myosins. Strip A was reacted with antibody to adult pectoralis MHC. This antibody also reacts with embryonic pectoralis MHC, but does not react with either SM_1 or SM_2 ALD MHC. Strip C was reacted with antibody to adult ALD MHC (ALD SM_2). This antibody cross reacts slightly with SM1 MHC but does not react with either embryonic or adult pectoralis MHC.

preincubation and others were stained with hematoxylin and eosin. Since both normal and dystrophic muscle were on the same slide, differences in reactivity of the dystrophic muscle could easily be observed and artifacts due to different reaction conditions minimized.

At 17 days in the embryo a population of cells (∿ 20%) that reacted with antislow myosin heavy chain and were positive for acid stable ATPase were observed. Many but not all of these cells

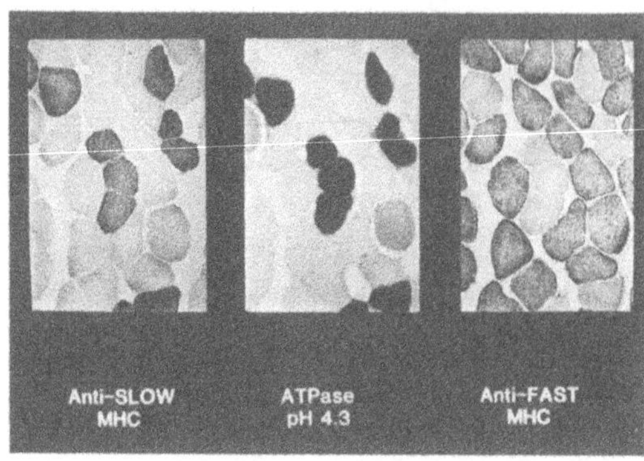

FIGURE 12: Immunocytochemical specificity of antifast and antislow MHC antibody. Cryostat sections of a mixed chicken leg muscle (medial gastrocnemius) were reacted with either antifast or antislow MHC antibody. A third serial section was reacted for histochemical ATPase at pH 4.3 which specifically stains slow MHC containing fibers. A recipropical staining pattern is observed with the antifast and antislow antibodies and those staining with the antislow antibody also stain with the ATPase reaction at pH 4.3.

also reacted with the antifast MHC antibody and exhibited alkali stable ATPase activity. The same pattern was observed in both normal and dystrophic muscle. At hatching this population of cells was greatly reduced and completely gone by 10 days ex ovo in the PLD from normal muscle but continued to be present in the PLD of dystrophic chickens. In older normal chickens no fibers (except for intrafusal fibers of the muscle spindles, see below) were positive for antislow MHC or acid stable ATPase. In contrast, muscle fibers which were positive for antislow MHC antibody and acid stable ATPase were reproducibly observed in dystrophic muscle. Two kinds of such fibers were routinely observed (Figs. 13 & 14). A large fiber with similar antibody and histochemical staining pattern as the Type I fibers of the medial gastrocnemius. These fibers make up 3-5% of the PLD in a 120d dystrophic chicken. In addition, very small fibers that react with the antislow MHC antibody and exhibit acid stable ATPase were seen in the dystrophic chicken at all ages studied. A majority of these fibers also exhibited ATPase activity after alkaline preincubation and were similar to the small fibers seen in embryonic and just hatched normal chickens. While these fibers were more prevalent than the larger fibers, because of their small size they account for less than 1% of the total muscle mass.

All muscle spindles contained at least 1 but often 2 or 3 intrafusal fibers that reacted with the antislow MHC antibody and contained acid stable, alkali labile ATPase activity. This was true in both normal and dystrophic PLD from 10d to 1 year.

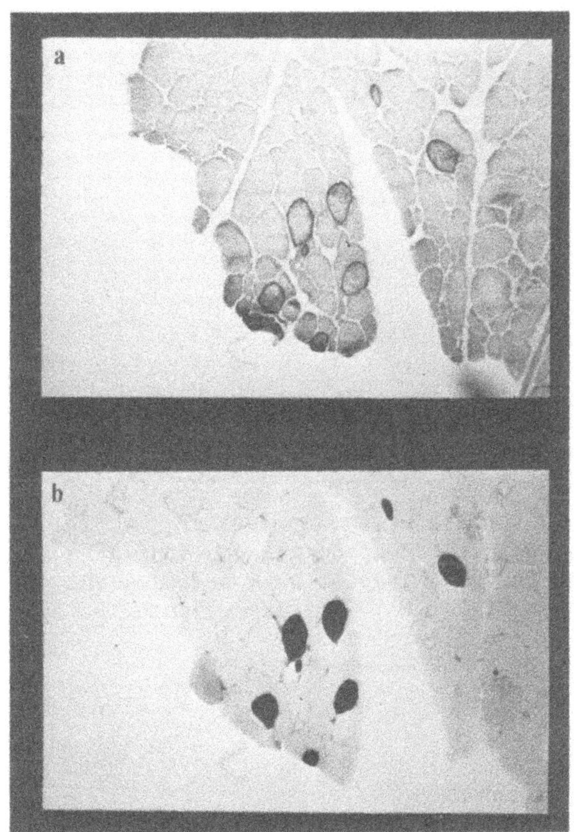

FIGURE 13: Large slow myosin containing fibers in the dystrophic PLD. Serial sections of a 120 day old chicken PLD were reacted with antislow antibody (a) and for acid stable ATPase (b).

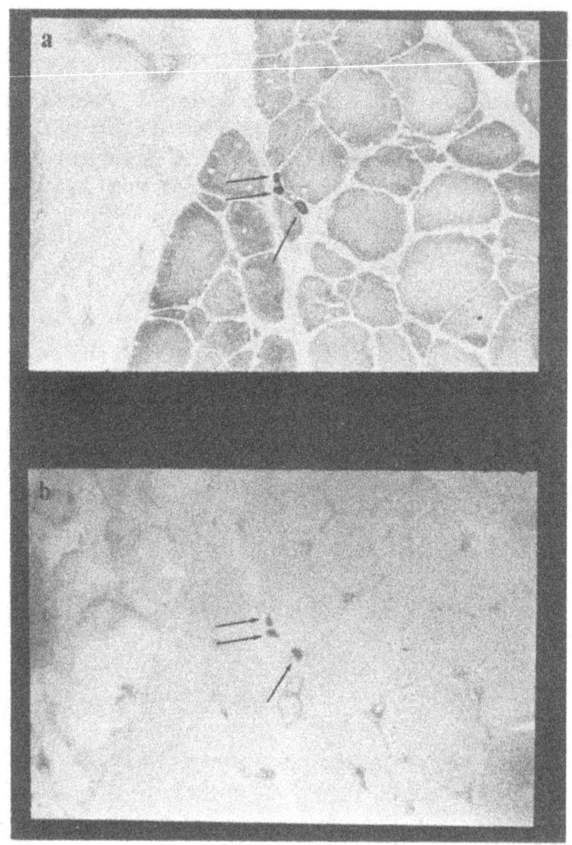

FIGURE 14: Small slow myosin containing fibers in the dystrophic chicken PLD. Serial sections of a 90 day old dystrophic PLD were reacted with antislow MHC (a) and for acid stable ATPase (b). The arrows point to small slow myosin positive fibers.

While these results could account for the presence of 5-6% slow myosin in the dystrophic PLD, calibration of gel scans of non-denaturing gels suggested that dystrophic muscle samples contained up to 20% slow myosin. Furthermore, the PLD of 1 month old normal chickens also contains up to 15% slow myosin, yet no slow fibers were observed at this age in normal muscles.

A possible explanation for these results comes from examination of the region where normal and dystrophic muscle can be observed in one field. After reacting the 1 year sample with antislow MHC it can be seen that all cells in the dystrophic muscle stain darker than those in the normal muscle. No differential staining is observed after reaction with antifast MHC antibody. A similar result was observed with the acid ATPase reaction. That is, all cells in dystrophic muscle were stained darker than those in the normal muscle. These results suggest that all cells may contain a small amount of slow myosin. Thus, it appears that in addition to the large and small Type I fibers the rest of the fibers in the adult dystrophic PLD also may contain slow myosin. Since normal neonatal PLD also contains slow myosin components, our results are consistent with the idea that avian muscular dystrophy inhibits muscle maturation in fast twitch muscles.

These observations may extend to other muscles in the dystrophic chicken. Unlike the medial gastrocnemius, the laterial gastrocnemius (LG) is a pure fast twitch muscle in the normal adult. Like the PLD, the LG contains slow myosin in the embryo and neonatal chicken. This slow myosin disappears from the muscle by 90-120 days. In the one year old dystrophic chicken, not only is the fast myosin isozyme pattern severely altered, but a significant amount of slow myosin is routinely observed. Immunocytochemical localization of slow myosin in the LG is currently underway.

It is possible that an altered activity pattern of fast twitch fibers rather than an inhibition of maturation is responsible for the expression of slow myosin in fast fibers of the PLD and LG. However, not all fast twitch muscles contain slow myosin isozymes. Although some slow light chains are present in the pectoralis major (PM) of 10-12 day old embryos, with the exception of a small red area in the adult, no slow myosin isozyme or slow myosin heavy chains have been observed in this muscle in dystrophic chickens.

In the pectoralis, most muscle fibers atrophy resulting in an inability of the dystrophic bird to right itself when placed on its back. Other fast twitch muscles (e.g., PLD) while showing clear morphological, histochemical and biochemical abnormalities are not as severely affected. A possible explanation for this observation may be that these muscles contain slow myosin components either as a result of inhibited maturation or as the result of an adaptive response to an altered activity pattern in dystrophic muscle. The inability of the pectoralis muscle to express slow myosin may be the reason that this muscle is so severely affected by avian muscular dystrophy.

DR. STREHLER: What is the clinical effect of the disease on chickens?

DR. BANDMAN: These chickens live a normal lifetime. They are capable of reproducing. The main manifestation of dystrophy is that the chicken can't right itself because its pectoralis muscle is almost completely atrophied.

DR. HOLTZER: Did you say the intrafusal fibers went along with the extrafusal in the muscle?

DR. BANDMAN: What I was trying to say is that we always see slow myosin in some of the intrafusal fibers in normal and dystrophic. There is no difference in normal and dystrophic chickens. Even normal chickens contain slow myosin in some intrafusal fibers in the muscle spindle. There are no differences between muscle spindles.

DR. WOOD: I wonder if you could comment on the idea of why some change in the myosin isoform pattern leads to or contributes to the weakness of these muscles. How do these data indicate any pathological development in these muscles at all?

DR. BANDMAN: We know very little about the properties of the isozymes of myosin certainly with respect to what that means when you are talking about a cross-bridge interaction with an actin filament. What interests me most about this particular system is that I think this is most likely a clear developmental disease. Why slow tonic muscle of the chicken is not affected by the disease yet the fast twitch muscle is affected by the disease may give us some understanding of the differences between those two muscles. The slow tonic muscles also undergo myosin isozyme transitions during maturation and for some reason those are not affected. Certainly in the pure slow tonic muscle of ALD, it is not affected. We haven't investigated what happens in a mixed muscle where in fact there may be some effect as a result of surrounding fiber degeneration in the fast fibers.

DR. LOWEY: Are you implying that these slow components in the PLD and dystrophic PM that are cross-reacting with your slow antibody are necessarily adult slow myosin?

DR. BANDMAN: That antibody presumably could be reacting with SM1 myosin isozyme. We might consider it a neonatal type of ALD heavy chain, but it doesn't react with the embryonic pectoralis myosin.

DR. LOWEY: The reason I bring this up is I have spent a lot of years isolating the component in the embryo pectoralis myosin that cross-reacts with the adult slow antibody. We actually isolated this very tiny fraction of the embryonic myosin that cross-reacted with the slow antibody. It in no way chemically, by peptide mapping, looked like adult slow myosin. So it is a distinct isozyme. I just want to caution everyone, we should be careful when we talk about slow myosin in either dystrophic or embryonic muscles, it may not and probably is not adult slow as we understand it.

DR. BANDMAN: That was one of the reasons for using the embryonic pectoralis myosin to absorb the adult antisera raised against the adult ALD. I was aware that it would indeed cross-react and did cross-react to some extent when it was first raised in rabbits; a primary sera would detect the small amount of embryonic pectoralis major myosin heavy chain, but after the absorption it no longer reacted with the component so those antibodies were presumably removed. The fact that we do see that adult slow myosin isozyme in our non-denaturing gels, I think, suggests and we could account for it by the presence of these fibers.

DR. PETTE: The point was just raised why is the ALD not affected. This is very naive. The ALD is always active whereas in the chicken which are not flying, PLD and pectoralis are not active. I just wondered what happens if one would fix mechanically the wing so that the ALD is not necessarily active.

DR. BANDMAN: I think people have shown if you do the cross-innervations then the ALD exhibits a dystrophic abnormality. If you did anything to induce the fast myosin program, whatever that is in that particular muscle, it starts to express those particular abnormalities, so it may be partly this large program that is being activated which results in the expression of the disease in that particular muscle.

DR. HOH: Are there any mechanical or physiological studies on dystrophic muscle.

DR. BANDMAN: There are very few physiological studies done on dystrophic muscle except for the PLD. People have looked quite extensively between PLD and ALD.

DR. WOOD: There are physiological data not all which have to do with myosin isoforms. I would like to make a very strong point that those data could be derived from changes in calcium release and/or change in calcium uptake or clearance and/or changes in troponin types.

DR. HOH: Large amounts of myosin implies that there ought to be a contribution of slow components within the muscle. In other words, an elevation of the slower component in the isometric twitch which in a whole muscle would summate with the form of the isometric which contributed fact finders. This becomes indistinguishable in terms of the relaxation rate.

DR. BANDMAN: Today is actually the first time I was made aware of the fact of a shift towards the slow myosin in the rats, humans and chickens. It seems to me it must be more than a coincidence in this variety of species which have a similar type of muscle affliction.

CHAPTER 6: SATELLITE CELLS IN NORMAL, REGENERATING AND DYSTROPHIC MUSCLE

Edward Schultz

Department of Anatomy
University of Wisconsin
Madison, WI

I will first present some background material on satellite cells including a review of some of our recent studies and then conclude with some observations which I hope will be a stimulus for further discussion.

I have included a picture of a satellite cell (Figure 15) to remind everyone that they are a population of mononucleated cells located on the surface of muscle fibers, usually in a slight depression on the myofiber surface. The cells are covered by the external lamina of the myofiber. There have been no junctional complexes found to be associated with satellite cell and the muscle fiber.

Satellite cells apparently are derived from the pool of myoblasts in areas of muscle formation. Such myoblasts must not fuse during the formation of myotubes, but rather remain on the surface of the myotubes. After maturation of the myotube to a muscle fiber, the associated single cells can be morphologically identified for the first time as satellite cells (144). For all practical purposes, therefore, they are of the same lineage as embryonic myoblasts. During postnatal myofiber growth, satellite cells continue to divide. After a mitotic division, one or both daughter cells fuse with the muscle fiber and donate a bit of cytoplasm and a new nucleus to the syncytium (225). In this manner the protein to DNA ratio is maintained at a stable level as the fiber enlarges. Thus, satellite cells have a very important role in postnatal growth. Their other important role is in muscle regeneration (225-226). When a muscle is damaged the surviving satellite cells are activated to recapitulate embryonic

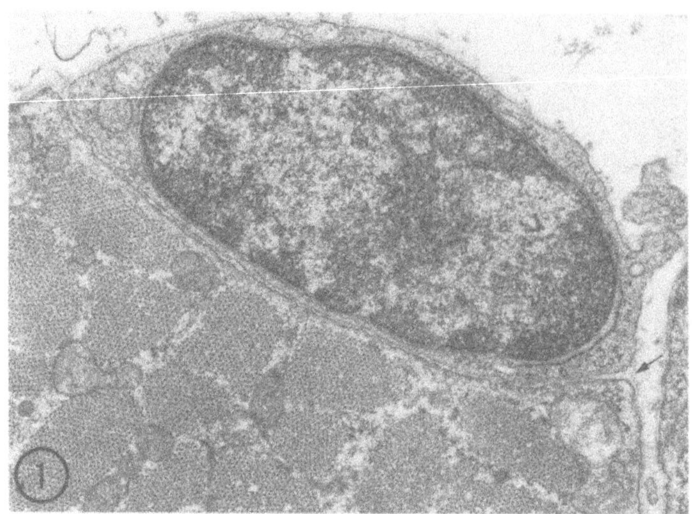

FIGURE 15: Satellite cell viewed in transverse section. Distinguishing features are the high nucleus to cytoplasmic ratio, paucity of organelles and heterochromatic nucleus. The external lamina of the muscle fiber (arrow) does not enter the interspace between cells. This satellite cell has a small cytoplasmic extension into the interstitial space.

myogenesis and give rise to new muscle fibers and/or repair existing fibers.

Because of their important roles in both muscle growth and regeneration, satellite cell nuclei have been counted by a number of investigators (227-234) and expressed as the percentage of the total nuclei counted (myonuclei and satellite cell nuclei). At birth and immediately after birth, satellite cells comprise a significant proportion of myofiber nuclei, generally reported to be at or around 30%. This proportion falls off rather rapidly with age so that adult animals commonly have only 4, 3 or 2% satellite cells. Some minor variability is evident between animals or between muscles of the same animal.

We recently reexamined these age-related changes in satellite cell percentages with a goal of understanding what permutations occur in the actual number of cells during postnatal growth and subsequent maturation. Whether satellite cell numbers increase, decrease or remain the same would be extremely important in our attempts to understand the processes of growth and potential for regeneration.

In our studies we used rat extensor digitorum longus (EDL) and soleus muscles because of the histochemical differences between the muscles (the EDL is glycolytic and the soleus is oxidative) and the observation that the percentage of satellite cells is always greater in the soleus (228-230) a difference which becomes greater with age.

Differences in Satellite Cell Number in Oxidative vs Glycolytic Muscles

We found a much larger population of satellite cells in the soleus than in the EDL (Table 3) even when the two muscles were compared, taking into consideration differences in size, number or length of fibers. Hence, muscles are not all equivalent with respect to satellite cell populations. The number of satellite cells actually increased in the soleus between 1 and 12 months, then declined between 12 and 24 months so there was no net change between 1 and 24 months. In the EDL we found a distinctly different pattern in which the absolute number of satellite cells gradually decreased with age. Therefore, although the relative number of satellite cells decreased in both muscles the absolute number of satellite cells paralleled that relative decrease only in EDL. We also examined how satellite cells were distributed on the different fiber-types in the soleus and EDL muscles. Both the soleus and EDL have Type IIA and Type I fibers but the EDL has, in addition, Type IIB fibers. We reasoned that differences in the number of satellite cells in the soleus and EDL muscles might be accounted for if the satellite cell population on Type IIB fibers was very small. We examined fixed sections of the entire cross-section of the EDL with the electron microscope. Once we found a fiber with a satellite cell sectioned through the nucleus, we marked the position of that fiber on a photographic montage of the whole cross-section stained with p-phenylenediamine (235) which has the same staining characteristics as SDH on frozen sections. Therefore, on the basis of SDH stainability we determined the fiber-type distribution of the soleus and EDL muscles in the general population and the fibers which had been selected for the frequency of satellite cells on their surface.

We observed that satellite cells are not found with equal frequency on all fibers (Table 4) and that the pattern of distribution is established by at least one month of age. Although the Type IIB fibers did have somewhat fewer satellite cells on their surface, we calculated that the decrease was not enough to account for the differences in total populations of the two muscles.

DR. KELLY: Are you suggesting that the EDL of the rat has 31.8% population of Type I fibers?

TABLE 3

Nuclear populations in soleus and EDL muscles

	Total Myofiber Nuclei ($x10^6$)		Absolute Number Satellite Cells ($x10^5$)	
Age	Soleus	EDL	Soleus	EDL
1 month	5.4	4.4	5.2	3.1
12 months	11.1	7.1	7.3	2.1
24 months	11.4	7.0	5.4	1.3

DR. WHALEN: The SDH doesn't correlate with ATPase, that is why there are differences.

DR. SCHULTZ: Yes, Dr. Whalen is correct. We have determined the distribution of satellite cells on fiber-types characterized according to SDH and not ATPase and the two methods do not exactly correspond. The point I would like to make is that our results indicate one cannot generalize regarding the distribution of satellite cells on the same fiber types between muscles. Type IIA fibers in the EDL have the highest percentage of satellite cells whereas the same fiber-type in the soleus has the lowest.

Local Control of Satellite Cell Concentration

In an effort to determine how the size of the reserve population of satellite cells might be determined in a muscle, we conducted a series of free graft experiments using the soleus and the EDL. The muscles were removed and then 1) returned to the original position, an orthoptic free graft, or 2) the muscles were removed and cross-transplanted, a heterotopic free-graft. As a result of severing all the nerve and vascular supplies, there is a necrosis of the myofibers leading to a complete degeneration/ regeneration of the muscle (236). We found that when the EDL muscle was placed in the soleus bed, the satellite cell percentage after regeneration was equivalent to that found in the soleus and alternatively the soleus regenerated in the EDL bed had a satellite cell percentage of the EDL (Table 5). There was no change in the satellite cell percentages of the orthotopically grafted muscles.

We have tentatively concluded from these experiments that the nerve, as it dictates fiber-types, also dictates in some way,

TABLE 4

Percentage Fiber Type Composition[1]

		1 Month			12 Months		
		General fiber population	Satellite-cell-fiber population	Satellite cell/general	General fiber population	Satellite-cell-fiber population	Satellite cell/general
EDL	Type IIA	34.9	42.0	1.20	14.1	23.8	1.68
	Type I	31.8	31.8	1.00	47.5	43.8	0.92
	Type IIB	33.3	26.2	0.78	38.4	32.5	0.84
Soleus	Type IIA	36.4	20.4	0.56	14.9	4.0	0.26
	Type I	63.6	79.6	1.25	85.1	96.0	1.12

[1]Chi square analysis of the data indicated that (1) fiber type composition changed significantly between 1 and 12 months in the general population of the soleus and EDL ($\alpha = 0.005$); (2) fiber type composition changed significantly between 1 and 12 months in the satellite cell-fiber population of the soleus ($\alpha = 0.005$) and EDL ($\alpha = 0.05$); (3) fiber type composition was significantly different between the general population and satellite cell-fiber population in the EDL at 12 months ($\alpha = 0.1$) and in the soleus at 1 and 12 months ($\alpha = 0.005$).

either directly or indirectly, the reserve population of satellite cells in a given muscle. Perhaps the satellite cell populations

TABLE 5

Percentage of Sattellite Nuclei

	EDL	SOLEUS
NORMAL	3.40	6.90
FREE GRAFT	3.45	7.50
CROSS-TRANSPLANT[b]	6.89	3.31

[a]The percentages are a mean from 6 muscles for each group except the free graft soleus in which 5 muscles were examined. Chi square analysis of the data demonstrated that the percentage of satellite cells was significantly different between (1) normal soleus and EDL muscles, (2) free graft soleus and EDL muscles, and (3) cross-transplants and their respective free grafts or normals. In each case, $p < 0.01$.

[b]Labeled as EDL or soleus according to their original position.

may somehow be related to the functions of a muscle since muscles that are engaged in continuous contraction, most of which are oxidative, have a very high percentage of satellite cells. Thus, the diaphragm and the soleus muscles have a very high percentage and population of satellite cells. Even within a muscle, the satellite cell distribution on fiber-types also follows the same pattern. Type IIA fibers, the most frequently recruited motor units in the EDL have the highest percentage of satellite cells. Conversely, Type I fibers, which are recruited most frequently in the soleus, have the highest population of satellite cells in that muscle.

Relation of Satellite Cell Number to Growth Rate

The results of our work also point to a possible correlation between the satellite cell percentage in a given muscle and growth rate of that muscle. For example, the rat soleus at maturity has about 11 million myofiber nuclei and the EDL has about 7 million. Despite the fact that there are so many more myonuclei in the soleus, it grows only for a period of 3 months, whereas the EDL is a much more slowly growing muscle, reaching its maximum over 10 months. The mere fact that satellite cells in the soleus must produce that number of nuclei in a shorter growth period requires a larger stem cell population.

We are also interested in quantitative aspects of the regeneration potential. Two common determinants of the success of a regeneration response are: 1) the number and the availability of stem cells; and 2) the ability of the individual cells to proliferate and take part in the response. From our quantitative studies we know the number of cells available to take part in a regeneration response in the rat and EDL and soleus muscles at 1-12 and 24 months. In order to determine the proliferative capacity of the cells we enzymatically removed and plated in culture the satellite cells from muscles of rats ranging in age from 1 week to 30 months. During the first two days in culture the position of individual myoblasts was marked on the underside of the culture dishes. Then on a daily basis we counted the number of cells in the colonies that arose from the individually marked cells.

Regeneration & Aging

I think it is quite evident (Table 6) that the cells from young muscle have a very high capacity for colony formation. With increasing donor age, however, the average size of the colonies decreased dramatically. The reductions in colony size between 1 week and 3 months donor age may be the result of satellite cell divisions required *in vivo* to supply additional nuclei to the growing muscle fiber. Reductions in colony size in older animals are more difficult to explain, although the reduction may relate to the fact that the rat is a continuously growing animal. In any case, this study shows that under identical *in vitro* conditions the ability of satellite cells to proliferate and form colonies is inversely proportional to the age of the donor animal.

DR. HOLTZER: Do all of your cells form definitive muscle cells, myotubes when you talk about satellite cells, clones, etc.?

DR. SCHULTZ: We have identified them on the basis of their morphology but nonetheless we feel quite confident that all of the cells we have included in the study are satellite cell-derived myoblasts. Marked cells in parallel cultures fused and formed myotubes.

The reduced proliferative capacity that we see as a result of increasing age, suggests that regeneration potential of the muscle decreases with age but, of course, the magnitude of that decrease depends upon the size of the reserve population of satellite cells. The total proliferative capacity of satellite cells in the soleus and EDL muscles is obtained by multiplying

TABLE 6

Mean Number of Cells Per Colony*

Donor Age	3	4	5	6	7	***p-Value
6 days	7.8±1.53	20.7±2.57	66.1±8.53	141.3±27.06	191**	0.01
15 days		15.6±1.76	60.2±7.93	74.0±12.2	87.1 ±16.03	0.10
1 month	10.6±1.28	16.3±1.46	43.1±5.98	57.4±10.9	58.6 ± 9.74	0.025
3 month	9.0±0.91	13.3±1.22	20.8±2.99	21.3±3.96	20.46±14.08	0.025
12 month	5.7±1.23	6.7±1.58	17.0±5.13	17.0±3.54	16.2 ± 3.07	
24 month	1.4±0.05	3.5±0.30	10.4±1.23	15.3±2.07	12.09± 1.73	
30 month	1.0±0.02	1.8±0.10	3.7±0.25	8.0±1.41	12.55± 1.41	

* Standard Error

** Estimate, colonies were too large to accurately count; p-value is based on 6 days *in vitro*

*** p-value is based on 6 days *in vitro*

the absolute number of satellite cells in the muscles at 1-12 and 24 months of age by the average number of progeny that each satellite cell is capable of generating. This provides a very crude indication of the regeneration potential of these muscles. Taking into account the existing myofiber nuclei population, one finds in very young animals, the ability to regenerate both EDL and soleus muscle several times over. With increasing age the regeneration ability of the satellite cell population is decreased to the extent that the EDL in old mature animals (24 months) cannot be completely regenerated.

I would like to propose the following scenario for discussion. In a normal growing muscle the satellite cells are continually dividing in order to provide additional myonuclei to the enlarging fibers. In the dystrophic situation, however, in the presence of degeneration and necrosis of existing fibers, satellite cells become engaged concurrently in regeneration of additional myotubes or for the repair of the existing fibers. Regeneration and growth can continue only until the proliferation potential of the cells is reached, after which the regeneration will simply fall apart. Rather than a primary defect in the satellite cells, therefore, I am advocating an exhaustion of the regeneration response in dystrophic muscle due to the phenotypic senescence of the satellite cells.

We have done several experiments that lend support to this scenario. When only a small portion of a fiber is damaged the activation of the satellite cells occur along the entire length of the fiber. Thus, even local lesions along the length of the muscle produce a general activation and response of satellite cells. I suspect if one were to quantitate the population of satellite cells at the onset of degeneration in dystrophy, one could find an elevation in the percentage of satellite cells. An increase in satellite cells has been reported in dystrophic muscles (234,237). Attempts to isolate satellite cells from dystrophic muscle at the onset of regeneration would produce ample numbers of cells for culture and very good myogenesis from the cells that had been liberated. However, a continued regeneration response would push the cells to the limit of their proliferation potential. At this point there would occur a reduction in the yield of cells from the diseased muscle and their ability to grow in culture.

An additional reason we think this is a reasonable scenerio is based upon the results of some recent experiments utilizing Marcaine injections of intact normal muscle. EDL muscles of normal young adult rats were twice injected with Marcaine (injections 30 days apart) to initiate a regeneration response (238). Thirty days after the second injection, the injected muscle and the uninjured muscle of the opposite leg were removed and prepared for culture. Our preliminary results demonstrate that the Marcaine injected muscle had a reduced number of satellite cells capable of producing large colonies. This preliminary study suggests a reduction in the total proliferation potential or premature senescence of satellite cells that were removed from the damaged muscle.

I think the important thing about advocating an early senescence of satellite cells in dystrophy is that it explains the decline of the regeneration response and, more importantly, separates the abortive regeneration from whatever primary defect causes death of existing fibers. We could thus infer that satellite cells themselves are spared from the dystrophic defect.

DR. STROHMAN: I would like to ask a question about some of the cell differences in the fibers you talked about in the different muscles. I understand that you are saying that the differences in the number of satellite cells cannot be explained on the basis of the difference in the fiber-types, but rather has to do with the functions of the muscle as a whole.

DR. SCHULTZ: I just don't think at this point we can make a general statement regarding the distribution of satellite cells on particular fiber-type muscles, other than to say they are not equally distributed. In both of the muscles we examined, the fibers most frequently used had the greatest number of cells. The fibers were not of the same type. The number of satellite cells in the EDL and soleus muscles also appeared to be related to the growth characteristics of those muscles.

DR. STROHMAN: When you did the transplanting experiments you said you thought you were studying the effect of the nerve. Why is it the nerve? Why couldn't it be the different vascularization pattern. I mention that specifically because in the next section we are going to come back to this at least theoretically to deal with growth factors; why is it nerve and not the circulation?

DR. SCHULTZ: The cross-reinnervation would help iron out some of those problems.

DR. STROHMAN: But it could be the circulatory pattern as well?

DR. SCHULTZ: Yes.

DR. PETTE: You might test this hypothesis with stimulation. If the nerve is responsible, you should be able to increase the number of satellite cells by stimulating the muscle.

DR. FISCHMAN: If I understand correctly, if the soleus of the right leg was damaged and caused to regenerate while the soleus of the left leg was left undisturbed. After repeated regenerations, you would predict that we should get senescent satellite cells on one side and not on the other. That is a clear prediction and I think it should be tested.

DR. SCHULTZ: We are presently examining induced senescence of satellite cells using Marcaine injections to initiate regeneration. Our preliminary results suggest a reduction in the proliferation potential of the satellite cells. The reduction is primarily due to an almost complete loss of the cells capable of giving rise to large colonies. In this sense the distribution of colony sizes from cells of the regenerated muscle resembles that of cells from older animals.

DR. YAFFE: You saw this dramatic regenerative capacity. Did you test it to see how many times you could regenerate an old muscle?

DR. BLAU: The experiment has been done by Bradley. He showed he could damage rat muscle and get it to regenerate 12 times over.

DR. SCHULTZ: In that particular experiment Bradley did not inject Marcaine directly into the muscle. I don't think he has really challenged the entire muscle to regenerate. The number of times a muscle can fully regenerate has yet to be tested.

DR. KEDES: Where you showed the number of doublings decreasing with age, the colonies were labeled as numbers of cells not numbers of doublings. The number of cells at the youngest age was 55, that is 6 doublings, then it went down to 15, that is only 4 doublings. Do you mean, therefore, that cells you isolate go through 6 doublings and 4 doublings, etc.?

DR. SCHULTZ: Prior to three months of age the donor cells had not reached their maximum number of doublings. Those were the number of doublings that took place during the time I looked at them.

DR. KEDES: I understand now, that means you didn't know what the complete doubling capacity of any individual colony was later, so you are really measuring the relative rate of the initial doubling. Is that correct?

DR. SCHULTZ: Yes, but at 3 months of age the cells of the donor reached a plateau and hence their maximum number of doublings. A minor population of colonies was still expanding at all ages we examined.

DR. YAFFE: Do you plate the cell and count the number of colonies?

DR. SCHULTZ: I plated out the cells and marked individual cells in the beginning of the experiment and then counted the colonies derived from the marked cells.

DR. YAFFE: How do you prevent them from fusing?

DR. SCHULTZ: For the first 7 days they do not fuse.

DR. KEDES: Are those cells from the late stages capable of fusing?

DR. SCHULTZ: Yes.

CHAPTER 7: EVIDENCE FOR DEFECTIVE MYOBLASTS IN DUCHENNE MUSCULAR DYSTROPHY

Helen M. Blau*, Cecilia Webster*,
Grace K. Pavlath* and Choy-Pik Chiu

*Department of Pharmacology
Stanford University School of Medicine
Stanford, CA

Duchenne muscular dystrophy (DMD) is a degenerative disorder associated with progressive muscle weakness. Affected children eventually die from respiratory or cardiac failure and rarely survive to adulthood. It is a genetic disease due to a defect at a single locus on the X-chromosome and is therefore transmitted by female carriers to their sons. The disease is relatively common; one in 4,800 males or a total of approximately 20,000 boys in the United States has DMD (239).

The hypothesis has been put forward that DMD is the result of a defective membrane in the mature muscle fiber (240). This was thought to be the cause of the characteristic hundred-fold elevation in serum levels of the muscle enzyme creatine kinase. Despite numerous studies, there is still little solid evidence to support this view (4), although differences between normal and dystrophic sarcoplasmic membranes have been demonstrated by electron microscopy (8).

The reason for the paucity of information regarding this disease is that muscle is a heterogeneous tissue containing adipocytes and connective tissue in addition to muscle cells. This heterogeneity is especially pronounced and problematic in diseased muscle tissue, in which the proportions of these other cell types is often increased and highly variable. Even different biopsies of the same muscle may differ in their cellular composition. Furthermore, upon cultivation of cells from dissociated muscle tissue *in vitro*, the problem may be further complicated; this is because the fibroblasts present in the cultures frequently outgrow the muscle cells. As a result, establishing consistent differences in morphological and biochemical parameters of muscle biopsies or the cultured cells derived from them is difficult due to the lack of a solid frame of reference.

To overcome these problems we developed a method for eliminating all other cell types and growing pure populations of human muscle cells in tissue culture. This permitted us to study the muscle cell itself under controlled conditions in order to determine whether there existed an intrinsic defect in that cell type. Although culture methods had been developed for chicken and rodent muscle, methods for cultivating human muscle cells were limited. We sought to extend the work of Dr. Hauschka (241,242) regarding the isolation and growth of human fetal muscle cells. Our methods were developed for postnatal human muscle tissue because we wanted to work with cells from patients with DMD; the diagnosis for this disease is not definitive until after birth (243). The cells we isolated from the muscle were the satellite cells, first defined by Dr. Mauro (144) as the myoblasts that lie between the sarcolemma and the basement membrane of mature muscle fibers. We established methods for obtaining large numbers of satellite cells (approximately 10^{12} cells per cell), freezing and storing them, and thawing them for use in numerous replicate cultures (244). This permitted us to compare systematically one sample with itself at different times, individual clones from the same sample, and different samples with each other.

In addition, we sought culture conditions which could be used to stimulate the muscle cells either to grow and proliferate or to fuse and differentiate. This was achieved by the use of different tissue culture media. As shown in Figure 16, upon exposure to a mitogen-rich medium, the cells actively divided; in a mitogen-poor medium, striated, contractile myotubes formed (244). We could also study the proliferative and differentiative properties either of a single myoblast and its progeny, or clone, or of numerous myoblasts derived from a number of pure muscle clones grown at high density.

Studies of Differentiated Myotubes

Our initial investigations were aimed at demonstrating the phenotype of the disease in differentiated myotubes obtained from pure muscle cultures isolated from the tissues of DMD patients. As show in Figure 17, the normal and dystrophic myotubes that formed in culture were morphologically indistinguishable. Upon fixation and staining, the typical striations characteristic of a mature muscle fiber were apparent and active contractions were observed in both types of muscle cultures (Figure 16).

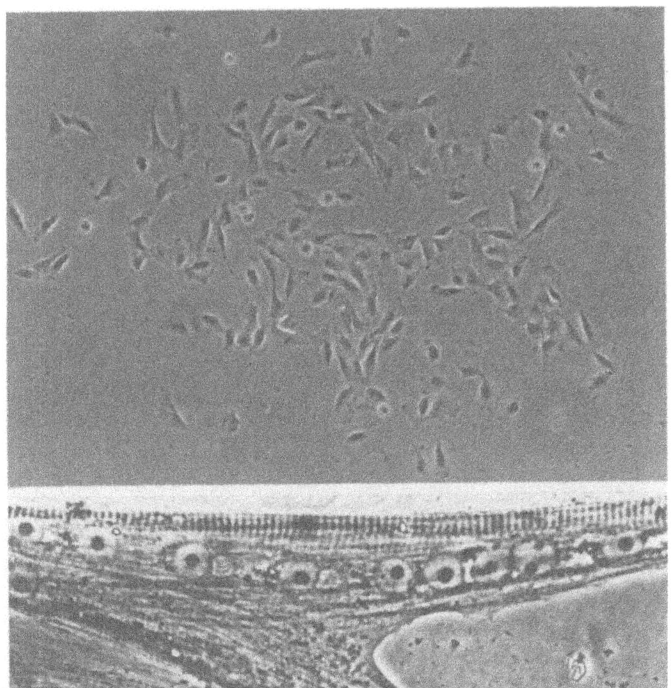

FIGURE 16: Growth and differentiation of human muscle cells in culture. Proliferating myoblast clone x 200 (upper). Striations are evident in well differentiated myotubes fixed in 2% glutaraldehyde in Hanks balanced salt solution for 20 min at 34°C and stained with 2% orcein in 45% propionic acid x 530 (lower).

DR. STROHMAN: There are some single cells there, too. Do these clones throw off in the course of differentiation, other cell types?

DR. BLAU: Those are not cell types; they are myoblasts. Like the muscle cultures of other species, e.g. rat, mouse, and chicken, not all of the human myoblasts fuse to form myotubes (245-247).

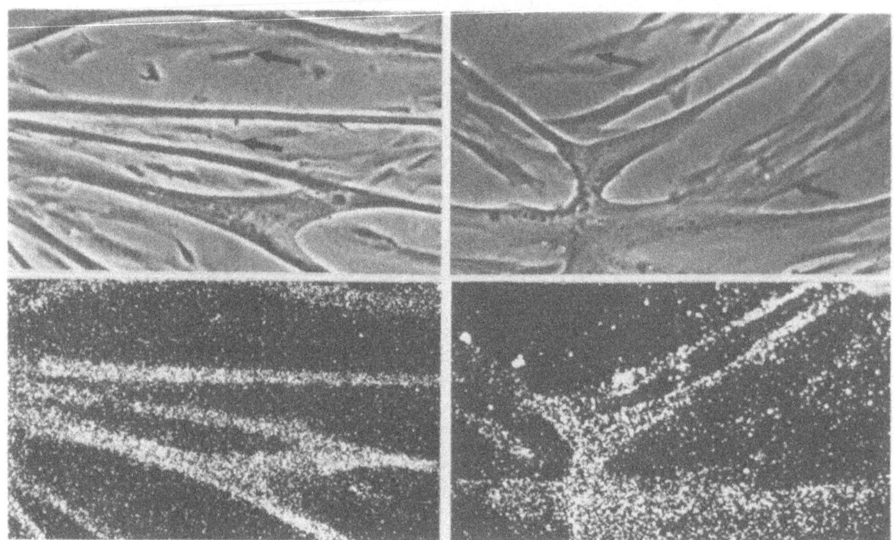

FIGURE 17: Morphology and distribution of acetylcholine receptors in normal and DMD muscle cells in culture normal (upper); DMD (lower). Differentiating myotubes are shown with phase-contrast optics (upper). Autoradiograms of the same myotubes as above are visualized in darkfield illumination to reveal the pattern of silver grains and the location of ^{125}I-α-bungarotoxin-labeled acetylcholine receptors (lower). Arrows indicate undifferentiated myoblasts which do not have receptors. X150.

We then compared a number of biochemical properties of the differentiated normal and DMD myotubes formed in culture (248,249). First, we examined the distribution, amounts, and kinetics of appearance of the acetylcholine receptor, a membrane glycoprotein essential to neuromuscular function. The receptor can be readily visualized using the ligand, α-bungarotoxin. We exposed the cultures to ^{125}I-α-bungarotoxin, performed autoradiography, and looked at the distribution of acetylcholine receptors along the myotubes (Figure 17). In both cases, receptors were not found on the myoblasts but only on differentiated myotubes, and no difference in the distribution of the receptors was apparent.

We then looked at the accumulation of acetylcholine receptors on the muscle cell surface as a function of time in culture. Again, the peak amount of receptor and the time course of accumulation were indistinguishable for the normal and dystrophic cultures studied (Figure 18).

We then focused our attention on another parameter of muscle differentiation, creatine kinase, since patients with DMD have greatly elevated levels of this enzyme in their serum. We examined the activity of creatine kinase as a function of time in culture and found that neither the kinetics of accumulation nor the peak values of creatine kinase activity differed significantly between Duchenne and normal myotubes (Figure 19). However, it was still possible that the DMD cultures were producing increased amounts of creatine kinase and that the enzyme was accumulating in the culture medium as a result of a membrane defect. We therefore examined the creatine kinase activity in the extracellular medium and compared it with the intracellular enzyme specific activity on different days in culture. Figure 20 shows the intracellular values for the enzyme at the peak and on subsequent days following the peak for Duchenne and for normal muscle. In addition, the percent of total intracellular creatine kinase activity which was extracellular is indicated. Using our assays, we could definitely detect creatine kinase activity in the medium, but it did not differ significantly between normal and Duchenne muscle and did not increase with time in culture. We concluded that there was no evidence of leakage of creatine kinase into the medium in cultures of Duchenne myotubes. Since a relative increase in the BB and MB isozymes of creatine kinase had been reported in muscle tissue extracts and in the sera of DMD patients (250,251), we examined the isozyme composition of the creatine kinase present in normal and DMD muscle cells as a function of differentiation in culture. Creatine kinase is a dimer composed of two subunits, B and M. Consequently, three different isozymes are possible. A transition from the BB to the MM isozyme is characteristic of muscle maturation. As shown in Figure 21, the transition from BB to MB to MM isozymes is apparent in both the normal and DMD cultures; there seems to be no problem with the regulation of expression of these genes during the maturation of DMD muscle in culture.

Finally, we compared the contractile proteins present in the normal and DMD myotubes by two-dimensional gel electrophoresis (252). Myosin light chains, actins and tropomyosins were synthesized and were similar in amount and relative proportion in both cell types. In summary, for all the various parameters of differentiation that we compared, we could see no difference between the Duchenne and normal myotubes which formed in tissue culture. These included a broad range of functions: a membrane glycoprotein, structural components of the contractile apparatus,

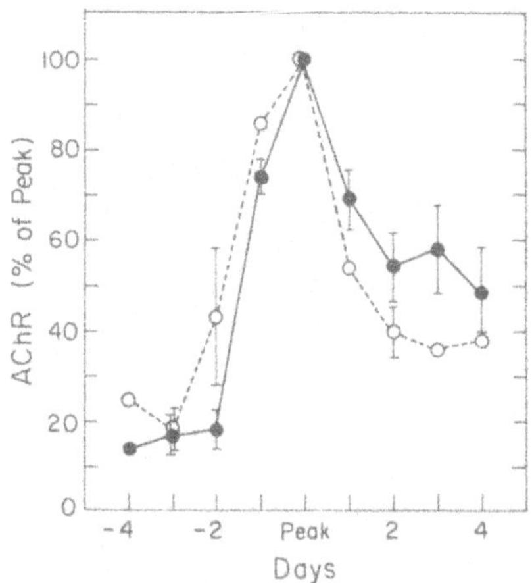

FIGURE 18: Accumulation of acetylcholine receptors on normal and DMD muscle fibers. ^{125}-I-α-bungarotoxin-labeled AChR is shown as a percentage of the peak AChR during differentiation in ●——●, normal; O---O, DMD cultures. Days indicate time before (-) and after (+) reaching peak level of AChR (fmole/mg protein). The means ± SE are shown. The results represent a total of seven experiments in which 72 individual muscle cultures were analyzed.

and an enzyme essential for generating the energy required for contraction.

These results differ significantly from those described by Ionasescu et al, (253) and by Thompson et al, (254). The differences can best be explained by the culture methods employed; both of these groups used a mixed population of fibroblasts and myoblasts. The presence of fibroblasts can significantly alter the extent of muscle differentiation. Since the proportion of fibroblasts is increased in DMD muscle (255), this cell mixture could be the cause of the observed altered myotube morphology (251,254,256), the decrease in specific activity of creatine kinase (253), and the relative increase in the synthesis of the BB isozyme (250,251). All of these findings could well be secondary to the heterogeneous composition of the culture system.

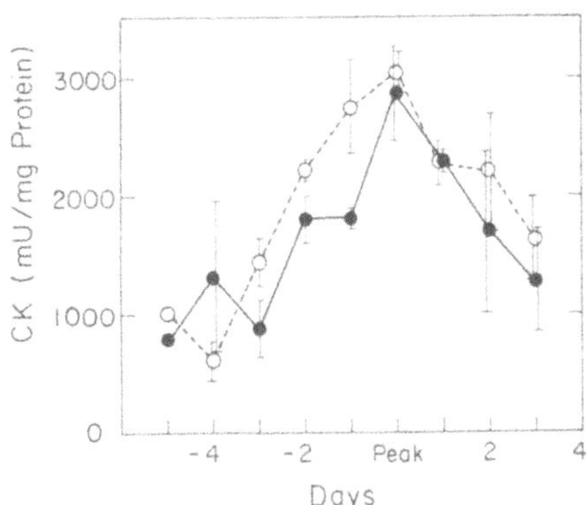

FIGURE 19: Accumulation of CK in normal and DMD cells in culture. CK activity is shown as a function of differentiation in ●—●, normal; O---O, DMD cultures. Days indicate time before (-) and after (+) reaching peak level of CK activity. The means ± SE are shown. CK activity was assayed spectrophotometrically and corrected for myokinase activity. The results represent a total of nine experiments in which one hundred individual muscle cultures were analyzed.

Studies of Myoblasts

Although no consistent difference between DMD and normal myotubes was detectable, a major difference in the precursor muscle cells, or myoblasts, was evident. A constant problem in studying DMD was the lack of muscle cells. Relative to normal controls, the yield obtained from a DMD biopsy was very small. We decided to focus our attention on this difference and examine the progeny of single mononucleated cells in culture. It was in these cells, the precursors of myotubes, that we found a defect. This defect was established from a study of nine patients with DMD and 13 age-matched normal individuals. The vastus lateralis muscle was biopsied in most cases. Control muscle samples were obtained from healthy children undergoing orthopedic surgery, usually for congenital hip dislocation. Therefore, they were uncomplicated by any neurological or muscular problems.

The first indication of a myoblast defect was the observation that the number of cells obtained per gram biopsy from a Duchenne sample was reduced by more than an order of magnitude. We then examined by morphology the types of cells obtained. We could

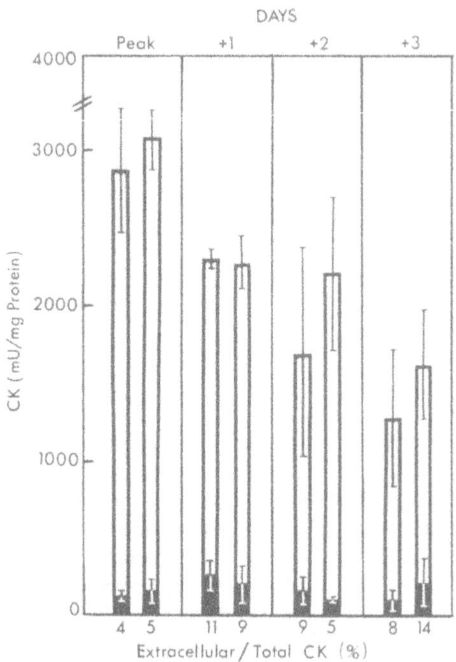

FIGURE 20: Intracellular and extracellular CK activities in normal and DMD cells in culture. Extracellular CK activity in medium (■) is shown relative to intracellular CK activity in normal (stippled bars) and DMD (□) cultures at peak, 1,2, and 3 days thereafter. The extracellular activity is shown as a percentage of the total intracellular and extracellular activity. Mean ± SE is shown in each case. The results represent a total of four experiments in which 56 individual cultures were analyzed.

readily recognize fibroblasts and myoblasts by their morphology (Figure 22), and we routinely tested this morphological distinction by exposing clones to a medium which induced fusion and differentiation. The presence of myotubes revealed definitively which clones were muscle. In addition, we detected a novel cell morphology among the clones derived from dystrophy samples. In Figure 23 normal human myoblasts which are triangular and refractile are compared with the cells with altered morphology seen among the clones obtained from Duchenne patients. We call this cell type a dystroblast, or D-cell. Dystroblasts are flat, distended cells with a prominent cytoskeleton. These cells are not another cell type, but an altered form of myoblast. Upon culture in fusion

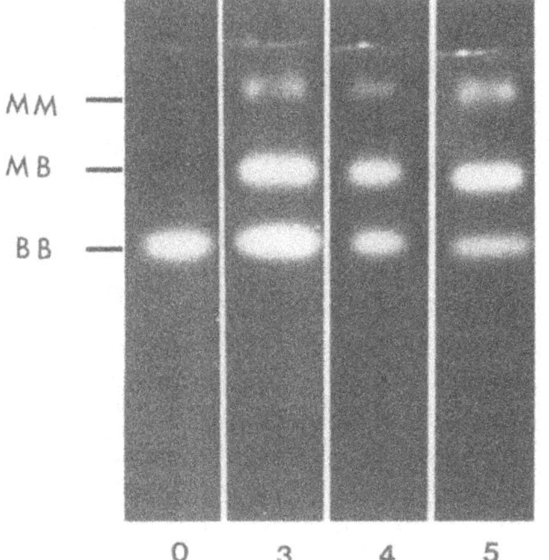

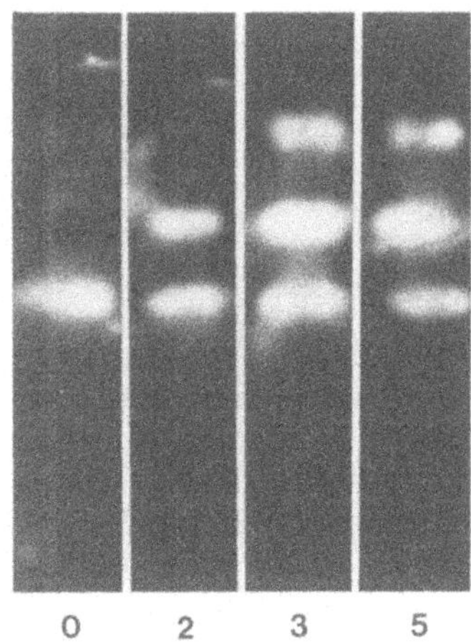

FIGURE 21: CK isozymes during differentiation of normal and DMD cells in culture. MM, MB, and BB isozymes for (left) normal; (right) DMD cultures were separated by electrophoresis on non-denaturing 12% polyacrylamide gels and visualized by the fluorescent product of a coupled enzyme reaction. Days indicate time after addition of fusion medium.

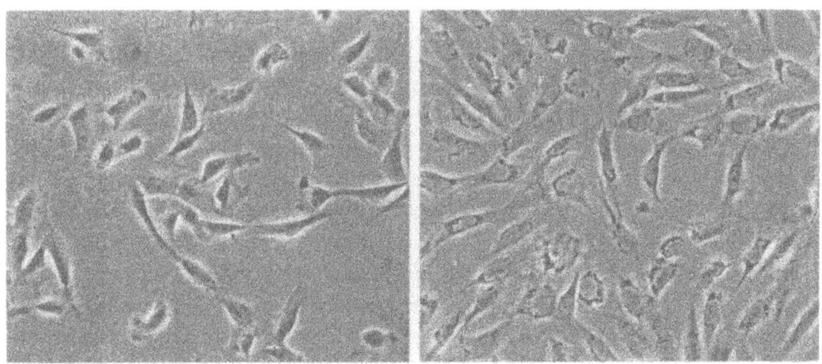

FIGURE 22: Morphology of myoblast and fibroblast cell types. Myoblasts are small refractile, triangular cells (left) that are easily distinguished from broad, flat fibroblasts with abundant dark perinuclear granules (right). Photographed in vivo with phase-contrast optics. (X70).

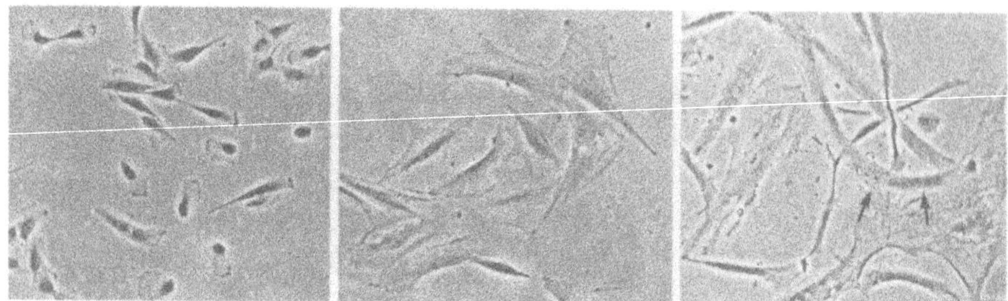

FIGURE 23: Morphology of DMD myoblast cell types. Proliferating myoblasts at clonal density are typically small, refractile, triangular cells that are actively dividing (left). The altered myoblast phenotype is characterized by large, flat, distended cells (center). These cells have limited proliferative capacity but can be induced to fuse and form multinucleated myotubes indicated by arrows (right). Photographed in vivo with phase-contrast optics (X120).

medium, the clones were induced to fuse and form multi-nucleated myotubes (Figure 23). Furthermore, like normal muscle cells, they bind a muscle specific monoclonal antibody (5.1H11), which recognizes a human muscle cell surface antigen (257), whereas fibroblasts do not (Figure 24).

We determined the relative proportions of myoblasts, fibroblasts and dystroblasts present in dissociated samples of normal and DMD muscle (Table 7). Normal individuals and DMD patients are both listed according to age. More than 1,000 clones were analyzed in each case. One of the first things we noticed was that for normal muscle the myoblast to fibroblast ratio remains relatively constant with age. Accordingly, the cell yield per 0.1 gram of muscle tissue averaged 5,000 for myoblasts and 150 for fibroblasts. The proportion of muscle cells obtained from normal muscle which had the dystroblast morphology was extremely low. Out of a total of 2,266 myoblast clones only two or less than 0.1% had cells with a flattened, distended morphology.

DR. STROHMAN: How long were the clones maintained before you assayed for the D-type cell?

DR. BLAU: For 25 days, or until the average cell number for a normal clone is 10^6 cells.

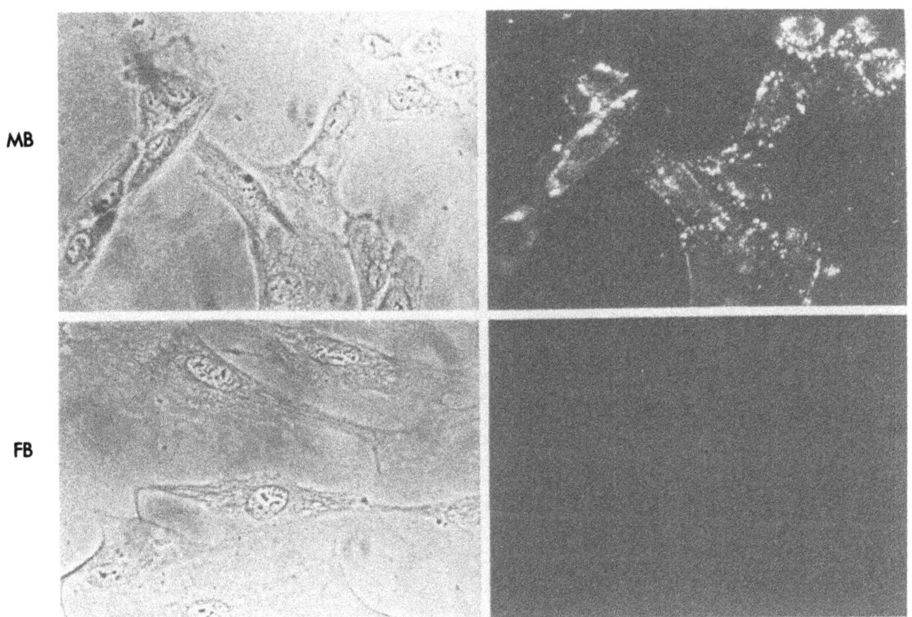

FIGURE 24: Specificity of 5.1H11 monoclonal antibody for muscle cells. Cultured human myoblasts (MB) and fibroblasts (FB) are shown in phase contrast (left) and in fluorescence (right) following fixation. The morphological difference between the two cell types seen in living cells (Figure 22) is not apparent when cells are fixed with methanol. However, the cells are readily distinguished following incubation with 5.1H11 and a second rhodamine-conjugated antibody.

By contrast with normal samples, in DMD samples the myoblast to fibroblast ratio changed remarkedly with age, from approximately 9:1 at age 2 yr to 3:7 by age 14. Thus, at young ages the ratio was comparable to that seen in normal muscle, but by older ages a shift had occurred so that the predominant cell type was the fibroblast. This change was not due to an increase in fibroblasts, since the yield of fibroblasts per 0.1 g biopsy was similar to normal. Instead, it was due to a decrease in the number of myoblasts, on average, only 5% of the normal yield of myoblasts per 0.1 g biopsy was obtained. Furthermore, the percent of total myoblasts which was dystroblasts was already 2% at age 2 yr and increased markedly to 93% by age 14 yr. Thus, even at the youngest

TABLE 7: Clonal Analysis of Cell Type by Morphology

Donor*	Age, yr	n[†]	M, %[‡]	F, %[§]	D/M, %[¶]	Yield per 0.1 g of tissue[‖] M	Yield per 0.1 g of tissue[‖] F
Normal							
L.S.	2	167	100	0	0.6	3,095	0
B.N.	2	170	96	4	0	13,370	575
K.D.	2	24	75	25	0	690	230
P.M.	2	229	85	15	0	15,000	2,615
M.C.	4	98	92	6	0	1,800	160
B.F.	5	73	86	14	0	1,210	190
B.M.	6	57	98	2	0	9,335	165
H.B.	7	384	100	0	0	1,485	5
S.W.**	8	329	100	0	0.3	3,705	0
A.B. (L)**	8	142	100	0	0	2,535	0
A.B. (R)**	8	533	100	0	0	5,860	0
C.B.	12	40	98	2	0	4,755	120
K.Z.**	19	20	100	0	0	—	—
Mean			96	4	<1	4,715	144
± SEM[††]			± 2	± 2		± 1,234	± 56
DMD							
P.D.	2	55	80	20	2	150	35
J.G.**	3	136	90	10	22	650	75
W.M.**	5	112	95	5	24	3,925	220
M.A.	6	26	39	61	70	60	95
J.L.**	8	247	62	38	67	215	130
P.A.	9	24	54	46	67	75	65
R.B.	12	133	27	73	56	250	675
S.L.**	14	273	27	73	77	105	290
M.B.	14	262	29	71	93	56	128
Mean			NA[‡‡]	NA[‡‡]	NA[‡‡]	215	143
± SEM[††]						± 77	± 31
Other							
R.B. (S)	12	184	72	28	41	2,290	875
B.L.	31	111	95	5	5	1,505	75
P.Z.	63	136	54	46	1	—	—
A.S.	77	10	40	50	0	—	—

* Samples were from the vastus lateralis muscle, with the exception of S.W. and K.Z., from whom the biceps femoris and thoracis spinales muscles were obtained, respectively. From R.B. both semimembranosus (S) and vastus lateralis muscles were obtained. From A.B., vastus lateralis muscles of left (L) and right (R) legs were analyzed. J.L. and S.L. as well as M.A. and P.A. are pairs of brothers. B.L. is an obligate carrier, the mother of J.L. and S.L. Donors P.Z. and A.S. were normal individuals from whom samples were obtained at autopsy following cardiac arrest. Normal donors consisted of four males and eight females; DMD donors were all males; and other donors were all male, with the exception of B.L.

[†] n is the number of total clones analyzed for each sample.

[‡] M is the % of total clones that were muscle (including D) (see text).

[§] F is the % of total clones that were fibroblasts.

[¶] D/M is the % of total muscle clones that had a diseased phenotype.

[‖] Yield of myoblasts (M) and fibroblasts (F) per 0.1 g of tissue was extrapolated from the number of clones obtained per size of tissue dissociated.

** Samples used in the analysis presented in Fig. 4.

[††] Trimmed means were calculated by eliminating the highest and lowest values in each case.

[‡‡] NA, not applicable because values changed with patient age.

ages studied, the proportion of D cells in dystrophic samples exceeded that in normal samples.

Further differences between normal and DMD myoblasts were seen when we examined the kinetics of growth of single clones during the first 10 days in culture. We did this by circling individual cells and then daily counting the number of cells associated with them.

Growth Kinetics of DMD and Normal Cells

As shown in Figure 25, normal myoblasts, regardless of the age of the individual from whom they were derived, consistently exhibit exponential growth kinetics. By contrast, the muscle clones even from a DMD patient of only 5 years of age, already show a heterogeneous pattern of growth. Some of the myoblasts divide at a normal rate for that period of time, whereas others already have poor growth kinetics and long doubling times. The myoblasts isolated from a 14 year old DMD patient all grow poorly. This finding is specific to the muscle cells; fibroblasts from DMD patients of all ages exhibit normal exponential growth kinetics similar to those observed with myoblasts and fibroblasts from control muscle samples.

The differences in growth kinetics and morphology are further demonstrated by an analysis of the data pooled from studies of 59 and 83 individual myoblast clones isolated from normal and DMD muscles, respectively (Figure 26). Normal myoblasts typically have doubling times of about 16 to 17 hours, as do fibroblasts from Duchenne patients. By contrast, the myoblast clones from the Duchenne samples had increased doubling times. We examined the proportion of myoblast clones exhibiting a doubling time of greater than 25 hours. Of the normal clones, only one exhibited altered growth kinetics; whereas more than 80% of the clones from a 14 year old DMD patient had prolonged doubling times during the first ten days in culture. The proportion of clones with altered dystroblast morphology showed a similar pattern. Of the 5,024 normal myoblast clones analyzed, only one had a dystroblast morphology, whereas from DMD samples, the proportion of myoblast clones with aberrant morphology increased with age to as much as 80% of the total clones analyzed.

DR. YAFFE: How do you tell whether it is a normal clone or not?

DR. BLAU: The normal phenotype is distinguished from the dystroblast phenotype on the basis of prolonged doubling times (greater than 25 hr), poor growth kinetics (non-exponential growth), and strange morphology (large, flat, distended cells) during the first ten days of growth in culture.

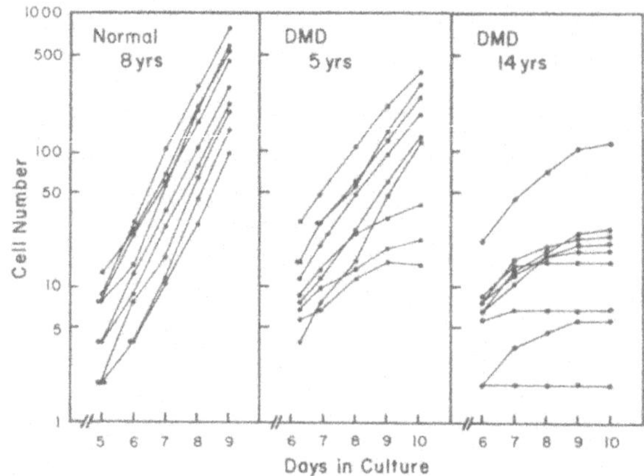

FIGURE 25: Clonal analysis of myoblast growth kinetics. Growth kinetics for representative myoblast clones of a normal (left) and two DMD samples (center and right) are shown. Growth of normal clones is highly uniform and typically exponential. Growth of DMD clones from a young patient is heterogeneous and often is not exponential. In older DMD patients, almost all clones exhibit defective growth kinetics. The normal clones were from S.W. and the DMD clones were from W.M. and M.B. of Table 7.

DR. HOLTZER: Does that mean your most abnormal clones still have rougly 70% of the cells in myotubes? You showed an earlier ratio.

DR. BLAU: When I spoke of a fusion index of 70%, I was referring to mass cultures of normal myoblasts at high density. In dystroblast clones of less than 1,000 cells, we obtain only a few myotubes. This is not unexpected, given the cell density and proximity within a small clone. It is sufficient to verify the myogenic nature of these clones. We have also confirmed this using a monoclonal antibody which recognizes a human muscle-specific cell surface antigen present on normal myoblasts and D-cells, but not fibroblasts (Figure 24).

Finally, we examined the total proliferative capacity, or longterm growth properties, of some of the clones from DMD samples which had appeared normal during the first ten days in culture.

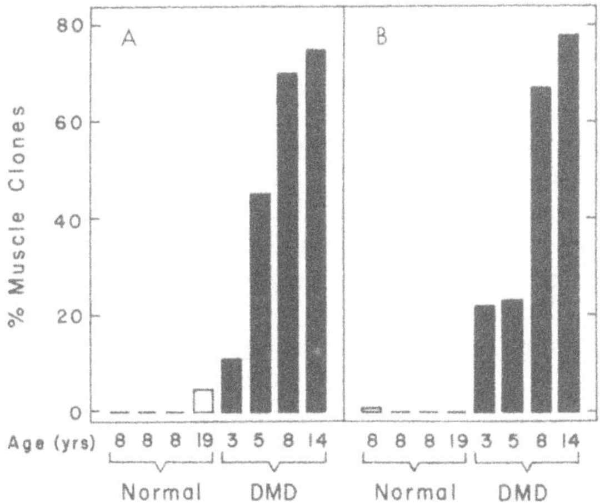

FIGURE 26: Clonal analysis of myoblast growth kinetics and cell morphology. The proportion of myoblast clones that had an altered phenotype was identified for normal (open bars) and DMD (closed bars) samples. As a function of age of donor, the proportion of clones with a doubling time >25 hr (left) and the proportion of clones with altered cell morphology (right) are shown for each sample. The samples used in this analysis are indicated by ** in Table 7. Growth kinetics are monitored for 59 normal and 83 DMD myoblast clones. Morphology was determined for 1,024 normal and 1,006 DMD myoblast clones. The difference between normal and DMD clonal growth kinetics was also examined by rank order analysis of doubling times and was found to be significant by the Mann-Whitney U test ($P < 0.01$).

Again, we observed a marked reduction in muscle cell number relative to normals. Thus, even DMD cells which initially appear normal, eventually exhibit the dystroblast phenotype and the total yield per cell is low. The difference in total growth potential is shown in Figure 27. Here we examined the number of cell doublings, or total cells which could be obtained per cell. From normal individuals, 40 doublings were obtained per myoblast. By contrast, the number of doublings per myoblast from a DMD patient of age 14 yr was only 10. This is really far greater than the 4-fold difference in number of cell doublings that is first apparent. It actually represents a difference in yield of 10^{12} and 10^{3} cells, or nine logs.

DR. FISCHMAN: If you extend the doubling time of normal myogenic cells, say you get them out to the 25-30th doubling, do they assume this abnormal morphology?

DR. BLAU: Not by the 25th or 30th, but by the 40th they do, and the senescent phenotype is a large distended cell.

DR. YAFFE: If you clone them later, will you get clones which have similar morphology to what you get in primary cultures?

DR. BLAU: We don't get the flat distended cell type until senescence.

DR. KELLY: Have you looked at other fibrosing myopathies?

DR. BLAU: We have looked at only one Becker's and it looks the same as Duchenne's. We also intend to study muscle from individuals with polymyositis.

DR. MIRANDA: In the initial studies you report that the population doubling times in the normal and Duchenne were the same. Does that mean that in those cases you looked at both stages?

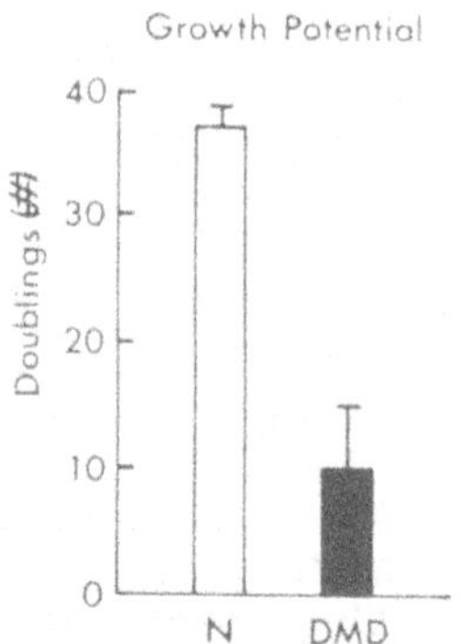

FIGURE 27: Comparison of the proliferative capacity of normal and DMD myoblasts. D myoblasts exhibit markedly decreased proliferative capacity _in vitro_. A normal cell typically undergoes 40 doublings and yields 10^8 cells. A DMD cell undergoes 10 doubles and yields 10^3 cells. This results in a difference in total growth potential for each cell of 5 orders of magnitude.

DR. BLAU: The average doubling time for clones from normals and from young DMD individuals during the first 10 days in culture is the same.

DR. MIRANDA: So you have to grow it for a long period of time.

DR. BLAU: We do not yet know whether there are differences in long term growth potential of muscle clones from patients. If you look at the clones from the older DMD individuals, you see the dystroblast phenotype very early, i.e., in the first few days in culture.

The major question of interest is: What is the basis for the dystroblast phenotype which is characterized by altered morphology, altered growth kinetics and decreased total proliferative capacity? It could be the result of a primary defect in the satellite cell. Thus, the satellite cell from Duchenne individuals would not be capable of growing as well as the satellite cell from normals. This would constitute a basic defect intrinsic to the myoblast itself. An alternate explanation for the dystroblast phenotype is that it is a secondary phenomenon resulting from the degeneration and regeneration of mature muscle fibers which themselves are defective. Thus, the inherently normal myoblasts would have exhausted their proliferative capacity in the course of replenishing these fibers and exhibit premature senescence.

We have two lines of evidence that suggest that the dystroblast is a primary defect in the myoblast. The first is the case of R.B., a 12 year old with DMD. Two different muscles were biopsied from R.B. One was the vastus lateralis, one of the first muscles to be affected by DMD, exhibiting both weakness and extensive histological signs of regeneration and degeneration. The other muscle we studied, the semi-membranosus, is usually affected considerably later in life. When we sampled these two muscles from R.B., the vastus lateralis muscle was severely affected and the semi-membranosus muscle was only moderately affected. As shown in Table 7, in the 133 clones analyzed from the vastus lateralis, a ratio of myoblasts to fibroblasts of approximately 3:7 was observed. In addition, the total cell yield was reduced by an order of magnitude in a manner characteristic of DMD. On the other hand, when we examined 184 clones isolated from the semi-membranosis of the same individual, we observed a ratio of myoblasts to fibroblasts of 7:3 and a cell yield more typical of normal muscle. These characteristics are in accordance with the histological and physiological findings that the semi-membranosis muscle had not undergone as much degeneration and regeneration as the vastus lateralis at this point in time. By contrast, the proportion of dystroblast clones present among the muscle clones isolated from these two different muscles was 56 and 41% and did not differ significantly. In other words, the proportion of cells which exhibited the dystroblast phenotype did not correlate with the extent of degeneration observed. That would suggest that this phenotype results from a primary defect and is not secondary to degeneration. We have since analyzed the same pair of muscles from another patient and made the same observations.

DR. HOLTZER: You are saying that your end point here is the dystrophic myoblast, you are not counting myotubes, just looking at the dystrophic myoblasts.

DR. BLAU: That is right. We are scoring the proportion of clones with the dystrophic phenotype.

Another case in point is that of the carrier, B.L., the mother of S.L. and J.L. She was 31 years of age and was among that one-third of carriers who are indistinguishable from normal. Two-thirds of carriers exhibit elevated creatine kinase activity in their sera and evidence of muscle degeneration in other biopsies. B.L. was exactly like a normal individual with respect to every available clinical assay. From the 111 clones analyzed from a sample of her vastus lateralis muscle, we observed a ratio of myoblasts to fibroblasts of 19:1, which is typical of normal. The total yield of myoblasts per 0.1 g biopsy was somewhat diminished, but more closely approximated that from normal than from DMD muscle samples. However, 5% of her muscle clones exhibited the dystrophic phenotype, as compared to the 0.1% frequency typical of normal muscle. As described below, this finding is in accordance with what one would postulate from the Lyon hypothesis. A female carrier of an X-linked disease should be a mosaic for any X-linked function. Thus, her muscle should contain two types of cells: one that manifests the normal phenotype and has normal morphology and poor growth. One would predict that a carrier who was asymptomatic, i.e., had normal serum creatine kinase levels and muscle histology, would have a lower proportion of dystroblasts than a carrier with detectable pathology. In both cases, the proportion of dystroblasts is likely to be significantly elevated over normal. That is what we found. It was important to demonstrate that these results are not due to B.L.'s advanced age. As shown in Table 7, among the clones isolated from samples of the vastus lateralis muscle of two normal individuals, 63 and 77 years of age, which were obtained post mortem, less than 1% had the dystrophic phenotype.

What is the significance of these findings? First, they fit well with our current understanding of the onset and progression of DMD. The disease is usually diagnosed between the ages of 2 and 6 yr. It has been shown in the rat and mouse and also in humans that the muscle increases 6 to 7-fold in mass in the first decade of life (229,258-261). Essential for this growth spurt is a constant nuclear to cytoplasmic ratio which requires the addition of nuclei to the developing muscle fiber. Where do these nuclei come from? It is well known that the nuclei inside of myotubes do not divide (262). Consequently, the only possible source of nuclei is the satellite cells or myoblasts, positioned adjacent to the muscle fiber. These myoblasts must undergo a significant number of cell divisions and fuse into the muscle fiber in order for the observed growth of muscle tissue to occur (224).

Hypothesis: DMD Results from a Primary Defect in Myoblast Growth

These observations have led us to develop the following hypothesis regarding the etiology of DMD: Dividing myoblasts are required for muscle growth and maintenance and the limited capacity of DMD myoblasts to grow is directly related to the progressive muscle degeneration characteristic of the disease. First, the yield of satellite cells from dissociated tissue plated in culture is only 5% that of normal. Second, each one of these cells has a markedly reduced proliferative capacity such that often only one millionth of the expected number of myoblasts available to contribute to growing muscle and the capacity of the defective myoblasts to form mature fibers is rapidly exhausted. As a result, the muscle cannot keep pace with the growth of the body during the first decade of life. It is at precisely this stage of development that the disease is usually diagnosed. The basis for this may be that stress from muscle use in early childhood leads to degeneration of existing muscle fibers which in turn leads to the release of the muscle proteins into the serum characteristic of the disease. We therefore postulate that the degeneration is secondary to inadequate muscle growth.

To determine definitively that the dystrophic phenotype we have identified in culture is due to a primary defect in the myoblast itself, we need to study additional obligate carriers of DMD. These carriers are required to establish that muscle clones with the dystrophic and the normal phenotypes are always present and that the proportion with the dystrophic phenotype is increased in carriers with detectable serum creatine kinase levels and aberrant muscle histology, as predicted by Lyonization. Evidence that the dystrophic phenotype is the result of a primary defect could best be derived from studies of obligate carriers of DMD who are also heterozygous for another X-linked marker such as glucose-6-phosphate dehydrogenase (G6PD). G6PD is a highly polymorphic marker present in high frequency in certain ethnic groups. For example, 10% of American Black women are heterozygous for two electrophoretically distinguishable forms of G6PD: A and

B. One approach would be to dissociate the muscle tissue from such a heterozygote who is also a carrier of DMD and analyze the progeny of each individual muscle cell obtained. Each of these clones would be tested for its G6PD isotype and for its morphology and total proliferative capacity. The prediction would be that if the clones that express G6PD A had normal growth capacity, the clones expressed G6PD B would have limited growth capacity. From this experiment it should be possible to determine whether the G6PD isotype invariably segregates with the dystroblast phenotype.

Of particular interest is the fact that the cellular defect in growth may provide a means for isolating the gene for DMD. To test this possibility we will attempt "cell rescue." We will determine whether the normal cell can rescue the dystrophic cell by complementation following cell fusion. Experiments of this kind would determine whether a missing or defective product in the Duchenne cell responsible for its poor growth can be provided by the normal cell. The assay of complementation would be the total growth capacity of the hybrids. For example, a D-cell known to be capable of producing a colony of only 10^3 cells, equivalent to the size of a pea, will be fused with a normal cell capable of giving rise to 10^{12} cells, equivalent to numerous T-75 flasks. This difference is readily apparent and will reveal which of the two cell types is dominant.

Cellular rescue will be followed by experiments utilizing normal DNA to rescue the defective D-cells. These experiments will be performed in collaboration with Dr. Kedes. If normal proliferative capacity is restored, this approach should lead to the isolation of the gene responsible for DMD. This is of interest because (1) it would provide a method for prenatal diagnosis and (2) it would make possible identification of the defective or missing gene product. This may lead eventually to prevention and treatment of the disease.

DR. FISCHMAN: Could it be simply explained that there is premature senescence in the myogenic population?

DR. BLAU: That could constitute a primary defect, too, i.e., premature aging. At this point we can't really distinguish between these possibilities. The finding is that the muscle cells from DMD patients cannot give rise to the total number of cells expected. The basis for it remains unknown.

DR. STROHMAN: It seems to me that the basic assumption here is that when you examine the very young dystrophic patient at age 2 or 3, there has really already been a very significant number of doublings in that muscle so that what you get out even at age 2 is a population which has a history of enormous numbers of doublings and what you've got left is simply a cell which has already gone 3/4 of the way down, its senescing pathway.

DR. BLAU: I think there may have been significant numbers of doublings by age 2 yr, but that there are many more which occur during the postnatal growth spurt. Furthermore, the D-cell phenotype is detectable in the 2 year olds and its frequency is significantly above normal.

DR. RUBINSTEIN: Have these already gone through 30 doublings whereas the normal satellite cell has gone through only 3 doublings?

DR. BLAU: That is the alternative hypothesis. However, the carrier data (B.L.) and the two muscles from the same individual (R.B.) which I described suggest that this second possiblity is unlikely. We don't know that definitively, but we think it is not due to senescence, but to a primary defect in the myoblast. Any cells that are growth-impaired have that morphology. If you add toxic drugs to cultures, the cells do not grow well. For example, if you add cytosine arabinoside to myoblasts they will look like dystroblasts. Consequently, it is not possible to determine whether the phenotype is due to senescence or to something else based on morphology alone.

DR. HOLTZER: If you were to irradiate a young animal on the basis of your proposition, you should be able to induce dystrophy or many of the characteristics of dystrophy. Would you agree to that? If you can keep an animal alive with no further divisions of its satellite cells then the wear and tear that you are postulating as being the cause, as I understand it, of dystrophy, you should be able to produce at will. If you are saying that what is happening here is a demand for constant fusion of young myoblasts, if you irradiate a very young animal, that is the end of the source of the young myoblasts. If you could keep that animal going by giving him all the blood cells he needs, theoretically, you should produce the symptoms and pathology characteristic of muscular dystrophy.

DR. BLAU: That is an interesting idea.

DR. WOOD: There is a disease, polymyositis, in which regeneration is enormous. The potential number of doublings of muscle cells from patients with this disease could be tested. If I heard right, you are testing this possibility. Is that correct?

DR. BLAU: That is exactly right and I'm glad you made that point. We have chosen polymyositis as a control for Duchenne because it is characterized by extensive degeneration and regeneration and occurs in early childhood.

DR. YAFFE: What is the distribution of the survival capacity of different clones from dystrophic muscle? If you compare the doubling time, the number of doublings you get from dystrophic muscle, do you get clones which are behaving like normal?

DR. BLAU: We need to test that; we need to analyze the total growth capacity, or number of doublings of individual clones from many more patients of different ages. Most of our results at present are based on early growth kinetics during the first two weeks in culture.

DR. BUCKINGHAM: The idea that one could use these cells as a test tube for the gene which causes the abnormality depends on one's ability to reverse the situation in vitro. What if the morphology of those cells is due to some kind of pre-conditioning which has taken place in vivo in the muscle, e.g., the influence of some kind of abnormal trophic factor which produced an irreversible change in the cells? Presumably one could test that by putting normal myoblasts into dystrophic muscle tissue and seeing if they then acquire a dystrophic morphology.

DR. BLAU: That is the kind of experiment we have in mind, but in vitro. By making a hybrid between a normal myoblast with normal proliferative capacity and a Duchenne myoblast we will test whether correction of the defect by the normal cell is possible. We don't know the answer to that question at this point.

DR. EASTWOOD: Is the cytoskeleton of these dystroblasts different from that of the normal myoblasts?

DR. BLAU: We haven't looked at that in detail. By phase contrast microscopy the cytoskeleton seems to be more prominent in the cells of dystrophic phenotype. It is possible that it is defective.

DR. SCHULTZ: I was wondering if Dr. Blau could test her hypothesis by adding additional dystrophic cells to a normal muscle.

DR. BLAU: I think the medical ethics committee might object to that kind of experiment in vivo! Although it will be hard to mimic the kind of stress that occurs in vivo in a culture dish in vitro, it is the best way we can do, given that Duchenne is a human disease.

DR. KUNKEL: Has anyone every transplanted normal muscle or Duchenne muscle back and forth between the two patients?

DR. STROHMAN: I think Ethel Cosmos has done that in chicks.

DR. EPSTEIN: I need a couple of points of clarification from Dr. Blau. I am not sure I fully understand your model. Is your model for Duchenne that there is an abormal population of satellite cells that never proliferates properly and falls further and further behind normal demands, or is it that on top of that it can't keep up with certain requirements in the disease, and falls further behind? I am not sure if it is both elements.

DR. BLAU: The hypothesis is that first there is a reduction in the number of satellite cells in the muscle: 5% of the normal level in the case of the vastus lateralis. In addition, those cells that are there have decreased proliferative capacity, so that one obtains only a small fraction of the total number of cells per cell. Consequently, as the body grows, there is not enough muscle tissue produced. There is an adequate amount of connective tissue, but a reduced amount of muscle which is not sufficient to support the needs of the body.

DR. EPSTEIN: But, in fact, you would argue that it has decreased muscle cells that you could measure even at that point or before that time.

DR. BLAU: The decrease is evident experimentally at the youngest ages examined.

DR. EPSTEIN: The difference between this and muscle from polymyositis is that the polymyositis muscle has a normal population of satellite cells even though it is always having to regenerate. In other words, it has a capacity which the Duchenne muscle could never have.

DR. BLAU: I think the comparison of Duchenne and polymyositis is very important for testing the validity of the growth hypothesis, and our preliminary results suggest that they are different.

DR. EPSTEIN: I seem to remember a number of years ago, Charles Epstein analyzed the question of Lyonization with respect to myotubes. There is no _a priori_ prediction you could make as to what you would expect for one genotype versus another. It could be anything for any given fiber, from almost 0 to 100%.

DR. BLAU: That is right.

DR. HAUSCHKA: The thing I'm worried about is your model at the end. The idea of a primary defect versus the explanation of the behavior of those remaining satellite cells just due to the proliferative stress that they have been put under. I would look at the data as being still in favor of a senescent model.

In terms of your model, you still have to explain the fiber degeneration. You have to postulate something wrong about those cells in order to continue to cause the fibers to degenerate and it seems to be like the observations we have about the behavior of the normal human myoblasts if pushed to extreme numbers of proliferations. Those cells all exhibited a senescent phenotype. It seems like you are disregarding an observation of normal cells, i.e. senescence.

DR. BLAU: I have read your papers on the myoblast from mouse dystrophy and they are a very nice parallel to what we are seeing in the human dystrophy. In fact, my interpretation would be that in your studies you may also have a growth problem due to a proliferative defect in the myoblasts. I don't see that your evidence can definitively rule out that possibility.

DR. KEDES: If I understand Dr. Blau's model correctly, to address the question Hauschka and Emerson were asking about, you have to understand what is happening to the fiber. I thought Dr. Blau said that quite clearly, at least to my way of thinking about it. If the muscle can't grow because it doesn't have enough proliferative capacity, and it is being asked to grow, those residual fibers which are there and are under stress are going to be damaged. They will break down. Furthermore, I think Dr. Holtzer's type of experiment has been done on humans. Many people have been irradiated. Radiation myopathy is well documented by pathologists. I would like to hear pathologists tell me what the effects of the X-ray on human muscle is.

DR. KELLY: I've done it in baby rats. If you leave it for a length of time you don't see very much in terms of morphologic change.

DR. FISCHMAN: I am puzzled here. How can we really say we have a satellite cell if we don't get a colony that forms muscle? Maybe we didn't have satellite cells. I was going to ask Dr. Holtzer whether one can identify every satellite cell or do we have other markers that would be independent of the proliferative cell and its final differentiative capacity that would give us another way of scoring the cells besides the ability to grow in a normal way?

DR. HOLTZER: You could identify a satellite cell the way Dr. Blau did in culture. You should be able to get those cells to form myotubes in culture.

DR. BLAU: As I showed you, we can get the defective myoblasts to form myotubes. In addition, we now have a monoclonal antibody which we obtained from Dr. Walsh that stains both dystrophic myoblasts and normal myoblasts, but not fibroblasts. I think that is definitive; it stains all clones in which there is fusion. I don't understand the question raised by Dr. Fischman regarding proliferative capacity. If, in clones isolated from control muscle, proliferative capacity is a highly reliable and reproducible measure, why shouldn't it constitute a means for characterizing dystrophy? It's value is in the comparison.

DR. MIRANDA: First, I would like to comment on Dr. Holtzer's idea of an _in vivo_ model. A major point that Dr. Blau spelled out very clearly is that the fibroblasts are not affected in Duchenne. If you irradiate an animal, you are going to kill the fibroblasts and muscle cells so you are not going to be able to reproduce the dystrophic process the way it exists in the animal. Second, I am always concerned about proliferating a muscle clone. With a mass culture, I can watch closely and split the culture anytime I don't want it to fuse. With a clone, it is a different situation. If I grow a clone for 3 weeks, even in a rich medium, by 3 weeks the medium is depleted to such an extent that the cells fuse. If the mitogens in the medium are not as high as in the medium I used last week, I am going to get small colonies that are fusing. I can't make the statement that these small colonies have less proliferative capacity; they just fuse earlier. The problem of counting cells and saying they look proliferative is tricky.

DR. BLAU: In order to promote proliferation and prevent fusion in clones, the media and feeding regimens used are extremely important.

DR. MIRANDA: We also need to look at the characteristics of controls. First we have to look at the normals, but then also look at all of the other dystrophies. When we look at polymyositis we have a different situation. This is an acquired myopathy. Myopathy can occur anytime in life. If Dr. Blau looks at someone who is 20 years old, the myopathy could have started at 19 which means the restoration of muscle by satellite cells has not been as long as in the Duchenne child. Therefore, you are going to have to look a little further and at populations later in life to see why it has a dystrophic phenotype.

DR. EPSTEIN: Is it possible when you are doing your cloning that you are cloning not only satellite cells but proliferating myoblasts?

DR. BLAU: I no longer make the distinction between a satellite cell and a myoblast. In the literature the satellite cell has so often been referred to as the cell responsible for regeneration. I think we have to change our views about that. There is so much muscle tissue growth going on and so much growth potential in the satellite cells. These cells are not likely to be just sitting there waiting for damage. As has been shown in the rat, they are actively involved in the development and growth of muscle (224).

PART III

REGULATORY INFLUENCES ON MUSCLE GROWTH

CHAPTER 8: TROPHIC INFLUENCES ON DEVELOPING MUSCLE

S. Hauschka*, R. Lim*, C. Clegg**, J. Chamberlain**
C. Bulinski** and T. Linkhart***

*Department of Biochemistry, University of Washington, Seattle; **Department of Biology, UCLA, Los Angeles, CA; ***Department of Mineral Metabolism, J.L. Pettis Veterans Hospital, Loma Linda, CA

The purposes of this talk will be to outline several general "rules" that are useful for studying myotrophic factors, and to provide a brief synopsis of the studies being carried out in our lab to determine how specific growth factors regulate skeletal muscle differentiation. In presenting these "rules," the hope is to provide a set of guidelines that may help to clarify the interpretation of data which is rapidly accumulating from the many different laboratories now studying myogenesis *in vitro*.

RULE 1 - All myoblasts are not identical.

The behavior of myoblasts derived from different species, embryonic stages, and muscle regions within a given individual are not identical. Comparative clonal analyses of embryonic human, chick, and mouse myoblasts indicate differences in both macromolecular substrate and media requirements and the colony behavior (263). For example, human muscle colony-forming (MCF) cells do not exhibit a strict dependence upon a collagen substatum for their growth and differentiation (264), whereas chicken MCF cells derived from comparable embryonic stages do (265). Permanent muscle cell lines from rat and mouse also differ with respect to their dependence upon an exogenously supplied collagen substratum; rat L-6 cells do not require collagen-coated surfaces(266), whereas mouse MM14 myoblasts do (unpublished observation). Perhaps the most emphatic example of species-specific differences in myoblast behavior has been that of the dependence of avian *vs* mammalian myoblasts on transferrin derived from the same animal classes (267-269). This topic.

is discussed in detail by Dr. Ozawa in an accompanying article. Other apparent species-specific differences in myoblast growth factor requirements are the mitogenic responsiveness of rat L-6 myoblasts to somatomedins (270-272) and the apparent lack of responsiveness of mouse MM14 myoblasts (273).

Examples of stage-specific differences in myoblast behavior within a single species have been observed during both human and chick embryonic development. MCF cells from early human fetuses grow equally well but differentiate poorly in media containing human serum as the sole macromolecular additive, whereas MCF cells from fetuses older than 50 days differentiate well in such media (274). Similarly, chick MCF cells from embryos earlier than day 6 will not grow in media containing fetal calf serum as the single macromolecular additive, whereas MCF cells from older embryos will grow in such media (unpublished observation). Finally, MCF cells derived from early and late stages of both human and chick embryos exhibit characteristic differences in clonal morphology which -- at least in the chick -- are heritable during sequential subclonal passages (274,275). Examples of differences in MCF cells derived from different anatomical regions have been reported for both chick and human embryos in which proximodistal gradients of early and late MCF cells are observed (274,276).

RULE 2 - Factors with different names may be identical, and factors with the same name may not be identical.

Although this "rule" may seem overly semantic, it is worth keeping in mind -- particularly during early phases of research on unpurified myogenic factors -- since it is during this period when operational terms may be applied to factors which have been characterized previously in quite a different context. A recent example of such confusion is seen in the studies of "muscle trophic factor" (277,278), "sciatin" (279), "neurotrophic factor" (280), and transferrin (269) on muscle growth and differentiation. When this confusion was sorted out by the careful work of Dr. Ozawa and his colleagues, it became clear that "muscle trophic factor," "sciatin" and "neurotrophic factor" were, infact, transferrin (269), and that transferrin itself could be replaced by iron (281).

The second part of rule 2 is also well exemplified by work from the Ozawa group in which it was clearly shown that transferrins exhibit class specificity (267,268). The important take-home lesson from these studies is that negative results from studies which attempt to apply polypeptide factors from one species to cells of another may be due to trivial species differences which have nothing to do with true physiological differences between cells of the two species.

RULE 3 - Semi-defined or defined factors required at high concentrations (μg - mg/ml levels) may mimic or contain ng/ml amounts of the physiologically "true" factor.

The first aspect of this rule is well illustrated in studies from Florini's laboratory on the role of somatomedins in muscle differentiation (270-272). In these studies with rat myoblasts it was clearly demonstrated that insulin concentrations which were 2-3 orders of magnitude higher than physiological could replace physiological concentrations of MSA as stimulators of myoblast growth and differentation. Presumably this is due to the ability of insulin to bind -- albeit poorly -- to the MSA (i.e. insulin-like growth factor - (264) receptor (282).

The second aspect of this rule -- that of the "true" factor being a minor contaminant of a "purified" factor whose required concentration differs from its normal physiological levels -- is well illustrated by the selenium requirement which has recently been established for many fully defined cell culture systems (283). Discovery of the selenium requirement came, in fact, from the recognition that an apparent thyroxine requirement was well beyond established physiological concentrations of thyroxine (284).

RULE 4 - The apparent requirement for a factor may be affected by the presence of other media components.

This rule is well illustrated by the response of rat L-6 myoblasts to dexamethasone and insulin. When fetuin is employed as a medium additive L-6 cells respond _independently_ to insulin and to dexamethasone (272) with respect to fusion; whereas when horse serum is employed as a medium additive, the response to dexamethasone _requires_ the presence of insulin (285). The implications of such observations are that the _total_ experimental environment should be considered with respect to conclusions as to factor activity.

RULE 5 - The activity of defined factors may differ from lot to lot.

While this rule may appear trivial, ignorance of this possibility could lead to premature conclusions as to a factor's effect and/or to its optimal concentration range. Experience from our studies of fibroblast growth factor (FGF) requirements for mouse myoblast proliferation have disclosed activity differences of nearly 100-fold over a 5 year period during which about 15 different commercial lots of FGF have been tested. A practical solution to this problem is to always design experiments so as to test factors over about an 0.03- to 30-X range of their reported activity optima. A second, and often ignored control experiment for situations in which a test factor appears to have "no" affect on one's experimental system, is to examine the same preparation for activity in a system it is known to affect. Upon observing a positive response, it is then safer to conclude that the negative result was a true indication of nonresponsiveness.

RULE 6 - Factor activity should always be interpreted relative to the total *in vitro* assay conditions employed.

Several of the more important conditions to keep in mind are: (a) effects due to residual media components from the preassay growth period, and (b) effects due to differences in cell density and growth state. For example, when log phase MM14 myoblast cultures are switched to media lacking FGF with or without two intervening rinses, many cells in the unrinsed cultures complete several cycles before differentiating, whereas cells in the rinsed cultures complete only a single cycle (unpublished data). Similarly, in situations where factors may become inactivated by mechanisms which are proportional to cell density, it is critical to pay strict attention to the related parameters of cell density, medium volume, and time since last feeding, since all of these can influence the apparent responsiveness to defined factors.

To summarize, the intent of specifying the aforementioned rules is not to limit the diversity of experimental approaches used in studying myotrophic factors. Clearly, this would be premature since our present knowledge of myotrophic factors is so limited that rigid constraints on experimental design would be counterproductive. Rather, the intent was to point out a number of considerations that should be kept in mind to avoid presently recognized pitfalls.

The second portion of this talk will concern a brief summary of current information pertinent to myotrophic factors. First, what is the present state of defined media for muscle growth and differentiation? Second, what is known regarding the mechanisms by which myotrophic factors affect muscle differentiation?

Considerable effort has been devoted toward developing fully defined media for muscle cell growth and differentiation. The goal has yet to be achieved with respect to growth media, but several labs have reported defined media in which myoblasts will differentiate. The first such media was devised for quail muscle cells (286) and consisted simply of a total replacement of serum and embryo extract with polyvinyl pyrolidone to maintain osmolality. A simple defined media containing only insulin and dexamethasone as additives have also been devised for rat L-6 cell differentiation (272). This medium also works well for MM14 mouse myoblasts, but these cells can, infact, initiate differentiation and remain reasonably healthy for up to 16 hours in a medium no more complex than Ham's F10 nutrients with calcium adjusted to 1.2 mM. Neither this medium nor Florini's defined medium will, however, support long term maintenance of mouse muscle cultures.

From these studies it is thus clear that muscle differentiation -- at least its initiation and early phases -- does not require the presence of media macromolecules after proliferating cultures are switched to defined media. It would be premature, however, to conclude that such muscle differentiation was occurring in a totally defined environment. For example, if the proliferating cultures had been grown in media containing serum and/or embryo extract, it is likely that one or more macromolecules from these additives would adsorb to the culture dish surface (263). This is clearly the case for fibronectin (287), and although fibronectin's major role may be in promoting myoblast attachement and alignment (288), it is conceivable that it -- or associated macromolecules -- play at least permissive roles during muscle differentiation. In conclusion it is worth recalling that despite the progress that has been made with defined media for muscle differentiation, no medium has yet supported truly long term survival of differentiated muscle culture; and the morphological quality of cultures maintained in defined media does not compare favorably with the quality of cultures maintained in media containing serum, and especially with the superb quality of muscle fibers co-cultured with nerve (289,290). There is thus still much to be accomplished.

Definition of the specific factors required for muscle cell growth is still in its infancy. Excellent progress has been made in terms of identifying factors required for rat L-6 cell growth; yet the same media have not worked for other myoblast types. The two published reports concerning L-6 media differ significantly in their composition. One media contains only insulin, dexamethasone, and fetuin as its "defined" additives (270,272). While fetuin is certainly more defined than whole serum and embryo extract, it is undoubtedly not homogeneous, thus this medium probably requires further refinement. The other medium contains insulin, transferrin, prolactin, growth hormone, fibroblast growth factor, angiotensin II, hydrocortisone, fibronectin, lithium and selenium as its defined additives (291). It is comparable to serum-supplemented media for L-6 cell growth, but it does not support the growth of either mouse MM14 myoblasts or human primary myoblasts (unpublished results).

Progress has also been made with respect to devising a defined medium for chicken myoblast growth (292). Similar to Hayashi's medium for L-6 cells, the chick myoblast medium contains fibronectin, insulin, transferrin, and fibroblast growth factor. This medium appears to support reasonable proliferation for several days when cells are innoculated at high density (5 x 10^5 cm dish). It does not, however, support clonal growth; and unlike Hayashi's medium, its support of proliferation is well below the maximal rate supported by the addition of serum and embryo extract. Interestingly, the transferrin used in the chick medium was of human origin. With the hindsight provided by Ozawa's studies of class-specific transferrin requirements (267-269), it seems likely that utilization of chicken transferrin might provide a more potent medium.

Clearly, much more extensive work is required to devise fully defined growth media for the myoblasts of various species. Such an effort is worthwhile since it will permit more uniform studies and more precise experimental manipulation of myogenic processes. It is important, however, not to overemphasize the usefulness of defined media. Many unanswered problems of myogenesis can be rigorously approached without recourse to defined media; thus the lack of such media is not an intellectual barrier to instructive studies.

At the conclusion of my presentation I would like to spend a few minutes summarizing information from our lab pertaining to the role of mitogens in regulating skeletal muscle differentation. These studies have been done with a permanent, clonally derived line of mouse myoblasts (MM14) which we established in 1978 (293). When feasible, results from MM14 have been verified with primary mouse myoblasts. _No_ discordancies between the behavior of MM14 and primary myoblasts have been observed.

The most important aspect of our studies has been the demonstration that muscle differentiation is regulated by a repression mechanism involving one or more polypeptide growth factors. Removal of specific mitogens (e.g. FGF) derepresses the myoblasts and terminal differentiation ensues (294). Mitogenic regulation of muscle differentiation is strictly cell cycle-dependent -- the "decision" to proliferate or to differentiate being made only during G_1 phase (295). The response of G_1 myoblasts to mitogen-depletion is an irreversible withdrawal from the cell cycle which we have called "commitment" to terminal differentiation. Commitment occurs within 3 hours of mitogen removal and is _not_ reversed by re-exposure to mitogens (295). Within 12 hours of a continuous exposure to mitogen-depleted conditions, the entire myoblast population has cycled into G_1 and has become committed to terminal differentiation. The process is thus synchronous within the time constraints of a single cell cycle. Muscle-specific messenger RNA (for M-creatine kinase) is first detected within 5 hours of mitogen removal (296); muscle-specific proteins such as acetylcholine receptor actin, M-creatine kinase, and myosin are first detected at 6 hours (296-298); and fusion commences in 12-14 hours. Although we are far from understanding these events in detail, several instructive insights have emerged from recent experimental studies.

a. An intervening cell cycle is and DNA synthesis not required between exposure of myoblasts to mitogen depleted media (DM) and activation of the commitment process.

Further evidence that commitment occurs during G_1 and that putative regulatory processes occurring in other cell cycle phases are not required was obtained by plating mitotically synchronized G_1 myoblasts directly into DM. All of the cells committed to a post-mitotic state and became AChR-positive without transversing another cell cycle. This observation may have important implications with respect to the mechanism of gene activation.

b. Repression of commitment by FGF is independent of proliferation.

To determine whether commitment to the post-mitotic state is controlled "directly" by FGF or "indirectly" via a signal coupled to proliferation, myoblasts were plated into media containing FGF but lacking sufficient serum to support proliferation. Under these conditions myoblasts became quiescent as they entered G_1 but failed to commit i.e. when serum was returned, they re-entered the cell cycle (297). This observation is consistent with the concept that commitment is repressed by an FGF signal and not secondarily by a signal due to proliferation. Since FGF is, however, also required for myoblast proliferation, it appears that the intracellular FGF signaling pathway must be bifurcate at some point so as to both stimulate proliferation and repress commitment.

c. Growth factor specificity for the stimulation of proliferation and repression of commitment.

Attempts to replace FGF with other (more purified) growth factors have been unsuccessful. EGF, MSA, insulin, and PDGF all failed to stimulate myoblast proliferation when added to serum-containing media; they were also unable to repress commitment (273). Interestingly, several types of variant myoblasts derived from the MM14 line will proliferate in response to mitogens other than FGF (e.g. EGF); and in those instances in which the variants maintain a capacity for muscle differentiation it is found that commitment can be repressed by these other mitogens (299).

d. Correlations between mitogen receptor behavior and commitment.

Since the earliest changes associated with commitment are withdrawal from the cell cycle and the acquisition of a post-mitotic phenotype, it seemed plausible that some component(s) of the mitogenic response mechanism might, itself, be involved in the commitment process. Unfortunately, little is known concerning the sequence of events in the signaling pathway of any mitogen; but since the signal is initiated by a mitogen-mitogen receptor interaction it seemed reasonable to analyze this process in myoblasts. Attempts to study FGF receptor behavior via ^{125}I-FGF binding have continued to yield tantalizing but basically uninterpretable results. The difficulties are that commercial FGF contains trace amounts of other proteins (which also become iodinated during the labeling procedure) and that FGF and/or the "contaminants" exhibit too high a level of non-specific binding to be sure that changes associated with commitment are due to changes in FGF receptor alone. As an alternative to studies of FGF receptor we have analyzed EGF receptor (EGFR) with the thought that its behavior might serve as a model for the behavior of other mitogen receptors during muscle differentiation. The initial rationale for studying EGFR was that it was the most thoroughly understood mitogen receptor. In addition, we had shown that EGF, while not mitogenic for normal MM14 myoblasts, was mitogenic for DD-1 cells, a differentiation-defect variant of the MM14 line (299), as well as for BUdR-treated myoblasts which become quiescent, yet fail to commit when exposed to DM (300). Thus under conditions in which commitment is inhibited, the seemingly "functionless" EGFR of normal myoblasts can initiate a functional mitogenic signal. The direct implications of eGFR data to FGF receptor behavior remain uncertain, but recent studies have strengthened the analogy.

A complete description of our EGF studies is contained in references (299) and (301), but the most critical observations are: (i) MM14 myoblasts exhibit specific ^{125}I-EGF binding and contain 3-4 x 10^4 EGFRs per cell; (ii) ^{125}I-EGF binding (EGFR) decreases to <5% of its level in proliferating myoblasts within about 20 h of their commitment to the post-mitotic state; (iii) an irreversible decrease in EGFR begins about 3 h after a media switch (the same time at which the first cells become committed) and continues in parallel with the kinetics of commitment; (iv) the decrease in EGFR occurs at the same rate (T 1/2 = 6.4 h) as the decrease in EGFR in proliferating cells caused by the inhibition of protein synthesis; and (v) the decrease in EGFR is correlated directly with commitment -- and not with withdrawal from the cell cycle or the G_1 phase -- because myoblasts arrested in G_0 (by serum deprivation in the presence of FGF) as well as mitotically synchronized G_1 myoblasts both exhibit high levels of EGF binding.

Evidence that these studies (which conern a growth factor which is not normally mitogenic in mouse myoblasts) may be relevant to the mechanism by which mitogens such as FGF regulate myoblast differentiation comes from studies of a myogenic revertant (DD-1α) of the MM14-DD-1 cell line. When DD-1α cells are switched to a low serum medium lacking EGF or FGF they differentiate, but if either mitogen is added, differentiation is repressed. Thus in DD-1α cells, EGF appears to have acquired the same ability to repress commitment as exhibited by FGF with the parental MM14 myoblasts.

Based on these observations we have proposed a model in which myoblast commitment to the post-mitotic state is closely coupled to an irreversible decrease in mitogen receptors. At present we do not know whether reduction of mitogen-receptors below some critical threshold level is the essential step in "causing" commitment to the post-mitotic state or whether this is an early consequence of the commitment process. In either case, it is clear that the irreversible loss of receptors is a mechanisticaly attractive process for converting a sub-population of cells within an environment -- which may be generally conducive to proliferation -- to an unresponsive state. How such a "selective" commitment process may be regulated *in vivo* remains to be determined.

Observations consistent with a mitogenic regulation of muscle differentiation have been reported for many other muscle cell culture systems including chicken and quail (306), rat (286, 302,303), lizard (304,305) and human (unpublished). In none of these cases, however, has a specific regulatory mitogen been identified. Although there appears to be general agreement that mitogens regulate muscle differentiation by repressing differentiation, not all myoblasts exhibit as rapid and/or irreversible a commitment to terminal differentiation as is exhibited by mouse myoblasts. In particular, at least some quail myoblasts which respond to mitogen depletion by withdrawing from the cell cycle and synthesizing muscle-specific proteins can be stimulated to cease myosin synthesis and to re-enter the cell cycle by refeeding the mitogen-rich medium (307). Studies with rat and mouse myoblast commitment and cell cycle mutants also indicate that the synthesis of muscle-specific proteins is not causally coupled to an irreversible withdrawal from the cell cycle (308,309).

Despite general unanimity among most investigators that mitogens can regulate the onset of muscle differentiation, not all investigators concur with the conept of an environmental regulation of muscle differentiation (310). It should thus be emphasized that this model does not fit -- at least easily -- all observations. How, for example, does the model explain the asynchrony of differentiation that is observed within single muscle colonies? Might there be microenvironments of mitogens -- perhaps adsorbed to the substrate -- which make even the microscopic region of mitogen receptors at the level of individual cells -- perhaps due to unequal segregation of receptors to daughter cells following mitosis? Answers to these questions will require further study. We thus wish to emphasize that while the mitogenic regulation model serves as a useful conceptual approach to how muscle differentiation is regulated, it would be premature to believe that the model provides a fully satisfactory explanation.

To summarize, and attempt to integrate our studies of the repressor-type regulation of muscle differentiation by specific growth factors with the initial two portions of my talk, we would propose that certain mitogens may act as "myotrophic" factors in the sense that their presence is required to maintain myoblasts in a proliferative state. This permits the initial myoblast population to expand and results -- indirectly -- in an elevated level of muscle differentiation once the growth factor(s) have been depleted below a critical level. One of the major values of devising defined media for muscle cell growth is that it would permit a more precise manipulation of environmental factors. Such studies could lead both to the identification of previously recognized "myotrophic" factors, and to more refined analysis of their mechanisms of action.

CHAPTER 9: TROPHIC AND MYOGENIC EFFECTS WITH SPECIAL REFERENCE TO TRANSFERRIN

Eijiro Ozawa

Division of Cell Biology
National Center for Nervous, Mental & Muscular Disorders
Tokyo, Japan

Chick myogenic cells grow and differentiate *in vitro* when incubated with a medium composed of Eagle's MEM, horse serum and a small amount of chick embryo extract (EE). However, they do not grow, when incubated with a medium composed of Eagle's MEM and horse serum (basal medium). This indicates that EE contains essential substance(s) for chick myogenic cell growth, which is contained in neither the artificial medium nor horse serum.

Our purpose is to isolate myotrophic substances from EE. Since the introduction of EE by Alexis Carrell 1913, (311), trials to obtain trophic substances which stimulate cell growth have been repeatedly challenged. But trophic substances with high molecular weight have never been isolated and characterized.

We have obtained a substance which promoted myogenic cell growth when added to the basal medium and identified it as transferrin (Tf). Since we have published most of the results concerning Tf, I would like only to summarize them here (312).

First, the active substance prepared from chick serum (313-314). It had molecular weight of 80K dalton, salmon pink color and the same antigenicity as serum Tf and ovo-transferrin. Its peptide maps of α-chymotrypsin and papain digests were almost the same as those of the latter two Tfs. All three fractions had myogenic activity. Their effective concentration was at the order of μg/ml. The activity was lost if Fe was removed from them.

The activity was restored increasingly in parallel with the increase in the ratio of the Fe-bound form to the sum of Fe-bound- and apo-forms. When their Fe binding was saturated, the activity ceased increasing by further addition of Fe to the solutions. Further the specific activities of these three on a protein basis were almost the same as one another (315,316). These show that the active substance is Fe-bound Tf.

We have also isolated a myotrophic substance from EE which was also identified to Tf by the same criteria (317).

Second, the activity is entirely dependent on the presence of bound Fe. Tf has been known to bind transition metals. Among the metal-Tf complexes, Fe-Tf was solely effective. Furthermore, Fe ion, either ferrous or ferric ion, alone was effective. But its effective concentration was about 200 times larger than that of Fe-Tf (318,319). This shows that what is needed for myogenesis is Fe, and the protein moiety of Fe-Tf seems to facilitate the entrance of Fe into the cells.

Third, Tf protein has specificity in its trophic activity

Species Specificity of Transferrins

for myogenic cells. Our basal medium contained nearly 450 μg/ml of horse Tf, about one-half of which is Fe bound form. Nevertheless, myogenic cells did not grow in the basal medium. This suggested that horse Fe-Tf did not work on chick myogenic cells.

To clarify this, we systematically studied the effects of various Fe-Tf on muscle cells from various animals (320,321). As shown in Table 8, chick, quail or duck myogenic cell growth was stimulated by chick, turkey or goose Fe-Tf, but not by horse, swine, rabbit or rat Fe-Tf. Inversely, rat or rabbit myogenic cell growth was stimulated by these mammalian Fe-Tfs but not by the avian Fe-Tfs. This relationship between animals who gave Fe-Tf and myogenic cells can be summarized as "class specificity." This specificity is the basis for the study of the effect of chick Fe-Tf in the presence of horse Fe-Tf. There were, however, a few exceptions. Dove and bovine Fe-Tfs stimulated the growth of some of the mammalian and avian cells, respectively.

Since myogenic cells have Fe-Tf receptors on their cell surface, it is reasonable to postulate that the specificity is due to the difference in binding affinity between Fe-Tf and receptor. Shimo-Oka in our laboratory showed that this was the case.

Lastly, what is the role of Fe-Tf in myogenesis? Fe-Tf stimulated myoblast proliferation. This effect has been shown with various kinds of cells (322,323). The number of Tf receptors

TABLE 8

CELL \ Fe-Tf	CHICK	GOOSE	TURKEY	DOVE	BOVINE	HORSE	SWINE	RABBIT	RAT
CHICK	+++	+++	+++	+	+	-	-	-	-
QUAIL	+++	+++	+++	+++	-	-	-	-	-
DUCK	+++	+++	+++	-	-	-	-	-	-
RAT	-	-	-	+	+	+++	+++	+++	+++
L_6	-	-	-	+	+	+++	+++	+++	+++
RABBIT	-	-	-	+	+	++	+++	+++	+++

Effectivity of Fe-Tfs from various animals on various myogenic cells. +++ : effective at about 1 μg/ml, ++ : effective at about 10 μg/ml, + : effective at about 100 μg/ml, - : not effective at 100 μg/ml.

in red cells diminishes as the cells mature (324). Cancer cells have a large number of Tf receptors. Therefore, TF is usually understood as a promoter of cell division. In the case of muscle cells Fe-Tf works in addition to keeping myotubes healthy. When Fe-Tf was removed from the culture medium, larger myotubes became slender, degenerated and finally died. But following readdition of Fe-Tf to the medium, surviving cells grew to form large myotubes again (325,326).

In the presence of Fe-Tf, myotubes continued to grow and at the same time they differentiated. They accumulated muscle specific proteins, such as myosin, actin and muscle type creatine kinase. They showed cross striations and spontaneous twitches. When stimulated electrically, they showed spike and plateau responses, followed by contraction. These hallmarks of differentiation also appeared if the cells were cultured with Fe ion in the place of Tf (327).

In the course of studying the effect of Fe-Tf on myogenic cells, EE was treated with anti-Tf-IgG to remove Tf from EE. Although the IgG treated EE (EE*) lost the myotrophic activity, EE* showed potentiating activity of Fe-Tf. In other words, myotrophic activity of EE was completely dependent on the presence of Fe-Tf, but EE* still contained some components which enhanced the effect of Fe-Tf (328).

As the potentiating substances, EE* contained heat stable and heat labile factors. Heat stable factors were eluted from a Sephadex G-75 column as high and low molecular weight fractions. The high molecular weight substance was RNA and the low molecular weight substances were purines and purine nucleotides. Using authentic substances, it became clear that the most potent stimulator of myoblast division was hypoxanthine among purine analogues. The effect of purine analogues was dominant in quail myoblasts but not in chick and rat myoblasts. RNA was, however, effective on all the myoblasts (329).

The heat labile substance was partially purified by the combination of ammonium sulfate salting out procedure and CM Sephadex and Sephadex G-75 column chromatographies. The molecular weight of the substance ranged from 16 to 20 K dalton determined by gel filtration. This substance is tentatively called myoblast proliferation factor (MPF) (330).

When quail myoblasts were incubated with a medium composed of 85% Eagle's MEM, 15% horse serum, 10 μg/ml chick Fe-Tf, and 10 μM hypoxanthine (BCMTH) to which a given amount of MPF was added, myoblasts continued to divide and remained as mononucleated cells for a while. Although they finally fused together to form myotubes, formation of myotubes was delayed compared with the control culture whose medium did not contain MPF. This concentration which gave the half maximum effect was 1 μg/ml.

It has been shown that myogenic cells cultured with conditioned medium fuse early whereas they remain mononucleated when bovine FGF is added to the medium (331). This effect of FGF was mimicked by MPF. Since the molecular weight of MPF is similar to that of FGF, MPF may be a related substance to FGF. When the concentration of FGF to give half maximal effect on qual myoblasts proliferation was compared with that of chick MPF, FGF was about 3 times more effective than MPF. This is probably due to impurity in MPF preparation.

In contrast to Fe-Tf, MPF showed less species specificity. MPF worked on chick and rat myogenic cells. The effects and effective concentrations in these cells were similar to what was needed for multiplication promoting effect on quail cells.

On these bases, the potentiating effect of EE* on Fe-Tf can be partly explained as follows: Purine analogues, RNA and MPF in EE* stimulate myoblast multiplication in the presence of Tf, and the larger number of myoblasts yields for the formation of myotubes of larger number and size.

However, the effect of EE is probably not completely replaced with the effect of combination of Tf, hypoxanthine and MPF. Since the maximum effect to promote cell multiplication of EE is larger than that when assayed in BCMTH, it is reasonable to assume that EE contains some factors other than those reported here.

CHAPTER 10: STIMULATION OF THE SYNTHESIS OF FRUCTOSE 1,6-DIPHOSPHATE ALDOLASE BY TRANSFERRIN

T.H. Oh*, G.J. Markelonis*, T. Dion Guidera*,
S.L. Hobbs* and L.P. Park*

*Department of Anatomy
University of Maryland School of Medicine
Baltimore, MD

The glycolytic enzyme aldolase (E.C.4.1.2.13) catalyzes the reversible cleavage of fructose 1,6-diphosphate to yield dihydorxyacetone phosphate and D-glyceraldehyde 3-phosphate. During embryonic development in skeletal muscle, this tetrameric enzyme undergoes a transition from a macromolecule composed primarily of C subunits to a homotetramer composed of A subunits (332-334). The work of Lebherz has shown that the steady-state concentration of aldolase and other glycolytic enzymes in "fast" and "slow-twitch" skeletal muscle fibers is regulated almost solely at the level of protein synthesis (334,335). During post-embryonic development, the synthetic rate of aldolase becomes four-fold faster in "fast-twitch" chicken breast muscle as compared to "slow-twitch" leg muscle (334-336). Thus, in terms of the glycolytic enzymes, fiber-type differentiation appears to progress via a transformation from a slow-type phenotype to a fast-type (335).

* The authors wish to express their thanks to Dr. D. Hoover, Mr. G. Holm, Mrs. J.L. Johnson and Mrs. F.F. Spaven for technical assistance and to Mrs. E. DeLong for editorial help. This work was supported by grants from the NIH (NS 16076-G.J.M. and NS 15013-THO), the MDA (T.H.).) and the Frank C. Bressler Research Fund of the University of Maryland (G.J.M.).

Reduction of Aldolase in Developing Dystrophic Muscle

Our interest in aldolase stems from the fact that the steady-state level of this enzyme in breast (fast-twitch) muscle is reduced by 50% in developing dystrophic chickens (336) or in denervated breast muscle from normal chickens (337). In either circumstance, the decrease in aldolase is due to a decrease in the number of aldolase molecules as a result of a reduction in the synthesis of the enzyme (336,337). The mechanism for decreased aldolase synthesis in dystrophic breast muscle may involve an alteration in the normal progression of fiber-type differentiation (336), while the results observed after denervation could reflect a partial "dedifferentiation" of the affected fast fibers (337).

We have shown that transferrin increases total protein synthesis (338) and the synthesis of acetylcholine receptors (339) in cultured embryonic chicken breast muscle. In view of these results, we decided to assess whether this iron-transport protein influences the genetic expression of the glycolytic enzyme, aldolase. In the present communication, we report that transferrin significantly increased the synthesis of aldolase-A molecules in cultures of embryonic breast muscle *in vitro.*

Cell Culture Technique

Trypsin-dissociated skeletal muscle cells were prepared from breast muscles of 12-day-old chicken embryos (Spafas Inc., PA) as previously described (340). Selective enrichment of myogenic cells was obtained by the method of Richler and Yaffe (341). The myogenic cells (5×10^5 cells) were plated on linbro plastic dishes (35 x 15 mm; FB-6-TC) that had been precoated with collagen (50 μg/dish, acid-soluble, Calbiochem). Cultures were maintained in the standard culture medium (SCM) at 37°C in a humidified atmosphere of 95% air and 5% CO_2. SCM consisted of 87.5% Dulbecco's modified Eagle's medium (DMEM), 10% horse serum (heat-inactivated) and 2.5% chicken embryo extract (EE). The culture medium was replaced every 3 days and no antibiotics were used. In some cultures, SCM was removed and replaced by SCM without EE (SCM-EE; 90% DMEM/10% horse serum). Transferrin (Tf) was obtained from Sigma (conalbumin, type II, diferric).

Synthesis of Aldolase by Muscle Cells in Culture

Proteins synthesized *de novo* in muscle cultures were labeled with 3H-L-amino acids or ^{14}C-L-leucine in a medium (DMEM) containing no L-leucine. Incorporation of tracers into protein remained linear for at least 3 h under the labeling conditions used (Figure 28). In studies on aldolase synthesis, shorter labeling periods were utilized.

In an initial set of experiments, myogenic cells were plated and grown continuously in SCM. On days 1 and 4 after plating, some cultures were treated with transferrin (30 μg/dish) while the untreated cultures served as controls. After 5 days in culture, newly synthesized proteins in myotubes were labeled in the presence of ^{3}H-L-amino acids. At time intervals, the radiolabeled A form of aldolase was precipitated from cell supernatants using the immunoprecipitation procedure described in Methods. Figure 29 illustrates that the rate of aldolase synthesis in transferrin treated myotubes reached 570% of the control rate within 60 min after isotopic labeling had been initiated.

In a second set of experiments, we assessed the effect of transferrin withdrawal from cultures of myoblasts and myotubes on aldolase synthesis. Such a protocol was used previously in studying the synthesis of acetylcholine receptors (339). In these experiments, myogenic cells were plated for 24 h in standard culture medium (SCM). Some cultures (myoblasts) were then grown in SCM containing no embryo extract (SCM-EE) in the presence or absence of transferrin (30 μg/dish) for 48 h. The remaining

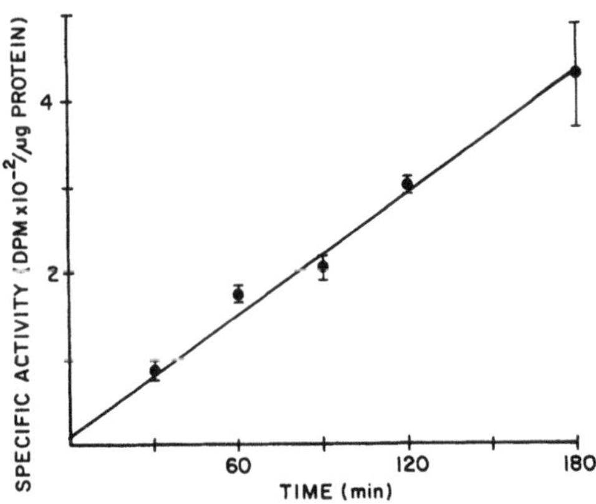

FIGURE 28: Protein Synthesis in Myotube Cultures. Muscle cells were growing in standard culture medium (SCM) for 5 days. At this time, the SCM was aspirated, cultures were washed thrice with HBSS and 1 ml of DMEM containing no L-leucine was added. Ten μCi of a ^{3}H-L-amino acid mixture was added to each dish, and the level of labeled amino acids incorporated into protein was determined at timed intervals by TCA precipitation as described in Markelonis (338). The values shown represent the mean ± SE of triplicate determinations. Incorporation remained linear for at least 180 min.

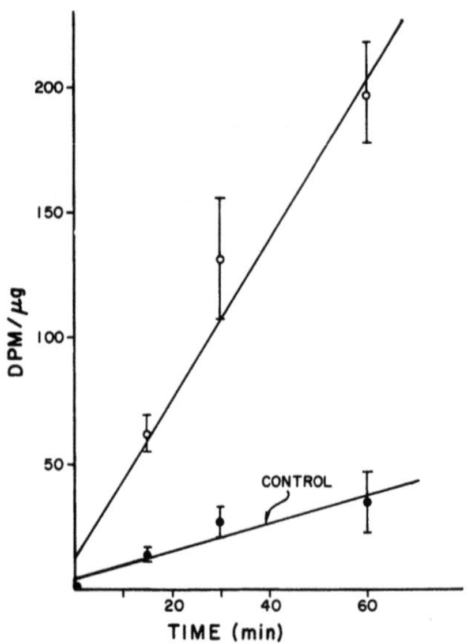

FIGURE 29: Effect of Transferrin on Aldolase Synthesis in Myotubes. Myogenic cells were plated and grown continuously in SCM. On days 1 and 4 after plating, some cultures were treated with Tf (30 μg/dish) while the untreated cultures served as controls. After 5 days in culture, cells were labeled with 10 μCi ^{3}H-L-amino acids as described in the legend to Figure 28. Incorporation of labeled amino acids into aldolase was assayed by immunoprecipitating ^{3}H-aldolase from the soluble cellular fraction with goat antialdolase serum as described in (339). Each value is the mean ± SE of triplicate determinations ● - control; 0 - Tf (30 μg/dish).

cultures (myotubes) were grown in SCM for 96 h at which time the medium was changed to SCM-EE ± transferrin for 48 h. Myoblast or myotube cultures were then labeled in the presence of ^{3}H-L-amino acids and aldolase was quantitated by immunoprecipitation. Figure 29 summarizes the effect of transferrin (Tf; 30 μg/dish) on the rate of aldolase A synthesis in myoblast or myotube cultures deprived of embryo extract for 48 h. The rate of aldolase synthesis in Tf-treated myoblast cultures (Figure 30a) was 220% of the control rate by 120 min. Similarly, the rate of aldolase A synthesis in Tf-treated myotube cultures (Figure 30b) was 174% of that in controls. Thus, an increased rate of aldolase synthesis in myoblasts or myotubes could be sustained in cultures deprived of embryo extract by the addition of Tf.

Control experiments showed that preincubation of Tf-treated

myotube cultures in the presence of puromycin (20 μmg/ml) for 4 h, or in cycloheximide (10^{-5}M) for 1 h diminished the 30-min incorporation of labeled amino acids into aldolase by more than 90% (transferrin: 397.7 ± 22.8 DPM/μg protein; puromycin: 29.9 ± 130 DPM/μmg protein; cycloheximide: 38.3 ± 15.9 DPM/μmg protein; mean ± SE of 3 determinations). Thus, the increase in the specific activity of aldolase as a result of treatment with Tf was due to de novo synthesis of the enzyme. Furthermore, an alteration in the intracellular pool of labeled amino acids could not explain the results obtained.

Turnover of Aldolase in Cultured Muscle Cells

Turnover experiments indicated that the rate of aldolase turnover in Tf-treated myotube cultures was not appreciably different from that in control myotube cultures. In Tf-treated cultures, ^{3}H-aldolase was degraded with a †1/2 of 9.1 h. Similarly, ^{3}H-aldolase in control myotube cultures was degraded with a half-life of 12.3 h. As Tf did not appear to appreciably alter the turnover rate of aldolase in treated muscle cells, the increase in the specific activity of aldolase following Tf-treatment appeared to result predominantly from increased de novo synthesis of the enzyme. This agrees with previous reports which showed that Tf increased total protein synthesis and the synthesis of the acetylcholine receptor in myotubes without appreciably affecting degradative rates (338,339).

Specificity of Transferrin Effect on Muscle Cell Aldolase

We have shown that transferrin induced a 2 to 5-fold increase in the rate of aldolase synthesis in treated muscle cultures (Figures 29,30). This increase in specific activity was abolished by inhibitors of protein synthesis, did not depend upon the presence of embryo extract in the culture medium (Figure 30), was not the result of an alteration in the intracellular pool of labeled amino acids and was not accompanied by an appreciable alteration in the turnover rate of aldolase. Thus, the increase in immunoprecipitated aldolase in Tf-treated muscle cultures appears to reflect the increased de novo synthesis of enzyme molecules. Furthermore, the increased synthesis of aldolase appeared to be confined only to muscle cells since the goat antibody used for immunoprecipitations did not cross-react with aldolase in fibroblasts. Therefore, transferrin appears to play a significant role in the genetic expression and regulation of aldolase and perhaps other glycoltyic enzymes in muscle cells in vitro.

The steady-state concentration of aldolase and other glycolytic enzymes in fast and slow-twitch skeletal muscle fibers in the chicken is regulated at the level of protein synthesis

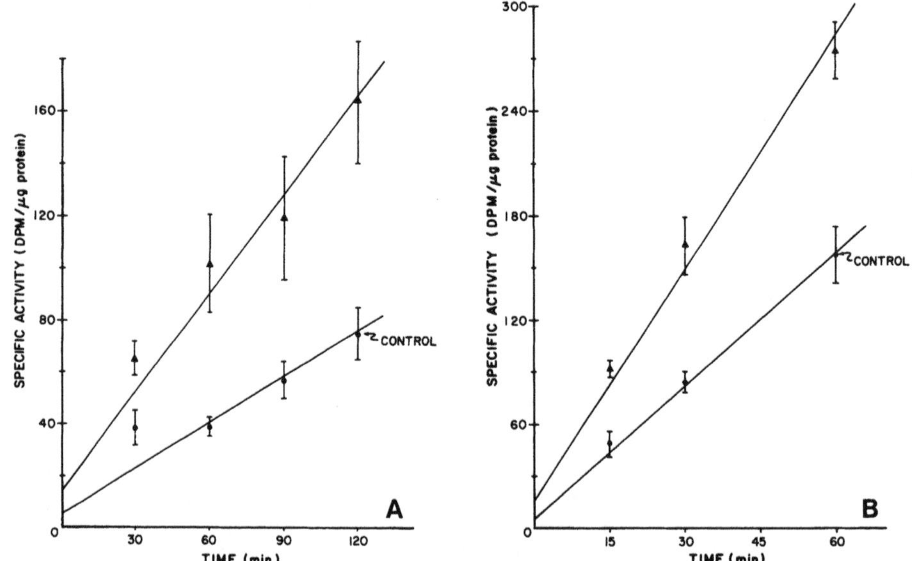

FIGURE 30: Effect of Transferrin on Aldolase Synthesis after Withdrawal of Embryo Extract. Myogenic cells were plated for 24 h in SCM. At this time, the culture medium in half the cultures was changed to SCM containing no embryo extract (SCM-EE). These cultures were then maintained in SCM-EE for 48 h in the presence (30 μg) or absence of Tf (myoblasts). The remainder of the cultures were grown in SCM for 96 h. At this time, the medium was changed to SCM-EE and the cells were grown in the presence or absence of Tf for 48 h (myotubes). The effect of transferrin on aldolase synthesis following withdrawal of embryo extract was then determined by isotopic labeling followed by immunoprecipitation (Methods). A. Aldolase synthesis in myoblast cultures. B. Aldolase synthesis in myotube cultures. Values shown represent the mean ± SE of triplicate determinations. ●-control; ▲-Tf (30 μg/dish).

(334-335). During post-embryonic development in the chicken, the synthetic rate of aldolase becomes 4-fold faster in fast-twitch breast muscle as compared to slow-twitch leg muscle (334-336). As a result, fiber-type differentiation in the chicken may progress via a transformation from a slow-type phenotype (slow glycoltyic enzyme synthesis) to a fast-type (rapid glycolytic enzyme synthesis) (335). It is interesting that transferrin, a ubiquitous serum protein, can mimic just such a shift in skeletal muscle cells in culture. Whether this protein is involved in the physiological "synthetic shift" observed *in vivo* remains to be determined.

The steady-state level of aldolase in chicken breast is reduced by 50% in developing dystrophic chickens (336) or in denervated breast muscle from normal chickens (337). This decrease in aldolase appears to be due to a decrease in the number of aldolase molecules as a result of a reduction in the synthesis of the enzyme (336,337). Whether transferrin plays a role in this reduction in aldolase synthesis is unknown. However, transferrin is known to be internalized by receptor-mediated endocytosis (342,343), and chicken myotubes are reported to have specific Tf receptors on their plasma membranes (334,335). Since membrane alterations are known to occur in dystrophic muscle (346,347) and in denervated muscle (348,349), a decreased ability to internalize Tf could conceivably result in an alteration in muscle aldolase synthesis *in vivo*. The immunocytochemical visualization of the Tf receptor in normal and dystrophic muscle could provide compelling evidence in this regard.

An intriguing question remains as to why transferrin, a protein which transports ferric ions required for oxidative enzyme synthesis should have such a dramatic effect on muscle aldolase, a glycolytic enzyme. Transferrin is known to have potent growth-regulating properties since blocking the Tf receptor of human tumor cell lines with antireceptor monoclonal antibodies dramatically reduces cell proliferation and growth (350). In fact, the expression of the transferrin receptor appears to be ubiquitous in neoplastic and rapidly-proliferating cell lines (342,351-356). Since tumor cells are known to express Tf receptors abundantly, and rely on glycolysis for their energy demands (357), it may be that Tf functions as a modulator which influences the expression of glycolytic enzymes in these cells. This hypothesis appears to be worthy of investigation.

CHAPTER 11: MYOTROPHIC FACTOR(S) IN NORMAL AND DYSTROPHIC CHICKEN SKELETAL MUSCLE

Ryoichi Matsuda* and Richard C. Strohman*

*Department of Zoology
University of California
Berkeley, CA

Transferrin is Selectively Accumulated in Skeletal Muscles

In our earlier work on satellite cell cultures (358) we noticed that slow muscle like the anterior latissimus dorsi (ALD) yielded a higher number of satellite cells than did the fast pectoralis major muscle (PM). We have now found that the ALD contains a high level of a muscle growth factor and we have identified this factor as transferrin (Tf) 359). In addition, Tf was found to be relatively low in normal PM muscle but elevated in PM muscle obtained from chickens with inherited muscular dystrophy (360). Finally, we have recently been able to show that the Tf fractions from ALD and dystrophic PM muscle contain a growth-promoting factor other than Tf which we have yet to identify. The Tf studies are published (359,360) and we will simply summarize them here with an attempt to relate the findings to normal and dystrophic muscle growth.

ALD Muscle Extracts Stimulate Muscle Growth in Culture

Extracts made from adult ALD but not from PM muscle stimulate protein synthesis, DNA synthesis and MHC accumulation in myogenic cell cultures of chick embryo PM myoblasts. This stimulation is dose-dependent and is observable at about 0.2 to 0.5 μg/ml muscle extract protein. This stimulation is observed even in the presence of complete medium (10% horse serum and 2% embryo extract) and is a roughly 4 fold increase in DNA and MHC. The ALD extract is added to the time of cell plating and the stimulation in muscle growth as measured by increased MHC accumulation is entirely due to a stimulation of myoblast cell division and therefore increased myotube number and/or mass.

If extracts are added to myotubes in the presence of embryo extract there is no stimulation of MHC accumulation.

The Stimulation Factor(s) is Identical to and/or Includes Transferrin

When ALD extracts are fractionated in DEAE cellulose we obtained a sharp zone of stimulation activity. The fractions carrying the activity were then subjected to SDS-PAGE electrophoresis. The active fractions contained Tf as judged by the presence of a band that co-migrated with purified chicken Tf and by the fact that a peptide map of the material in this band matched a similar map of purified Tf.

Active Extracts Contain a Growth Factor in Addition to Transferrin

The fractionated material was assayed for activity in cultures that did not contain embryo extract and yielded 100 fold increases in growth. This was to be expected since in the absence of embryo extract there is practically zero growth and embryo extract can be completely replaced by Tf (361). We then compared the growth stimulus obtained with our factor to that obtained with purified Tf. In the presence of embryo extract our extract always yielded a higher level of growth stimulation than could be accounted for on the basis of its Tf content. This led us to believe that the active extracts contained a growth factor in addition to Tf. In order to determine if a factor in addition to Tf was present we tested out ALD extract for its ability to promote growth in the rat L6 muscle cell line. It has been shown previously that chicken Tf will not support growth of rat cells and generally that mammalian Tf will not support growth of avian cells in culture (361,362).

Our ALD extracts and active fractions gave a growth stimulation in rat L6 cells of greater than 2 fold. In addition, purified chicken Tf gave no growth response in these L6 cultures. We are confident, therefore, that ALD muscle of adult chickens accumulates not only Tf but another factor that perhaps works synergistically with Tf in promoting myoblast division. It appears therefore that we are in good agreement with Dr. Ozawa (this volume) in that the growth factor he isolates from serum also appears to contain active material in addition to Tf.

Transferrin is Localized in Skeletal Muscle Predominately in the Extracellular Matrix Surrounding Muscle Fibers

We obtained an affinity-purified antibody to chicken Tf and used it in a series of immunocytochemical localization studies in ALD and PM muscles We are able to show that Tf is heavily localized in the interstitial space between muscle fibers. The ALD interstitial areas of the ALD are much more extensive than those of the PM and the levels of Tf-antibody binding to material in these areas is also much more extensive in the ALD than in the PM. The extracellular matrix itself may be a kind of "sink" for Tf or the Tf may be concentrated by connective tissue cells of the interstitial space. In any case it appears that a muscle like the ALD which appears to have a greater number of satellite cells than the PM also shows a higher accumulation of growth factors like Tf.

It is interesting to speculate on the relationship between Tf levels in the muscle extracellular space and the requirement for growth factors in the muscle satellite cell population. As Dr. Schultz has pointed out in this meeting (363), slow muscles like ALD tend to be active over long periods and perhaps because of their high levels of activity result in a higher rate of turnover of intracellular structure. One has higher levels of satellite cell activity in these muscles and the presence of high levels of Tf and perhaps other growth-promoting molecules in the spaces adjacent to satellite cells would be consistent with his observed higher satellite cell number.

Transferrin is Accumulated in Dystrophic but not in Normal PM Muscle

While Tf and growth promoting activity are both very low in the PM muscle of normal chickens they are significantly present in PM muscle from dystrophic chickens. In a developmental study of PM muscle, Tf levels are found to be high during embryonic development but fall quickly after hatching so that by 2 weeks posthatching there is little or not Tf or growth promoting activity present in the PM. In the dystrophic bird however the situation is quite different. Instead of falling after hatching, the PM Tf levels remain quite high and extracts of dystrophic PM muscles show quite high levels of growth promoting activity when tested on standard muscle cell cultures either from the chicken (360) or from the rat (362).

Speculation: Growth Factors, Satellite Cells and Dystrophic Muscle

Dr. Blau (this volume) has provided us with a very interesting theory that relates at least one form of dystrophy to a defect in the satellite cell itself. But unexplored still is the relationship between satellite cell growth and the factors in (or outside of) the muscle which control that growth. Our observations on dystrophic chicken PM muscle are interesting from the point of view of this relationship.

When dystrophic muscle is examined by immunocytochemistry using the Tf antibody the same intense staining of the extracellular space is seen that we see for the ALD but not the normal

PM. The dystrophic PM muscle has a much more elaborate extracellular space or endomysium than does the normal PM and Tf binding is correspondingly much more intense in the dystrophic than in the normal PM. A causal relationship between high levels of growth factors in the muscle endomysium on the one hand and the presence of large number of single cells, presumably including satellite cells, on the other is not proven. A growth response in muscle, however, will almost certainly involve a stimulation of the muscle fiber's satellite cell population (364). The enlarged interstitial space may represent a storage capacity for growth factors and under appropriate conditions, injury, trauma, increased intracellular turnover, etc., the satellite cell would be exposed to these growth factors and stimulated to initiate division. This model would predict that extracellular matrix of dystrophic muscle or of the slow muscles discussed by Dr. Schultz, which bear increased numbers of satellite cells, would also yield high levels of growth factors on appropriate extraction and/or would show high affinity binding for factors capable of stimulating satellite cell division.

CHAPTER 12: CONTROL OF MYOSIN ISOZYMES DURING MYOGENESIS IN THE RAT

Neal A. Rubinstein*, Gary E. Lyons*, Brigitte Gambke* and Alan Kelly**

*Department of Anatomy; **Department of Pathobiology
University of Pennsylvania School of Medicine
Philadelphia, PA

Like most contractile proteins, the myosin molecule exists in a number of polymorphic forms which show specificity among muscles (365,366) and among muscle fibers (367,368) with different physiological and metabolic properties. For example, fast and slow twitch fibers contain both different myosin heavy chain and myosin light chain complements; and among the fast twitch fibers, IIa and IIb fibers contain myosins with qualitatively distinct myosin heavy chains, but similar myosin light chains (369,370). These distinct properties within individual adult fast and slow fibers are partly the result of innervation by different types of motoneurons, since cross innervation of fast and slow muscles causes a reciprocal transformation of the muscles' properties (371). Eccles et al (372) have demonstrated that fast and slow motoneurons have different frequencies of impulse activity; and in fact, the effects of cross innervation of a fast muscle with a slow motoneuron can be mimicked by chronic stimulation of the fast muscle's own intact motoneurons at 5 - 10 Hz, the frequency of activity of a slow motoneuron (373,374).

* This work was supported by NIH grants HL 15836 to the Pennsylvania Muscle Institute and NS 14332 and by a grant from the Muscular Dystrophy Association of America. N.A.R. is an established investigator of the American Heart Association.

Thyroid hormones are also important in determining the properties of different muscle types. Treatment of experimental animals with thyroxine increases skeletal muscle mitochondria and mitochondrial enzymes. These changes occur even after denervation (375). Thyroid hormones also increase the myosin ATPase activity and shift the light chains from the slow to fast types (376). Hypothyroidism has the opposite effect: it causes a marked slowing of contraction and half-relaxation times of the already slowly-contracting soleus muscle, a total conversion of fast to slow twitch fibers, and the disappearance of fast myosin light chains (377,378).

Influence of Thyroid Hormones on Muscle Fiber Types

Changes in fiber types and myosin isozymes also occur during development. Initially, a muscle generates a homogeneous population of fibers, all synthesizing a myosin heavy chain unique to the earliest stages of development (379,380). Maturing fast-twitch fibers sequentially synthesize this embryonic myosin heavy chain, then a neonatal myosin heavy chain, prior to the synthesis of the adult fast myosin heavy chain characteristic of the adult muscle (381,382). Slow muscles similarly synthesize the embryonic and neonatal myosin heavy chains prior to the synthesis of adult slow myosin heavy chains (383). This sequence of myosin types is characteristic of both mammalian and avian muscles (384-386).

The neural and hormonal control of embryonic or neonatal myosin isozymes during development is currently being investigated. Earlier, we demonstrated that the initiation and maintenance of adult slow myosin light chains is dependent on innervation (387). In the absence of motoneurons, a developing slow muscle synthesizes only the light chains characteristic of adult fast myosin. Fast myosin light chains are unaffected by denervation. Because of the subsequent discovery of embryonic and neonatal myosin heavy chains prior to the appearance of definitive adult myosin heavy chains, we have investigated the factors responsible for transition in synthesis from one myosin heavy chain to another during development.

Control of Myosin Isozymes During Development

Combinations of myosin heavy and light chains result in native myosin isozymes which can sometimes be distinguished by their mobility on pyrophosphate gels. Figure 31a shows computer enhanced scans of myosin isozymes of the developing fast EDL of the rat after pyrophosphate gel electrophoresis. To obtain this data, myosin isozymes were subjected to electrophoresis on pyrophosphate slab gels; the gels were stained, destained, and digitized in a two-dimensional matrix on a microdensitometer with a step size of 37.5 microns. The resolution of

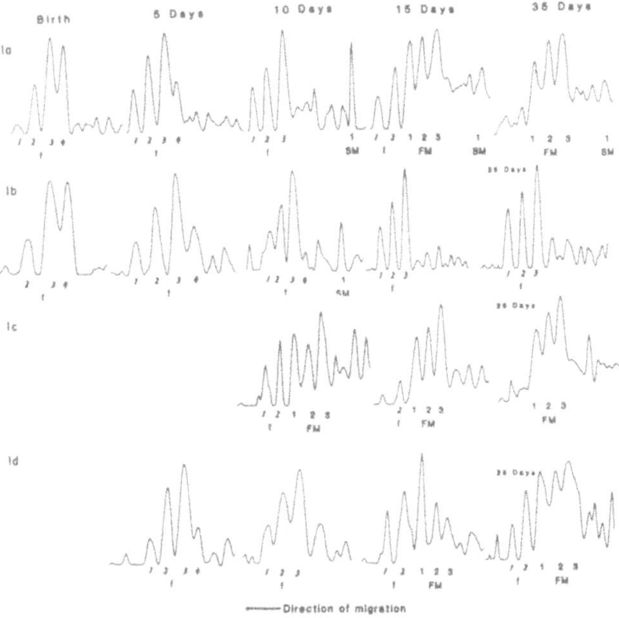

FIGURE 31: Myosin Isozymes of the developing fast-twitch EDL muscle. Myosins or actomyosins were analyzed by pyrophosphate gel electrophoresis on slab gels according to Lyons et al (383). Gels were stained, destained, and digitized in a two-dimensional matrix on a microdensitometer with a step size of 37.5 microns. The resolution of the band peaks was enhanced using a computer program for a constrained iterative deconvolution scheme (388). (a) Isozymes from the developing EDL at 0, 5, 10, 15, and 35 days postpartum. Isozymes containing the embryonic or neonatal myosin heavy chains are labeled f1-f4, while adult fast myosin isozymes are labeled FM1-FM3. Between 10 and 15 days postpartum, the muscle switches from predominantly neonatal to predominantly adult fast isozymes. (b) Isozymes from the developing EDL of animals made hypothyroid from 13 days gestation onwards. This hypothyroid muscle fails to make a significant transition from neonatal to adult fast isozymes. This inhibition is reversible. (c) Isozymes from the developing EDL of animals made hyperthyroid from 3 days postpartum onwards. These muscles undergo a precocious transition from neonatal to adult fast myosin isozymes. (d) Isozymes from the developing EDL of euthyroid animals after denervation of the muscle at birth. The lack of innervation does not prevent the muscle from synthesizing adult fast isozymes. (Figure reprinted from FEBS Lett., Gambke et al (391)).

the band peaks was enhanced using a computer program for a constrained iterative deconvolution scheme (388). During the first two weeks postpartum, the EDL contains predominantly four myosin isozymes, labeled f1-f4 after the convention of Fitzsimmons and Hoh (389). Immunoblots and immunoprecipitations of these samples using our monoclonal antibody - 2B6 - specific to the embryonic myosin heavy chain (390) has revealed that f4 and a fraction of f3 and f2 are isozymes containing the embryonic myosin heavy chain. The remainder of f3 and f2 plus all of f1 represent isozymes with the neonatal myosin heavy chain. With increasing maturation, the scans show a steady decrease in f4 and a changing stoichiometry of f3, f2, and f1. This represents a decrease in synthesis and accumulation of embryonic myosin heavy chains and a concomitant increase in neonatal myosin heavy chains. Between 10 and 15 days postpartum, adult fast isozymes FM1-FM3 appear and the developmental isozymes begin to disappear.

The developing slow-twitch soleus muscle (Figure 32a) shows a similar series of changes in embryonic and neonatal isozymes. In this muscle, however, the decrease in embryonic myosin heavy chain is less rapid, a result confirmed by radioimmunoassay with monoclonal antibody 2B6 (390). Also, the soleus contains two isozymes, labeled s1 and s2, which are precursors to adult slow isozymes and may represent combinations of slow myosin heavy chains with fast myosin light chains. By 15 days postpartum, these isozymes have attained the mobility of SM1 and SM2, while the developmental isoforms are decreasing. In the adult, SM2 is the predominant isozyme.

Because our earlier studies suggested a dependence of slow myosin light chain synthesis on innervation, we examined the isozymes of these two muscles after denervation of the distal hindlimb at birth. Changes in fast myosin light chains of the EDL were

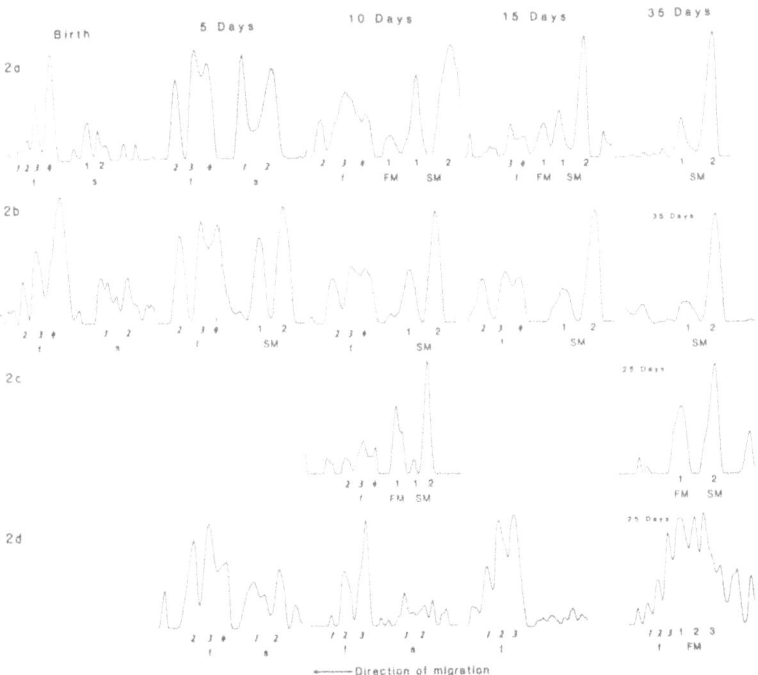

FIGURE 32: Myosin isozymes of the developing slow twitch soleus muscle. Myosins from the soleus muscle were analyzed as described in the legend to Figure 31. f1-f4: isozymes containing either embryonic or neonatal myosin heavy chains; s1, s2: isozymes present during the immediate pre- and post-natal period in the soleus; these may be hybrids of fast light chains and slow heavy chains or some precursor slow myosin; SM1, SM2: adult slow myosin isozymes. (a) Isozymes of the developing soleus. At 10 days postpartum, isozymes with the mobility of the definitive adult slow isozymes, SM1 and SM2, are seen. In the adult, SM2 is the dominant isozyme. (b) Isozymes of the developing soleus of animals made hypothyroid from 3 days gestation onwards. Hypothyroidism hastens the appearance of definitive adult isozymes, which can be seen already in the 5 day animal. (c) Isozymes of the developing soleus of animals made hyperthyroid from 3 days postpartum onwards. The transition from neonatal to adult slow isozymes is not affected. The adult hyperthyroid animal contains SM2 plus a fast isozyme, FMS. (Figure reprinted from FEBS Letts, Gambke, et al (391).

independent of innervation. Figure 33 shows the light chains of the EDL at birth (Figure 33a), 25 days postpartum (Figure 33c), and 25 days postpartum after denervation at birth (Figure 33e). The changes normally seen between birth and 25 days postpartum are a disappearance of the embryonic light chain (lemb) and an increase in fast light chain 3f. These changes are independent of innervation.

The soleus of the newborn also contains a predominance of fast light chains, plus slow light chain (1s) and the embryonic light chain, (lemb) (Figure 33b). By 25 days postpartum, however, the muscle has accumulated equal proportions of fast and slow light chains and the embryonic light chain has disappeared (Figure 33d). After denervation, however, slow light chain accumulation ceases and the slow light chains already present begin to disappear (Figure 33f). The muscle continues to accumulate only fast light chains. The disappearance of the embryonic light chain is unaffected by denervation.

Analyses of native isozymes after denervation reveal a similar dependence of slow, but not fast, myosin on innervation. In the developing EDL (Figure 31d), the muscle progresses from embryonic to neonatal to adult fast isozymes regardless of the state of innervation. In the soleus, however, denervation results in a suppression of slow myosin isozymes (Figure 32d). The muscle ultimately synthesizes only fast isozymes. Preliminary data has suggested that the denervated soleus is synthesizing a fast-red myosin heavy chain, while the innervated and denervated EDL muscles synthesize a fast-white myosin heavy chain (382).

Effect of the Thyroid on Myosin Synthesis in the Adult

Altered plasma levels of thyroid hormones affect myosin isozymes in adult animals: hypothyroidism leads to an increase in slow myosins, while hyperthyroidism favors fast myosin synthesis. We examined the role of thyroid hormones in the progression of myosins during development (391). In our radioimmunoassay of plasma thyroxine levels, the rat was essentially hypothyroid at birth (i.e. levels were below the limit of detectability, 1 ng/ml). Between 5 and 15 days postpartum, levels increased from 2 to 45 ng/ml before decreasing to the adult level of 35 ng/ml at 35 days postpartum. Thus, rapidly increasing plasma thyroxine levels coincide with the switch from neonatal to mature isozymes. We

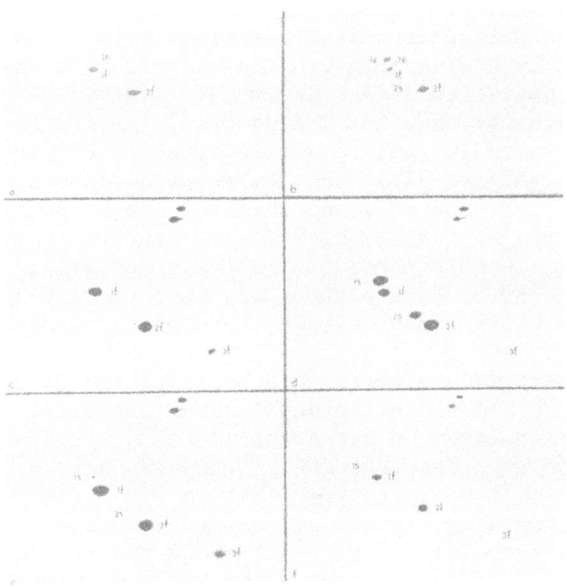

FIGURE 33: Myosin light chains of the developing soleus and EDL muscles. Myosin light chains were analyzed by two-dimensional electrophoresis using a pH gradient of 4-6 in the first dimension and 17% acrylamide-SDS gels in the second dimension. 1f, 2f, 3f: fast myosin light chains; 1s, 2s: slow myosin light chains; lemb: the embryonic myosin light chain. Light chains were analyzed from the EDL (a) at birth, (c) at 25 days postpartum, (e) at 25 days postpartum after the muscle had been denervated at birth. Normal changes between birth and 25 days postpartum include the disappearance of the embryonic myosin light chain and an increase in fast light chain 3f. These changes are not affected by denervation. Light chains were also analyzed from the soleus (b) at birth, (d) at 25 days postpartum, (f) at 25 days postpartum after denervation at birth. Normal changes between birth and 25 days postpartum include the disappearance of the embryonic light chain and large increases in slow light chains 1s and 2s relative to the fast light chains 1f and 2f. Fast light chain 3f does not increase. Denervation at birth prevents the increase in slow light chains 1s and 2s, although the disappearance of the embryonic light chain is unaffected. The denervated muscle accumulates predominantly in the fast light chains 1f and 2f. Light chain 3f is not seen in large quantities.

examined the effect of altered thyroxine levels on this myosin transition. Animals were made hypothyroid from three days gestation onwards by adding propylthiouracil (PTU) to the drinking water of pregnant rats and to the water of newborn pups. Animals were also maintained on a low iodine diet. In the fast muscles of hypothyroid animals, adult fast isozymes do not appear between 10 and 15 days (Figure 31b), and the neonatal isozymes f1-f3 continue to be the only isozymes at least until 60 days. Unlike neural changes in cretinism, this inhibition to adult fast myosin synthesis is reversible. If hypothyroid animals are removed from PTU and the low iodine diet at 35 days postpartum, they rapidly synthesize adult isozymes FM1-FM3 and degrade the neonatal isozymes.

Animals were made hyperthyroid by injecting 25 ug thyroxine on days 3, 5, 7, and 9. At 10 days, serum thyroxine levels were above the maximum level of detectability of our radioimmunoassay, 1 μg/ml. By 10 days the fast EDL already was accumulating large quantities of adult fast isozymes (Figure 31c). This precocious transition to adult myosin can be confirmed by peptide maps of the myosin heavy chains. Figure 34b shows the peptide maps of myosin from the fast gastrocnemius muscle of a euthyroid neonatal animal (lane a) and from an adult euthyroid animal (lane f). Myosin from 10 day hyperthyroid animals (lane b) also showed the adult myosin peptide pattern.

The soleus is less responsive to changes in the plasma thyroxine levels. In the soleus of hypothyroid animals (Figure 32b), SM1 and SM2 appear by 5 instead of 10 days postpartum. In the hyperthyroid muscles, SM2 appears normally, although SM1 is replaced by an adult fast isozyme (Figure 32c).

As demonstrated above, fast muscle denervated at birth still makes the transition from neonatal to adult fast myosin isozymes. This can be confirmed by peptide maps of the fast gastrocnemius muscle after various perturbations. Figure 34b, lane a, shows a peptide map of the neonatal myosin dominating the muscle at 5 days

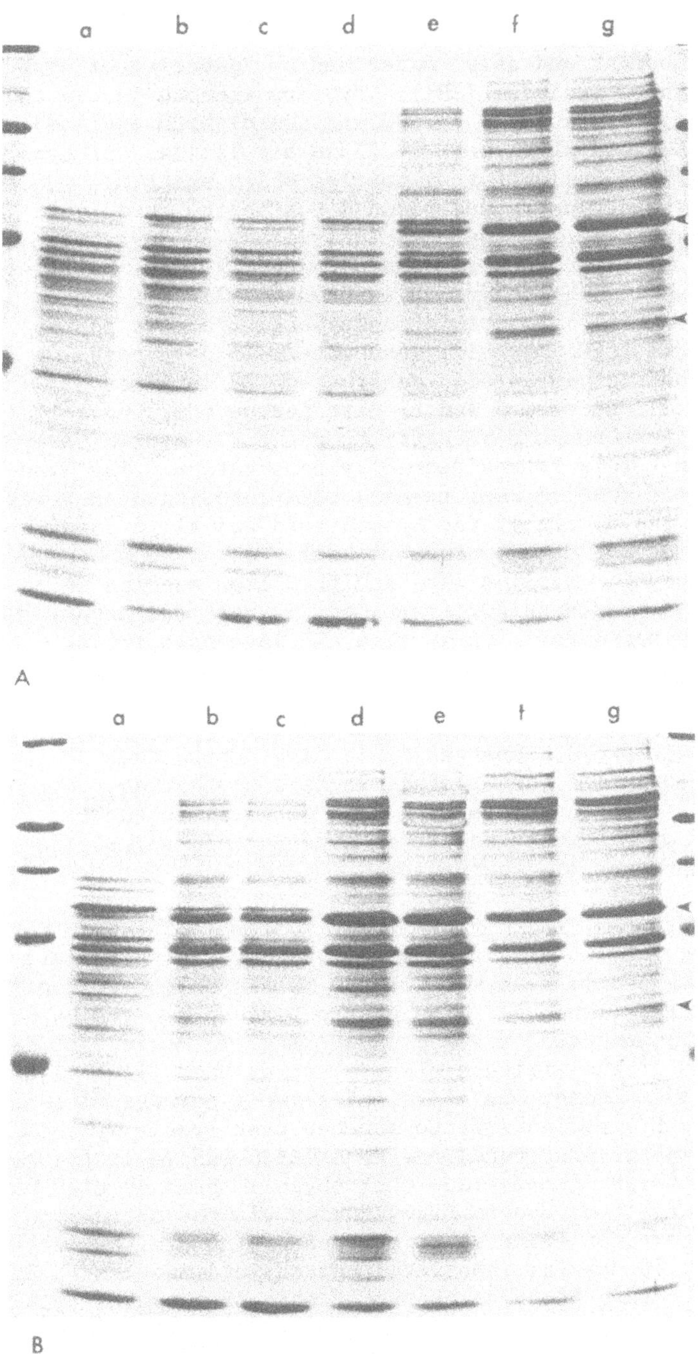

Figure caption on p. 150.

FIGURE 34: Peptide maps of myosins from the fast-twitch gastrocnemius muscle. Myosins were column-purified from the gastrocnemius muscle during normal development and after experimental induction of hypo- or hyperthyroidism (391). Myosins were subjected to limited proteolysis in SDS and the digests analyzed on SDS gels which were 12.5% in acrylamide. A: Myosins were analyzed from muscles which were (a) euthyroid, innervated, 5 days postpartum (neonatal myosin); (b) hypothyroid, innervated, 10 days postpartum; (c) hypothyroid, denervated, 10 days postpartum, (d) hypothyroid, innervated, 25 days postpartum; (e) hypothyroid, denervated, 25 days postpartum; (f) euthyroid, innervated, 25 days postpartum; (g) euthyroid, denervated, 25 days postpartum. Between 5 and 25 days postpartum, the animal switches from the neonatal to the adult myosin heavy chain. This is unaffected by denervation. The hypothyroid muscles fail to make this transition; however, when the muscle of the hypothyroid animal is denervated, it does begin to synthesize adult fast myosin heavy chains. B: Myosins were analyzed from muscles which were (a) euthyroid, innervated, 5 days postpartum; (b) hyperthyroid, innervated, 10 days postpartum; (c) hyperthyroid, denervated, 10 days postpartum; (d) hyperthyroid, innervated, 25 days postpartum; (e) hyperthyroid, denervated, 25 days postpartum; (f) euthyroid, innervated, 25 days postpartum; (g) euthyroid, denervated, 25 days postpartum. The precocious transition from neonatal to adult fast myosin which occurs in hyperthyroid animals is independent of innervation.

postpartum. By 25 days postpartum peptides characteristic of adult fast myosin can be seen whether the muscle is innervated (lane f) or denervated (lange g). The gastrocnemius from the hyperthyroid animal also undergoes a precocious change to adult fast isozymes regardless of the presence (lane b) or absence (lane c) of innervation. Hence, one effect of thyroid hormone must be a direct action on the muscle fiber to enhance fast myosin synthesis. Our peptide maps of innervated and denervated muscle in the hypothyroid animal, however, demonstrate that thyroid hormones also have an indirect effect on myosin heavy chains via the motoneuron (Figure 34a). Innervated (lane b) or denervated (lane c) hypothyroid muscles at 10 days or innervated hypothyroid muscles at 25 days (lane d) contain peptides characteristic of neonatal myosin, a result confirming the pyrophosphate gel analysis (Figure 31). In the 25 day hypothyroid muscle which has been denervated at birth, however, adult fast myosin heavy chain has begun to accumulate.

This suggests that the immature motoneuron inhibits the transition from neonatal to adult fast myosin and that this inhibition can be relieved in either one of two ways: by adding thyroid hormone to promote maturation of the peripheral nerves or by removing the nerve and its inhibitory effect altogether.

Diversity among muscle fibers begins at an early stage of development. Both immunohistochemical studies of rat myogenesis with anti-myosin antibodies (379) and histochemical myofibrillar ATPase reactions of chicken muscles (392) suggest that differences among fibers can be detected as early as 2 days after the initial formation of myotubes from a muscle primordium. The initial myosin detected in bulk hindlimb muscle contains the embryonic myosin heavy chain described by Whalen et al (381). Immunohistochemical studies in our laboratory with a monoclonal antibody specific to mammalian embryonic myosin heavy chain initially shows a uniform distribution of embryonic myosin heavy chain in all fibers, regardless of their ultimate destiny (390). Diversity among fibers can be detected when a subset of fibers begins to react with a polyclonal antibody against adult slow myosin heavy chain (379). Whether this antibody is recognizing true adult slow myosin heavy chains or a closely-related species of myosin heavy chain is uncertain; however, the distribution of this myosin heavy chain is not uniform, but is limited to the primary generation fibers in most muscles. Since the slow soleus muscle contains a larger proportion of primary generation fibers than do developing fast muscles, clear distinctions in the staining capacity of fast and slow muscles are seen very early (379,380). These differences have been confirmed by pyrophosphate gel electrophoresis of native isozymes, as well as by peptide maps of isolated myosin heavy chain from soleus and EDL at 18 days gestation (380).

Effects of Thyroid vs Nerve in Regulating Isozyme Transitions

With increasing maturity, differences among fibers are accentuated and the stage at which adult staining characteristics are attained appears to be muscle specific. In a series of papers, we have examined the myosin isozymes responsible for the diversity for fiber types defined by immunohistochemistry in the rat and the factors contributing to changes from one myosin type to another (379,382,383,390). Myosins from the developing fast-twitch EDL and gastrocnemius muscles and from the slow-twitch soleus of the rat were analyzed by pyrophosphate gel electrophoresis of native myosins, two-dimensional electrophoresis of light chains, peptide mapping of heavy chains, and immunoblots and radioimmunoassays with 2B6, our monoclonal antibody specific to the embryonic myosin heavy chain. Initially at 15-16 days gestation when antibody staining with 2B6 shows a uniform distribution of embryonic myosin heavy chain among the fibers of the rat hindlimb, only two isozymes with mobilities of f4 and f3 are seen on pyrophosphate gels

(383). By 18-19 days gestation, both soleus and EDL contain isozymes with the embryonic myosin heavy chain as well as those with the neonatal myosin heavy chain; the soleus additionally contains isozymes with slow or precursor-slow myosin heavy chains. Differences in the stoichiometry of embryonic versus neonatal isozymes exist between these two muscles during the first two weeks postpartum. Between 10 and 15 days postpartum, both muscles reveal the presence of adult isozymes.

The control of these isozyme transitions has been examined in detail. The progression from embryonic to neonatal to adult fast isozymes in the fast EDL and gastrocnemius muscles is unaffected by denervation. In the hypothyroid animal, however, the disappearance of embryonic myosin heavy chain is retarded severely and the transition from neonatal to adult fast myosin does not occur. Alleviation of the hypothyroid condition reverses the block to adult fast myosin accumulation. Hyperthyroidism causes a precocious accumulation of adult fast myosin and accelerates the disappearance of embryonic and neonatal myosin heavy chains.

The transition from neonatal to adult slow isozymes in the slow soleus is controlled differently. Changes in plasma thyroxine concentrations do not qualitatively affect the switch. This transition, however, can be completely disrupted by denervation. If the soleus is denervated at birth, the muscle progresses from neonatal to an adult fast set of isozymes, rather than a set of adult slow isozymes. Both heavy and light chains respond to denervation in this way.

Although thyroid hormones are clearly important factors for the synthesis of adult fast myosins in distal hindlimb muscles, the fact that all muscles do not synchronously initiate the synthesis of fast myosin makes it certain (a) that fibers have a wide range of sensitivity to thyroid hormones and (b) that these hormones are not the unique cues for adult fast myosin synthesis. We have shown, for example, that newborn rats are essentially hypothyroid, with thyroxine levels below the limit of detectability of our radioimmunoassay. Despite the hypothyroid condition of rat pups _in utero_, some fibers in the diaphragm initially synthesize adult fast myosin as early as 18 days gestation (390). Either this synthesis is independent of thyroid hormones or the fiber responds to thyroid hormone concentrations below the detectable limit. A second wave of adult fast myosin accumulation occurs during the first 10 days postpartum, an accumulation that _is_ sensitive to thyroxine levels. In the animal made hypothyroid from three days gestation onward, then, the diaphragm contains approximately equal amounts of adult fast myosin and neonatal myosin. Immunohistochemical studies suggest that two populations of fibers exist, one sensitive and one insensitive to thyroid hormones for their synthesis of adult fast myosin.

Effects of the same Stimulus on Different Muscles

Muscles of mastication show a different response to thyroid hormones (390). These muscles make the transition from neonatal to adult fast myosin at a later stage than do the limb muscles, perhaps because their use is not demanded prior to weaning. The transition to adult fast myosin occurs, then, after the peak thyroxine levels have been reached. Thus, thyroid hormones at the peak levels present during the second week postpartum are insufficient to force a muscle to switch to adult fast myosin synthesis. Since hypothyroid masseter muscles, however, fail to synthesize adult fast myosins, thyroid hormones must play some role in the transition even in this late developing muscle. Possibly, a level of maturation must be attained prior to the development of thyroxine sensitivity.

The testosterone effect on the myosins of the temporalis muscle of the guinea pig also indicate the heterogenous response of different muscles to the same stimulus (393). The fast-white myosin heavy chain synthesized by the male temporalis is under the control of testosterone. In castrated males it is not accumulated: and in testosterone supplemented females it is synthesized in the temporalis muscle. This same myosin, however, is resistant to testosterone control in other fast-white muscles.

It is still too early, then, to determine what combination of hormonal, neural, and myogenic factors are actually responsible for movement from one myosin type to another during development. The factors responsible for these transitions, however, probably vary from muscle to muscle.

CHAPTER 13: INFLUENCES OF TESTOSTERONE ON CONTRACTILE PROTEINS OF THE GUINEA PIG TEMPORALIS MUSCLE

A. Kelly*, G. Lyons**, B. Gambki** and N. Rubinstein**

*Department of Pathobiology; **Department of Anatomy
University of Pennsylvania School of Medicine
Philadelphia, PA

We have recently shown in the rat that the switch from neonatal to adult fast myosin is orchestrated by thyroid hormone (391); it is delayed in hypothyroid animals and switches precociously in hyperthyroid animals. In view of this hormonal effect on the development of fast muscle, we have been interested in other hormonal effects on myosin gene expression.

Testosterone is known to stimulate protein synthesis and influences muscle growth. However, comparatively little is known about androgenic influences on muscle structure or the contractile proteins. In the guinea pig, striking effects of castration and of testosterone administration have been described (394) on the size and metabolic enzymes of the fast twitch temporalis muscle. Gutmann et al have reported that this muscle can be classified as "fast white" (low oxidative enzyme concentration) in the mature male and "fast red" (high oxidative enzyme concentration) in the mature female (395). This suggested to us that testosterone may alter the expression of myosin isozymes in the male temporalis since it is widely believed that the subdivision of fast fibers into fast red and fast white phenotypes is correlated with differences.

* The authors wish to thank Ms. J. Collenberg and Mrs. Z. Paltzmann for their expert technical assistance during the course of this study. Supported by the PHS grants HL 15835-011 to the Pennsylvania Muscle Institute, NS 14332 and by a grant from the Muscular Dystrophy Association of America. N.R. is an established investigator of the American Heart Association. G.L. is supported by the predoctoral training program in cardiovascular research, HL 07502.

in forms of myosin. For these reasons, and because the transition from IIa to IIb fibers has not previously been studied biochemically, we investigated the myosin isozymes in the male and female guinea pig temporalis, and have followed the development of this sexual dimorphism from late fetal life to maturity. The myosins in these muscles are compared with the myosin isozymes in two other testosterone sensitive muscles, the psoas and the masseter of the guinea pig.

The Course of Fiber Type Development

At birth, a fundamental pattern of specialization emerges in both the male and female temporalis. With the myosin ATPase reaction virtually all fibers stain well after alkali preincubation (pH 10.4) (Figure 35a). After acid preincubation (pH 4.5) there is a continuous range of staining intensities between IIa, IIb and darkly stained IIc fibers (Figure 35b). As a consequence, discrimination between fiber types is difficult. Approximately 40% are IIa in type, 40% IIb and 20% are intermediate and IIc fibers. Small numbers of type I cells are also present. They are also found in the masseter at this stage and are presumably transformed into type II fibers soon after birth for they are rare in both muscles at 50 days and in the adult. There are no IIm fibers (396).

We have examined the early stages of fiber differentiation using a monoclonal antibody, 2B6, to rat embryonic myosin. This antibody cross reacts with an embryonic myosin in all mammals we have studied (390). In the neonatal temporalis there is a spectrum of fiber staining intensities with this antibody (Figure 35d), which is consistent with the myosin ATPase results, and suggests that the heterogeneity of ATPase fiber staining at birth is due to the coexistence of varying proportions of embryonic and adult fast myosins within each of the developing fiber types. Antibody staining is most intense in small IIb and IIc fibers suggesting that IIa fibers are the first to differentiate and that hypertrophy is correlated with elimination of embryonic myosin. By 5 days of age, only occasional fibers react with the monoclonal antibody.

Sexual dimorphism first becomes evident by 30 days, and by 50 days the male and female temporalis are clearly distinct in terms of fiber size (Figure 36) and histochemical differentiation. In the female, IIa and IIb fibers are approximately the same size in cross sectional area. The relative proportions of these two fiber types are comparable to the ratio at birth. Type IIc fibers are infrequent. The guinea pig grows throughout life with the result that the temporalis slowly hypertrophies (Figure 36) in both sexes. However at 18 months of age the pattern of fiber differentiation is approximately the same as at birth and 50 days in the female (Figure 37). This stability of specialization

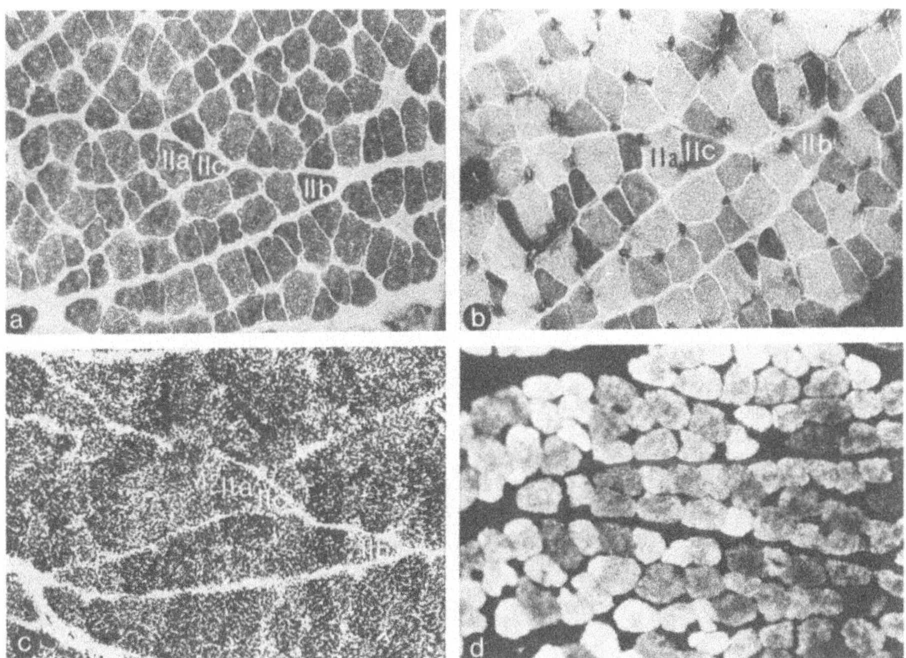

FIGURE 35: Serial sections of the guinea pig temporalis muscle at birth stained for myosin ATPase activity after alkali preincubation (a) and acid preincubation (b) and with DPNH for mitochondrial enzyme activity (c). Figure (d) is from a comparable area stained with a monoclonal antibody 2B6 to embryonic myosin. There is a spectrum of fiber staining intensities with the antibody which is consistent with the myosin ATPase results. These results suggest that the heterogeneity of ATPase staining is due to the coexistence of varying proportions of embryonic and adult fast myosins within each of the developing fiber types. Antibody staining is most intense in small IIb and IIc fibers magnification x200.

suggests that with growth, there is a constant relation between body size and temporalis muscle and that the frequency of fiber usage necessary to achieve mastication, does not significantly change with age in the female.

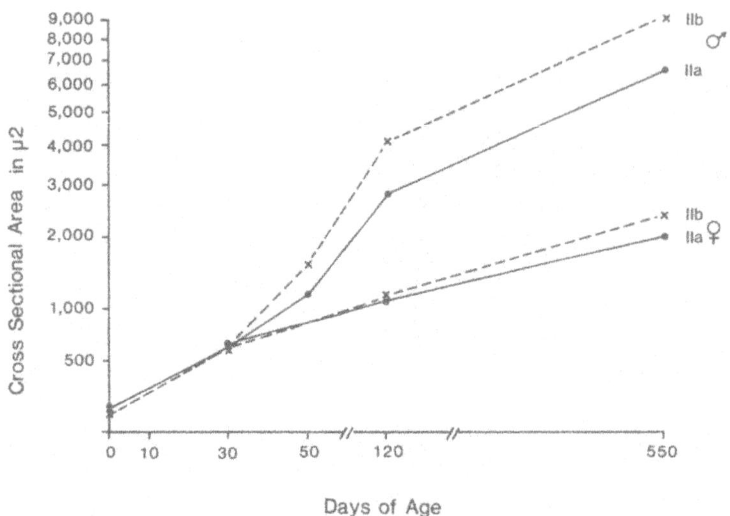

FIGURE 36: Cross sectional areas of IIa and IIb fibers at successive stages of development in the male and female guinea pig temporalis.

The male guinea pig enters puberty at approximately 30 days of age and completes adolescence at 60 to 65 days (397,398). Both type IIa and IIb fibers are slightly larger in the male than in the female at 30 days and this distinction is clearly evident at 50 days (Figure 36). This hypertrophy is accompanied by a shift towards the IIb phenotype so that at 50 days, IIb and intermediate fibers respectively comprise, approximately, 55 and 25% of the total fiber population and reciprocally, proportions of IIa fibers are reduced to 20%. By 18 months of age the majority of fibers stain homogeneously as IIb. Intermediate and IIa fibers together represent less than 15% of the fiber population (Figure 37).

As hypertrophy proceeds in the male, the level of mitochondrial enzyme staining progressively declines in both IIa and IIb fibers. Thus there appears to be a general correlation between fiber size and level of mitochondrial enzyme activity. This change toward a more fatigue sensitive muscle suggests that as bite strength increases in the male, individual motor units are recruited less frequently during mastication. As IIb fibers are predominantly glycolytic in metabolism these results are consistent with the studies of Beramini showing that testosterone stimulates glycogen synthesis in the androgen sensitive, rat levator ani muscle (399).

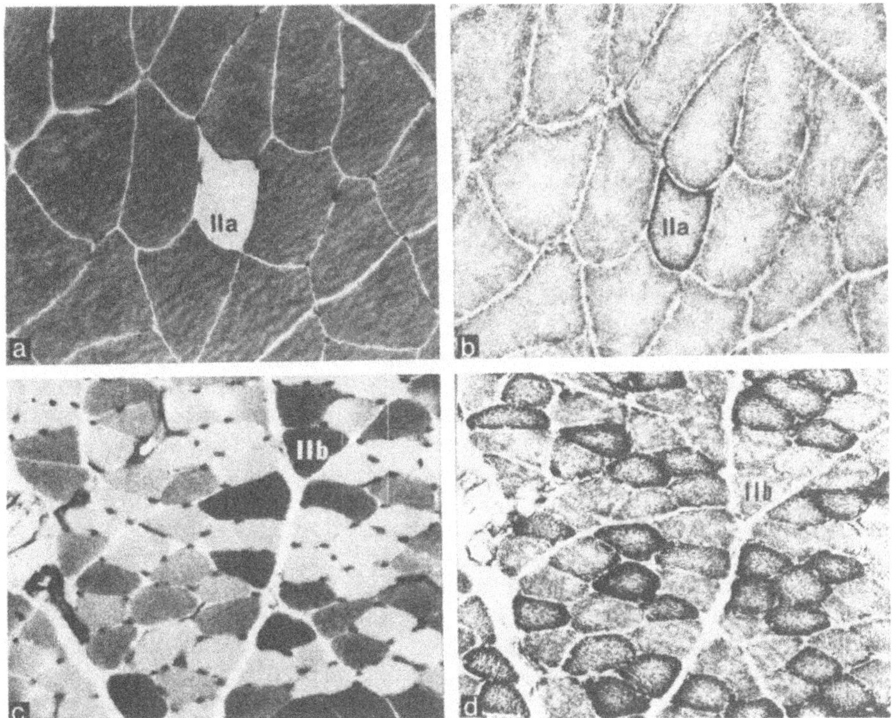

FIGURE 37: Serial transverse sections of adult male and female temporalis muscle at 18 months of age. In the male almost all fibers are IIb in type. In the the female there is a range of staining intensities with myosin ATPase (pH 4.5) including IIa, intermediate and IIb fibers. Compared to the male, mitochondrial enzyme staining is high in all fiber types. Magnification x85.

Myosin Heavy Chains

Heavy chains of column purified myosin were partially digested with chymotrypsin and run on 12.5% acrylamide SDS gels according to the method of Whalen et al. (380). Peptide maps from the mature male temporalis, longissimus dorsi and psoas muscles (Figure 38, lanes g, h and i, respectively) are remarkably similar. They demonstrate a cleavage pattern which is characteristic of muscles predominantly composed of IIb fibers and reveal that, although these muscles have different developmental programs and different embryologic origins, they contain very similar, if not identical, myosin heavy chains. In Figure 38, lanes e and f are the cleavage products obtained from the female temporalis and the masseter. These peptide maps are characteristic of muscles which are rich in type IIa fibers. The distinctions between muscles predominantly composed of either IIa or IIb fibers suggest that there are differences in primary structure of myosins from these two forms of muscle. These results are consistent with the studies of Dalla Libera, et al (369).

Lanes a, b, c and d of Figure 38 are maps of the masseter a), temporalis (b), longissimus dorsi (c), and psoas (d) from the guinea pig at 2 days of age. Cleavage products from the psoas and longissimus dorsi at this stage are identical to those of the adult (compare lanes c and d with lanes h and i). The 2-day temporalis and masseter also contain heavy chain peptides characteristic of IIa muscle but maps of these myosins are distinct from those of the adult, particularly in the high molecular weight region of the gel. Peptides labeled (n) which are prominent in the 2-day masseter and temporalis are either not present or present in only small proportions in these muscles in the adult. Similar high molecular weight peptides are present in the fetal posas and longissimus dorsi but are eliminated at birth. Thus, myosin from the IIb psoas and longissimus differentiates rapidly and achieves a mature configuration at birth. By contrast, myosin from the IIa masseter and from the temporalis matures more slowly, and does not achieve the adult cleavage pattern until after 50 days of age. This distinction in IIa and IIb muscle differentiation is not unique to the muscles of mastication for Brooke et al found that IIb fibers differentiated significantly earlier than IIa fibers in hind limb muscles of the rat (400).

Peptide maps of the heavy chain from the male and female temporalis are identical at 5 days (Figure 39, lanes f and g). Thereafter, peptide maps of the heavy chain of the female temporalis are modified only in the high molecular weight region of the gel. As the male matures, however, rearrangements in the pattern of cleavage products are more extensive (lanes h and j), and we interpret these as a replacement of IIa by IIb myosin heavy chain. This process consists of changes in the proportions of peptides such that some, present in very small amounts at 5 days, are greatly amplified while other, originally major bands, become minor constituents in the adult.

Castration experiments show that this heavy chain transformation is absolutely dependent upon testosterone. In males castrated at 120 days and examined at 230 days, there is regression towards the IIa, female phenotype (Figure 39, lane c). This is accompanied by fiber atrophy. The result indicates that testosterone must be continually present to maintain the male phenotype. Finally, in mature females treated for 3 months with testosterone proprionate (100 μg/kg) in sesame oil (401), there is substantial transformation to the IIb phenotype (Figure 39, lane a).

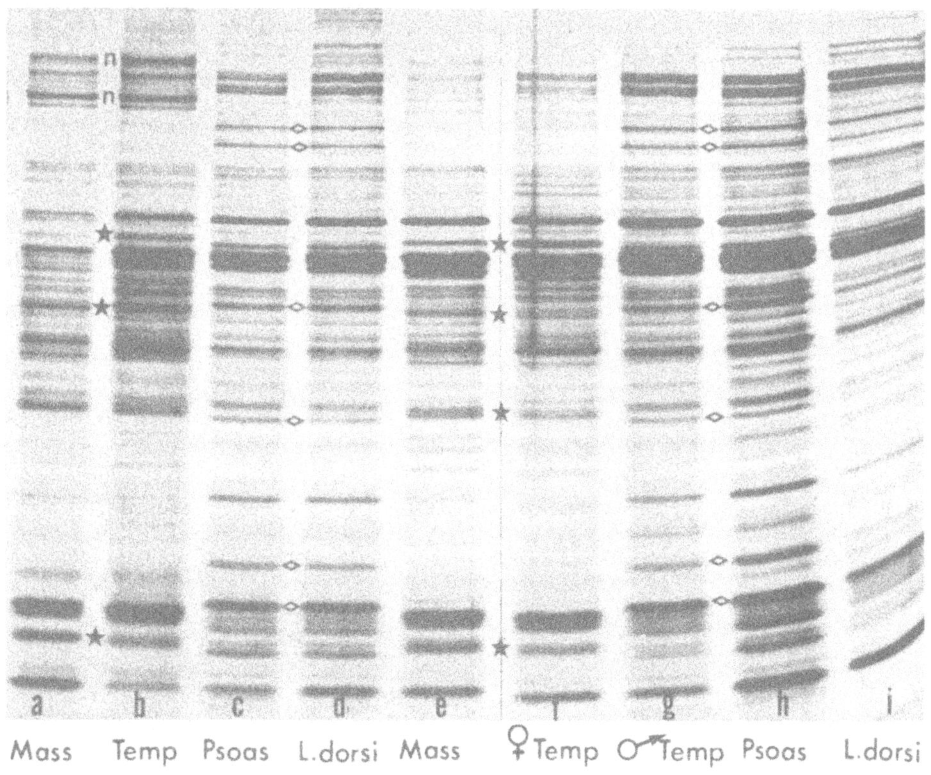

FIGURE 38: Peptide maps from adult masseter and female temporalis muscles (lanes e and f), which are rich in IIa fibers, and from the male temporalis, psoas and longissimus dorsi, which are rich in IIb fibers, lanes g, h and i. Difference peptides are labeled by stars and diamonds. Maps from the adult male temporalis, psoas and longissimus dorsi are remarkably similar. Cleavage products from the adult psoas and longissimus dorsi are almost identical to those at 2 days of age (compare lanes c and d with h and i). Peptide maps of the adult male and female temporalis and masseter are distinct from those at 2 days of age particularly in the high molecular weight region of the gel (compare lanes a and b with lanes e and f). Peptides labeled (n) present at 2 days are either absent or present in only small proportions in these muscles in the adult. Similar high molecular weight peptides are present in the fetal psoas and longissimus dorsi but are eliminated before birth.

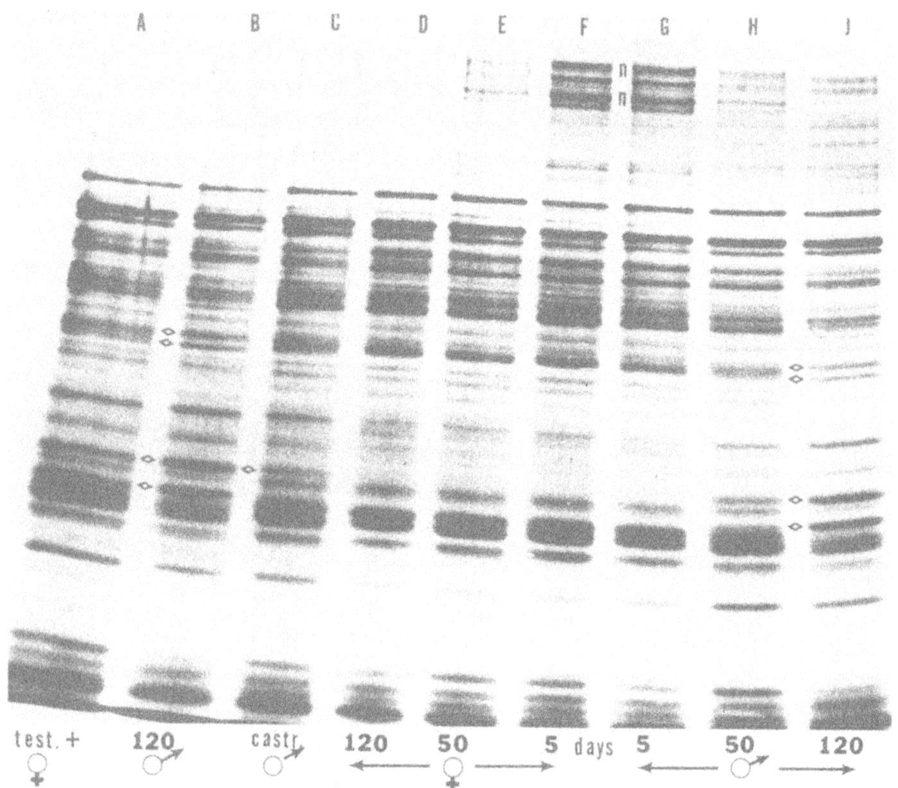

FIGURE 39: Peptide maps from male and female temporalis during development. Adult, 50-day and 5-day male temporalis, lanes g, h and j; 5-day, and 50-day and adult female temporalis, lanes f, e and d. Castrate male, control male and testosterone treated female, lanes c, b and a. There is a progressive replacement of IIb for IIa heavy chains in the male temporalis. Difference peptides are marked with diamonds. Peptides labeled (n) are eliminated from the temporalis of both genders with age.

These qualitative changes were not seen in the androgen sensitive masseter and psoas after castration or testosterone treatment. Peptide maps of these muscles from adult male and female guinea pigs are identical (Figure 40). As the masseter is significantly larger in the male than in the female guinea pig, testosterone must promote ongoing synthesis of IIa myosin in this muscle.

From birth to maturity all muscles contain the three fast light chains in approximately equal proportions (Figure 41). In the fetus, the beta subunit of tropomyosin is predominant in all muscles. At birth there is a change to approximately equal proportions of alpha and beta subunits (Figure 41), and the female temporalis, as well as the psoas and longissimus dorsi, retain this stoichiometry of subunits to maturity. By contrast, the male and female masseter (not shown) and the male temporalis gradually switch to only the alpha subunit. In the masseter, the switch is completed by 120 days. In the temporalis, the switch is slower, and is complete by 1 1/2 years of age. This appears to be a consequence of testosterone secretion, for in the androgen treated female the relative proportions of the alpha subunit are increased.

Myosin Light Chains and Tropomyosins

Native myosins from the adult male and female temporalis were run on 4.5% acrylamide gels under nondissociating conditions according to the method of Hoh et al. (402) as modified for use with slab gels by Lyons et al. (403). Isozymes from the fast type IIa, female temporalis have a faster mobility than isozymes from the IIb male temporalis (Figure 42b). The mobility of the male temporalis isozymes is the same as the psoas and longissimus dorsi. This is consistent with the heavy chain peptide maps. Mobilities of the masseter and female temporalis isozymes are identical. These results compare with the studies of Mabuchi et al. (370), showing that as myosin ATPase IIb fibers in the rabbit are changed to the IIa phenotype by electrical stimulation, there is an alteration in the mobility of native myosin isozymes.

Native Myosin Isozymes

Isozymes are labeled according to the system of nomenclature introduced by Fitzsimons and Hoh (389). The female isozymes are FM_1 to FM_3 in order of decreasing mobility; the male isozymes are FM_2', FM_3' and FM_4. These differences in myosin isozymes correlate with the heavy chain distinctions (Figure 39) between IIa and IIb muscle. In view of this, FM_2 and FM_3 are distinct isozymes in IIa and IIb muscles.

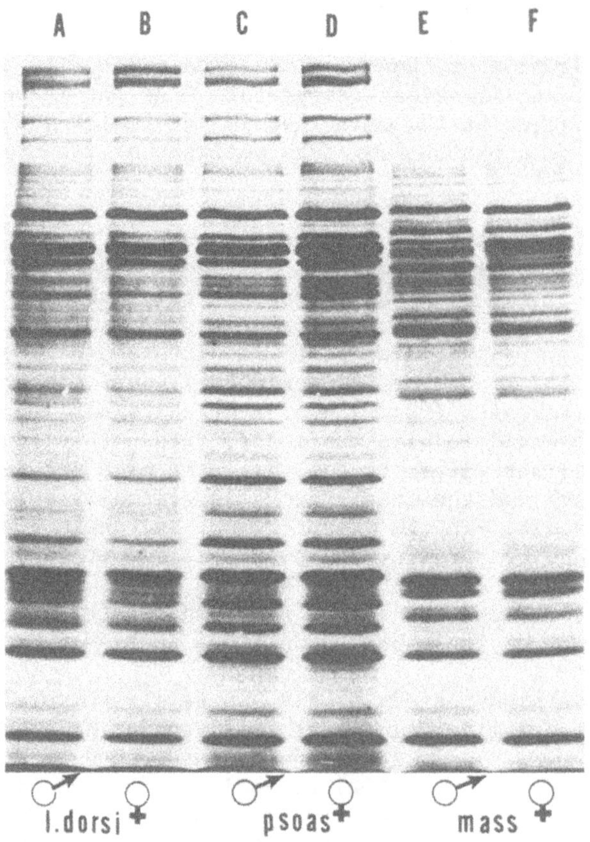

FIGURE 40: Peptide maps of mature male and female masseter, lanes e and f; male and female psoas; lanes c and d; male female longissimus dorsi lanes a and b. In each muscle the cleavage products from the male and female are identical.

In the 55-day fetal temporalis, four isozymes, f1 to f4, (Figure 42a) which have a faster mobility than either of the mature isozymes. A switch occurs at birth. At 5 days post partum, isozymes from the male and female temporalis have the same mobility and comprise FM_1, FM_2 and FM_3. This pattern persists in both genders at 50 days, and the male configuration of isozymes emerges fairly abruptly between 60 and 70 days of age. This result is surprising since switching to the IIb phenotype is evident both by peptide mapping of the myosin heavy chain and by histochemistry at substantially earlier stages of development. In this system then pyrophosphate gel analysis of native myosins is a less sensitive index of myosin switching than the other techniques.

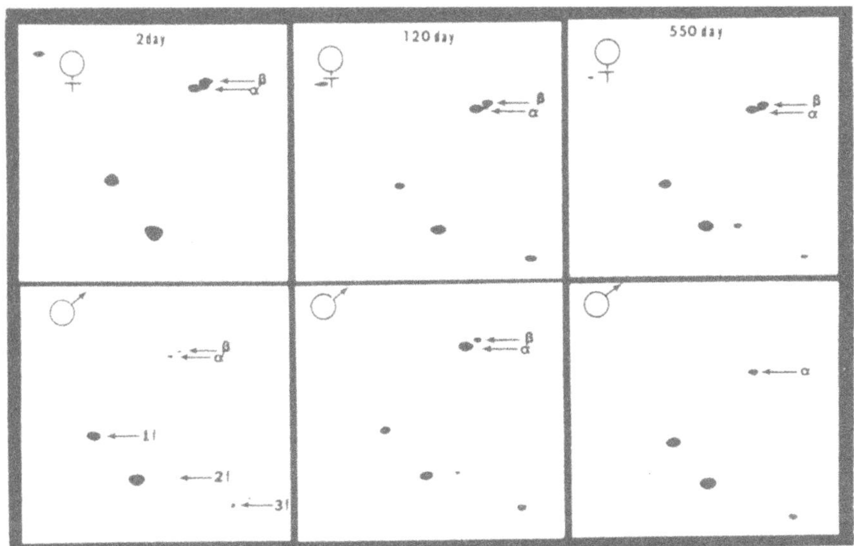

FIGURE 41: Myosin light chains and tropomyosins of the male and female temporalis during development. At 2 days postpartum the proportions of fast myosin light chains 1f, 2f and 3f and α and β tropomyosins occurs in the male and at 18 months only tiny amounts of the beta subunit remains. The proportions of tropomyosin subunits do not change in the female. The only other muscle we have studied which shows a complete shift to alpha tropomyosin is the masseter, which is homogeneously composed of IIa fibers.

Western Blots

Native myosin isozymes from fetal temporalis, masseter and psoas (lanes a, b and c, Figure 43) were run adjacent to isozymes from 5-day psoas, 5-day masseter and adult temporalis (Figure 43, lanes d, e and f) stained with Coomassie blue for reference. An identical series of native myosins run on the same pyrophosphate gel were transferred to

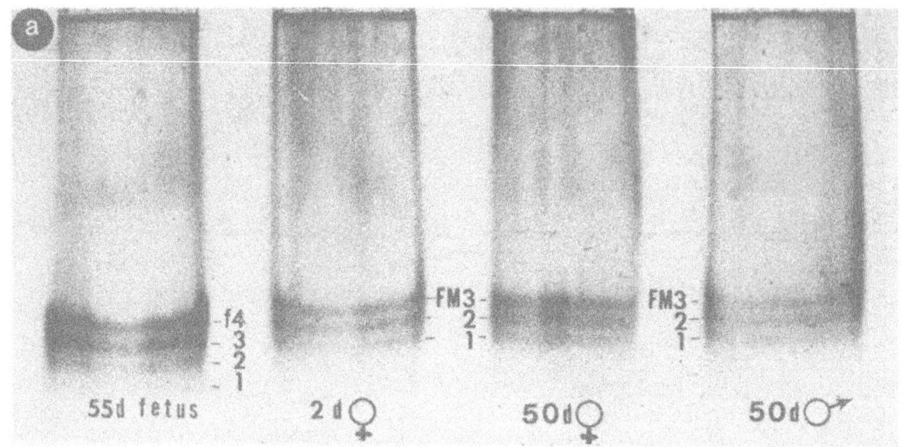

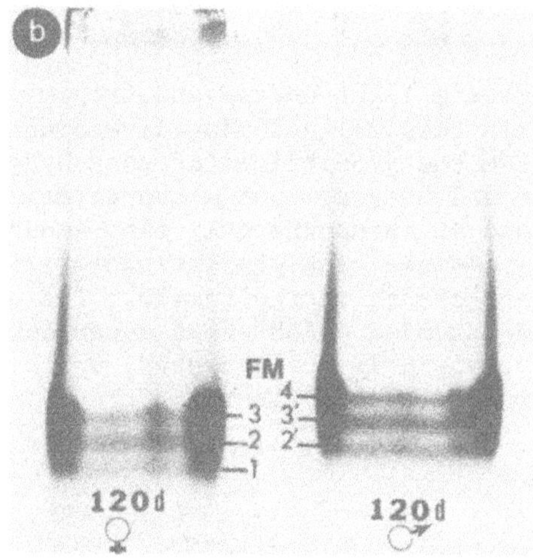

FIGURE 42a: Native myosin isozymes of the developing temporalis. Native myosins from successive stages of the developing temporalis muscle electrophoresed on 4.5% acrylamide pyrophosphate gels. In the 55 day fetus, four myosin isozymes are evident, labeled f1-f4 in order of decreasing mobility. In the neonate, there is a shift to the mature, IIa complement of isozymes (FM1-FM3). This is caused by a switch in the myosin heavy chain (See Figure 43). At 50 days the mobilities of the male and female are identical. Beginning at 60 days a second shift occurs in the mobility of the male but not the female temporalis isozymes. This switch is completed by 120 days (42b).

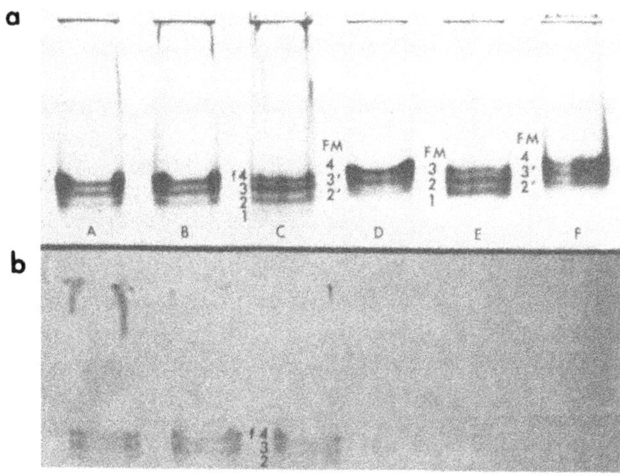

FIGURE 43: Pyrophosphate gel electrophoresis of fetal and adult native myosins (a) followed by Western blotting (b). Native myosin isozymes from 55 day and term fetal temporalis (A and B) term fetal masseter (C), 5 day psoas (D), adult masseter (E) and adult male temporalis (F) were run on a 4.5% acrylamide slab gel under nondissociating conditions. In the fetus, temporalis and masseter isozymes, labeled f1-f4 in order of decreasing mobility, are identical. Isozymes of the 5 day psoas and adult male temporalis have the same mobility and are labeled FM_2', FM_3' and FM_4. These have slower mobilities than isozymes from the fetus and the adult masseter. The adult masseter isozymes are FM_1-FM_3. They have the same mobility as the female temporalis. The same sequence of native myosins as in lanes A to F were run on the same slab pyrophosphate gel, transferred to nitrocellulose paper and stained with a monoclonal antibody to fetal myosin heavy chain. Fetal isozymes in lanes A, B and C react with this antibody whereas isozymes from the postpartum muscles, lanes D, E and F do not. This result supports the immunochemical results in figure 35d, and shows that the difference in mobility of isozymes between fetal and postpartum temporalis, Figure 42, are the result of differences in the myosin heavy chain.

nitrocellulose paper and stained with a monoclonal antibody, 2B6, the heavy chain of fetal myosins(390). Figure 43 demonstrates that the antibody cross reacts with the fetal isozymes but not with the 5-day or adult isozymes. This result supports the finding that the differences in mobility of isozymes in fetal and mature muscle are the result of differences in the myosin heavy chains.

Summary

The present study outlines the changes in contractile proteins which occur during sexual differentiation of the guinea pig temporalis muscle. This is an androgen sensitive muscle, which in the female progresses from a fetal phenotype to a muscle rich in IIa fibers, and in the male, undergoes a further switch to an almost pure IIb fiber phenotype. We show the IIa to IIb transition in the male involves a change in myosin heavy chain synthesis (Figure 39), a corresponding change in the mobility of native myosin isozymes run on pyrophosphate gels (Figure 43), and changes in the proportions of the alpha and beta subunits of tropomyosin (Figure 41). Myosin light chains appear to be unaltered in this transformation.

CHAPTER 14: ALTERATIONS IN PHENOTYPE EXPRESSION OF MUSCLE BY CHRONIC NERVE STIMULATION

Dirk Pette, Annegard Heilig, Gary Klug, Heinz Reichmann
Udo Seedorf and Walter Wiehrer

Faculty of Biology
University of Konstanz
D-7750 Konstanz, West Germany

The experimentally induced transformation of adult mammalian fast-twitch muscle by chronic nerve stimulation has been established during the past years in our laboratory as a model for studying neural regulation of phenotypic gene expression in skeletal muscle. As was originally shown by Salmons and Vrbová (404), fast-twitch muscles of the rabbit are transformed into slow-twitch muscles by chronic indirect stimulation with a frequency pattern naturally occurring in nerves to slow-twitch muscles. This transformation affects the muscle fiber as a whole and concerns every functional, morphological and molecular property studied so far. The stimulation-induced transformation process has been investigated thoroughly in tibialis anterior (TA) and extensor digitorum longus (EDL) muscles of the rabbit with regard to the three main functional systems of the muscle fiber, i.e. energy metabolism, sarcoplasmic reticulum and proteins of the myofibrillar apparatus.

Chronic stimulation induces pronounced increases in myoglobin (405) and in mitochondrial content (406-408). This "white" to "red" transition is also reflected by elevated enzyme activities of pathways of aerobic substrate oxidation,

Energy Metabolism

such as the citric acid cycle, fatty acid oxidation, ketone body metabolism and respiratory chain (405,406,408-413). The increase in enzyme activities of the citric acid cycle, fatty acid oxidation and respiratory chain occurs in parallel so that the proportions of these enzymes are maintained. A higher and therefore disproportional increase is found for the enzymes of ketone body utilization (β-hydroxybutrate dehydrogenase, ketoacid-CoA transferase). In addition to the increase in mitochrondria, these changes indicate qualitative alterations of the mitochondrial population (408). Changes in the enzymatic composition of the inner mitochondrial membranes are furthermore suggested by altered proportions of succinate dehydrogenase which increases, and of glycerolphosphate oxidase which decreases slightly (405,408,410).

Contrary to the increase in aerobic substrate oxidation, chronic stimulation decreases the capacity of anaerobic energy supply. Except for the increased activity of hexokinase, cytosolic activities of glycogenolytic and glycolytic enzymes are strongly reduced (405,406,408-410,412,413). In the case of lactate dehydrogenase the decrease in activity is paralleled by an isozymic M to H subunit transition (405,406,413).

Taken together, the quantitative and qualitative changes in the enzyme pattern of energy metabolism indicate a thorough rearrangement of the metabolic properties. As judged from the extent of these changes, chronic stimulation leads to a complete metabolic conversion of an originally "glycolytic" muscle to one which can be classified as "oxidative." As is evident from the activities of selected reference enzymes in Table 9, stimulation-induced changes in the enzyme activity pattern tend to exceed quantitatively the phenotype of a typical "red" muscle (soleus) which is composed almost exclusively of slow-twitch type I fibers. The stimulated originally "fast-glycolytic" muscle is thus transformed into a muscle with "super-red" metabolic properties.

TABLE 9

Effects of 54 d continuous (24 h/d) nerve stimulation (10 Hz) on key enzymes of energy metabolism in rabbit tibialis anterior (TA) muscle

	Control TA	Stimul. TA	Normal Soleus (n=4)
	Activity (U/g w.wt.)		
Glyceraldehyde-P dehydrogenase	381	107	115 ± 14
Lactate dehydrogenase	542	152	110 ± 16
Citrate synthetase	3.1	15.2	6 ± 2
3-OH-acyl-CoA dehydrogenase	1.7	10.8	6 ± 2
Ketoacid-CoA transferase	5.6	34	12 ± 2

Sarcoplasmic Reticulum

Chronic stimulation induces a transformation of the sarcoplasmic reticulum (SR) from that of a fast-twitch into that of a slow-twitch muscle (Figure 44). The densitographs of the electrophoreses of SR from a 30 d stimulated TA muscle and from normal slow-twitch soleus muscle are nearly indistinguishable in Figure 44. The most obvious changes induced by the stimulation consist of decreases in the 115,000-M_r subunit of the Ca^{2+} -pumping ATPase and in calsequestrin as well as of increases in 55,000-M_r peptides (high affinity Ca^{2+} -binding protein, glycoprotein?) and in a 30,000-M_r (NADH cytochrome b5 reductase?) peptide (413-417). The pronounced decrease in amount of activity (413-417) of Ca^{2+}, Mg^{2+} -dependent ATPase leads to a strongly reduced Ca^{2+} - uptake capacity (415,416,418) similar to that of SR from a slow twitch muscle. In addition to the changes of intrinsic and extrinsic membrane proteins, the transformation of the SR is evident also from qualitative and quantitative alterations in the phospholipid matrix of the SR membranes (419).

Parvalbumin

As was recently observed, parvalbumin decreases rapidly in chronically stimulated fast-twitch rabbit muscles and is no longer detectable after 28 d of stimulation (420). This finding is another example of the fast to slow transformation elicited by chronic nerve stimulation. It has been shown that parvalbumin is present in mammalian muscles only in fast-twitch but is devoid in slow-twitch fibers (421,422). The reduced potential of Ca^{2+} -sequestration by the converted SR is thus accompanied in the transformed muscle by a substantial decrease in parvalbumin and therefore in the capacity of Ca^{2+} -binding in the sarcoplasm. The nearly identical time curves in Figure 45 of the changes in the parvalbumin content and in the 115,000-M_r subunit of the Ca^{2+} -pumping ATPase suggest a close functional correlation of these two compounds.

Myofibrillar Proteins

Prolonged stimulation results in a progressive decrease in the maximum rate of tetanic tension development which is obviously caused by changes in the properties of myosin. These changes consist in a reduced activity of Ca^{2+} -activated myosin ATPase (370,418,423) and in a fast to slow type conversion of myosin as reflected by transitions in the myosin light chain pattern (370,410,418,423-425). Long-term stimulation induces an almost complete replacement of fast by slow myosin light chains. In stimulations up to 150 d a complete change was observed of the fast with the slow DTNB light chain and of fast alkali light chain 1 by the corresponding slow light chain (425). Alkali light chain 2 of the fast type was reduced but could still be detected in the 150 d stimulated muscle (425). Decreases in N-methylhistidine content point to a transformation also of the

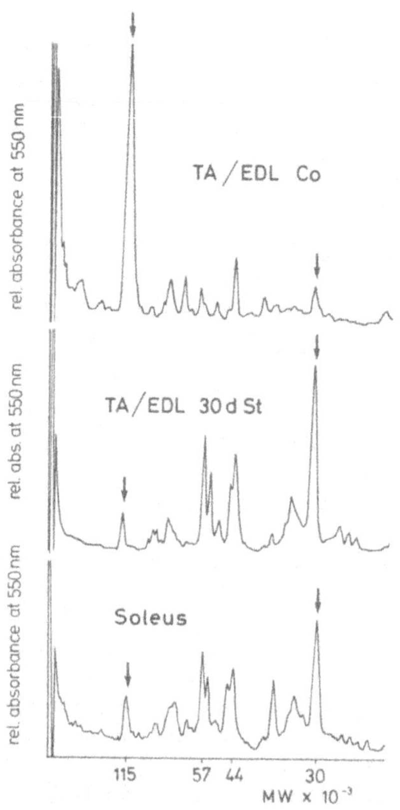

FIGURE 44: Densitographs of polyacrylamide gel electrophoresis of sarcoplasmic reticulum prepared from contralateral (top) and 30 d (24 h/d) stimulated (10 Hz) TA and EDL muscles (center) and from normal slow-twitch rabbit soleus muscle (bottom). Arrows mark peaks corresponding to the 115,000-M_r subunit of the Ca^{2+} -pumping ATPase and to the 30,000-M_r peptide.

myosin heavy chains (426).

Transformations in the myofibrillar protein composition are not restricted to the thick filament. Changes in the ratio of α- and β-tropomyosin subunits have been interpreted as a fast to slow transition (427).

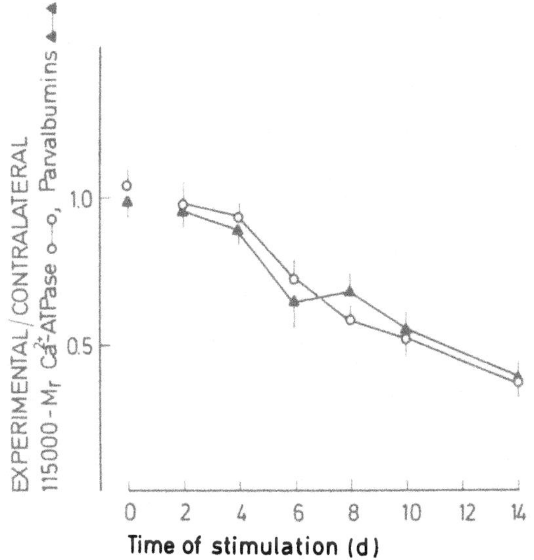

FIGURE 45: Time course of changes in the concentrations of the 115,000-M_r subunit of the SR Ca^{2+}-pumping ATPase and the cytosolic parvalbumin during chronic (10 Hz, 12 h/d) stimulation of rabbit TA muscle. Data were obtained from densitometric evaluations of electrophoreses (413). Results are expressed as ratios of the values obtained from the experimental versus those from the contralateral muscles. Each time point represents the mean value from 3-5 animals ± S.E.M.

It may be suggested that the majority of the aforementioned alterations is due to qualitatively and quantitatively altered transcriptional activities.

Changes in Transcription

Chronic stimulation increases the total RNA content of rabbit TA to the level of soleus muscle within 8 d (428). Figure 46 shows the time course of the increase in total RNA in chronically stimulated EDL. The levels reached after 14 d (1260 ± 74 µg/g w.wt., n = 3) exceeds (580 ± 89 µg/g w.wt., n = 13). Most probably, the increase in total RNA is mainly due to an elevation of mRNA. Qualitative changes in mRNA have been detected by _in vitro_ translations of poly (A) mRNA isolated from stimulated muscles (428,429). Thus, considerable amounts of myosin light chains LCs1 (alkali 1) and LCs2 (DTNB) were translated _in vitro_ from mRNA of 28 d stimulated

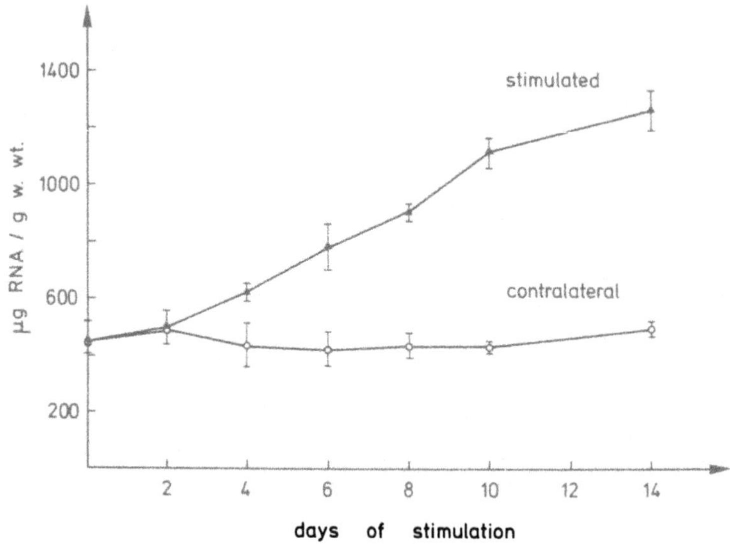

FIGURE 46: Time course of increases in total RNA content of chronically stimulated (10Hz, 12 h/d) rabbit EDL muscle. Each time point represents mean values ± S.D. obtained from three animals.

TA (429). However, changes in mRNA composition are detectable earlier already. Preliminary data obtained from *in vitro* translations of poly(A)mRNA from 15 d stimulated TA indicate that mRNA specific for parvalbumin is greatly reduced. The observation that parvalbumin is reduced by 60% (Figure 46) at a time (14 d) where specific mRNA was not detectable, suggests that the protein is no longer synthesized and that the remaining parvalbumin is subjected to normal degradation.

The available data cannot exclude the possibility that the expression of specific proteins in muscle is controlled also post-transcriptionally. Thus, considerable amounts of *in vitro* translated slow type myosin light chains are seen also in the contralateral muscles. Coomassie-blue stained two-dimensional electrophoreses of myofibrillar extracts prepared from these muscles contain only traces, if at all, of the slow myosin light chains. This might indicate post-transcriptional control. On the other hand, rabbit TA contains between 5-10% of slow-twitch fibers. If these fibers have a higher protein turnover than fast-twitch fibers (430), they should contain higher levels of mRNA for specific proteins. This would result in higher amounts of the respective proteins in the in vitro translation assay. Obviously, this point needs further clarification.

The observation that fast and slow type myosins coexist in the same muscle fibers during the process of transformation (424,431) has ruled out the possibility that preexisting fast-twitch fibers are replaced by newly formed slow-twitch fibers. The fast to slow transition of the stimulated muscle is due to a true transformation of the preexisting fibers (424).

Time Course of Transformation

Different time courses of stimulation-induced changes suggest a sequential transformation of the muscle fiber. The decrease in parvalbumin, the changes in composition and function of the SR as well as transitions in the enzyme activity and isozyme patterns of energy metabolism (413) precede the changes in tropomyosin (427) and myosin (418,418,425). It is obvious therefore that early changes in contractile properties. especially increases in half relaxation time and in time to peak of isometric twitch contraction (410,415) which precede the changes in myosin, are mainly due to the early alterations in Ca^{2+} -uptake and probably also Ca^{2+} -release.

The transformation of the fiber as a whole appears thus to result from a set of transition processes which affect different functional systems in a timely ordered sequence. This sequential transition has been studied in detail for the exchange of fast with slow type myosin light chains (425). It was shown that DTNB (phosphorylatable) and alkali light chains follow different time courses. Thus, the exchange of the fast type DTNB light chain with its slow type counterpart precedes that of the replacement of the fast light chain 1 (alkali 1) by the respective slow type light chain.

The underlying sequential changes in gene expression point to the existence of different thresholds. Furthermore, the question arises whether or not early changes create conditions which induce successive events in this chain of transformations. An early intracellular signal may be an increased Ca^{2+} -concentration. A dramatic but transient increase in total intracellular Ca^{2+} was observed during chronic stimulation (24 h/d) of rabbit TA by Sréter et al. (432). Despite the fact that the elevated Ca^{2+} -concentration declined after 3 d of stimulation, a persistent elevation in free Ca^{2+} may result from the described reduction in parvalbumin (413,420). The concentration of parvalbumin in rabbit fast-twitch muscle is in the range of 0.05 - 0.1 mM (420) which corresponds to a potential binding of 10^{-4} -2 x 10^{-4}M Ca^{2+}. The stimulation-induced disappearance of parvalbumin might thus increase considerably the sarcoplasmic concentration of free Ca^{2+}. This is stressed by the observation that there is simultaneously a decrease in the Ca^{2+} -pumping and Ca^{2+} -binding capacities of the SR (414-417).

A role of Ca^{2+} in regulating protein synthesis and degradation is generally accepted. It has also been suggested that a high concentration of sarcoplasmic Ca^{2+} might suppress the synthesis of the Ca^{2+} -pumping ATPase of SR (433). The initial and transient increase in total intracellular Ca^{2+} in the stimulated muscle (432) might thus initiate reductions in Ca^{2+} -binding and -pumping proteins, most probably by decreased synthesis. It cannot be excluded that an increase in free Ca2+ would activate in addition Ca^{2+} -dependent proteases so that some of the observed reductions of specific proteins might also result from an increase in protein degradation.

DR. WOOD: Does this imply that at some point at some time during the transition from a fast and slow type, that you have what amounts to a hybrid cell with slow type metabolic processes? What is the twitch relevation time?

DR. PETTE: We observed there are not changes in myosin but we saw the twitch change occurring after 4 days. There is increase after stimulation which is then followed by a second increase. When we stimulate up to 3 weeks we see no real change in the myosin, especially the heavy chain. You will find changes in the contractile velocity also.

DR. WOOD: I think this is an extremely important model as to what the composition of the cell is.

DR. PETTE: We have pointed out on our first paper when we saw that we have changed the condition of SR without having touched the myosin.

DR. WHALEN: With respect to the comment about time to peak, the first change in the heavy chain composition that occurs will occur before the slow myosin heavy chain comes in, is that a change over in the types of fast heavy chains from what seems to be a 2B type to a 2A type. Do you think that would accept the time to peak value which should reflect the myosin composition more so than the half relaxation that may reflect the SR change?

Secondly, the time course of our experiments was at least twice as fast. In other words the conversion transformation was complete as yours by 10 weeks of stimulation where you go beyond 20.

DR. PETTE: We see changes in time course occasionally. The position of the electrodes may be different. We also readjust the amplitude by palpitation of the muscle and so on, but we have no explanation for such a difference.

We kept the conditions as constant as possible, but we have published data where we show different fast and slow responses of the enzymes. Recently we have done a complete study of the change of the SR, the enzyme pattern. We saw there was a complete agreement in time of these changes.

CHAPTER 15: INDUCTION OF INCOORDINATE SYNTHESIS OF MUSCLE PROTEINS BY THE TUMOR PROMOTER TPA AND THE CARCINOGEN EMS

H. Holtzer, S. Forry-Schaudies, P. Antin,
G. Dubyak and V. Nachmias

Departments of Anatomy and Biochemistry-Biophysics
University of Pennsylvania Medical School
Philadelphia, PA

Introduction

Combined cytoimmunofluorescent, electron microscopic, and biochemical studies have repeatedly demonstrated the following about normal myogenesis: (1) That the switch in differentiation programs from replicating presumptive myoblasts to their daughter postmitotic myoblasts occurs prior to fusion; (2) That this switch requires DNA synthesis, but not cytokinesis; (3) That 6-12 hours after their last mitosis, both daughter definitive myoblasts initiate the coordinate synthesis of muscle-specific myosin heavy and light chains, tropomyosin, C-protein and M-band protein and at about this time become fusion competent. This switch in differentiation programs also involves the initiation of the synthesis of the muscle-specific intermediate filament protein, desmin; (4) That this sequence of events begins in chick myotomes at stages 14-15 and in chick limb buds at stages 20-21; (5) That there is a lag phase of hours between the earliest detection of these muscle-specific isoforms in mononucleated postmitotic myoblasts and their assembly into myofibrils. During this lag period, myofibrillar proteins and desmin appear to be widely distributed throughout the sarcoplasm. Only much later in development is the widely distributed desmin confined to, and integrated with, definitively striated myofibrils (434-438).

Recently we reported that the co-carcinogen TPA and the carcinogen EMS reversibly blocked the synthesis of many myofibrillar proteins without affecting the synthesis of desmin in myogenic cultures. In this report, this observation is further described at both immunofluorescent and biochemical levels. What is apparent from these studies is that the mechanisms linking the synthesis of desmin with that of the myofibrillar proteins in control cells have been reversibly uncoupled by TPA and EMS (439-441).

Because of their compact geometry, postmitotic mononucleated myoblasts are unfavorable material for studying many aspects of myofibril assembly. However, TPA and EMS transform elongated, thick myotubes into either multinucleated myosacs or very flat myosheets which lack most myofibrillar proteins. These inordinately attentuated structures prove to be ideal for correlating the topographical relationships between (1) microfilaments, intermediate filaments (IFs), and nascent myofibrils, and (2) loci of synthesis of the monomeric contractile proteins and their subsequent assembly into thick and thin filaments.

Myogenic cultures were prepared from dissociated muscles of 12 day chick embryos. Day 3 cultures were treated with TPA for 48 hours and then allowed to recover in normal medium or 10^{-6} M Colcemid (439, 440). Day 1 cultures were treated with EMS for 3 days and then allowed to recover in normal medium (441). The distribution of muscle-specific myosin heavy chains, nonmuscle myosin heavy chains, α-actin, vimentin, and desmin was followed by using rabbit monospecific, polyclonal antibodies (434,437,442-444). Rhodamine-phalloidin was used to detect F-actin. Bisbenzamid was used to visualize the spatial relationships between nuclei and the cytoplasmic domains occupied by Ifs and emerging myofibrils.

Materials & Methods

The protein synthetic pattern of control, treated, and recovered cultures were followed with two-dimensional SDS-PAGE and with Western blots. In each case, proteins were labeled with ^{35}S-methionine for one hour prior to being harvested. Whole cell samples were prepared, run on first dimensional isoelectric focusing gels according to O'Farrell, and subsequently on second dimensional SDS gels. Gels were fluorographed, dried and exposed appropriately.

Control Myogenic Cultures

Control day 5 muscle cultures contain elongated, multinucleated myotubes, postmitotic myoblasts, replicating presumptive myoblasts and fibroblasts. Over 85% of the definitive myogenic cells in such day 5 cultures were born between day 1 and day 4 *in vitro*. The myofibrillar proteins in these definitive myoblasts and myotubes have been assembled into typical striated myofibrils (Figure 47a). At this stage of maturation vimentin and desmin colocalized, being organized primarily into longitudinally-oriented 10nM filaments which coursed between and parallel to individual myofibrils (434,443-445). The Ifs also occupied the growth tips and the fine short, pseudopodial processes that anchor myotubes to the substrate. Myofibrillar proteins were absent from these areas. In some of the more mature day 5 myotubes, anti-desmin localized not only to the longitudinally oriented Ifs, but also to the I-Z region of individual myofibrils. This spatial redistribution of desmin to the I-Z band became more pronounced with further maturation (438,444,446).

TPA promptly blocked fusion of fusion-competent postmitotic myoblasts. However, cell replication was not blocked by TPA (438,447).

TPA-Treated Myogenic Cultures

Consequently, day 5 cultures exposed to TPA from day 3 to 5, displayed myotubes that had fused prior to treatment, newly born postmitotic myoblasts, and enormous numbers of replicating presumptive myoblasts and fibroblasts. Most mononucleated cells in these cultures were elongated and bipolar. Morphologically, these presumptive myoblasts and fibroblasts were indistinguishable.

TPA produced profound changes in the morphology of myotubes and in the distribution and synthesis of their myofibrillar proteins. After 48 hours in TPA, previously elongated myotubes collapsed into multinucleated myosacs. These myosacs varied in the number and extent of their processes and in their overall morphologies which ranged from being roughly isodiametric to being more anisodiametric. The number of nuclei in such myosacs varied from several to over 100. These nuclei tended to cluster in the myosac center and commonly assumed a ring-like arrangement (Figure 47 d,f).

The amount of anti-LMM binding and its localization varied from myosac to myosac. Many myosacs were totally negative, whereas others displayed diffuse patches of different sizes and degrees of fluorescence. Nothing suggestive of striated myofibrils was observed in these TPA-induced myosacs. Intense LMM-positive patches were often located in the center of rings of nuclei (Figure 47 c,d). These myosacs were rich in autophagosomes (439,440).

In contrast to the great reduction of light meromyosin, the muscle-specific IF protein desmin was abundant in TPA-treated myosacs. Double-staining with both anti-desmin and anti-vimentin suggested coextensive distribution of these IF proteins. The staining intensity in different regions of the same myosac differed greatly, and commonly these IF antibodies were strongly bound to regions just peripheral to the clustered nuclei (Figure 47 e,f). Low power views did not reveal any details as to IF patterns. However, higher magnification allowed the fluorescence to be resolved into a web of poorly aligned filaments of indefinitive length (>100nm). The numerous neurite-like processes that characterized the irregular outline of TPA-induced myosacs invariably bound both anti-vimentin and anti-desmin; these processes did not bind anti-LMM.

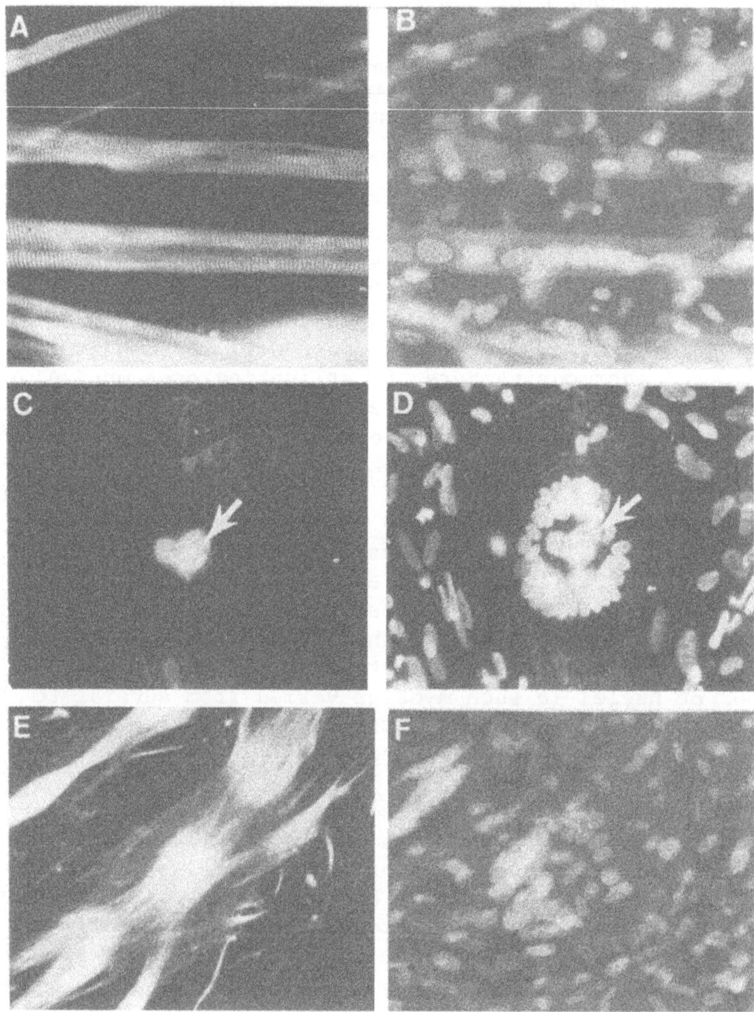

FIGURE 47: (a,b) Identical fields of day 5 control muscle stained with: (a) anti-LMM, and (b) anti-LMM plus bisbenzimid. (370X) (c,d,e,f) Identical fields of day 5 muscle treated with TPA from days 3-5. (c) Anti-LMM staining and (d) anti-LMM plus bisbenzimid show the great reduction in myosin as well as the circular nuclear arrangement common in TPA-treatment. Note that under these staining conditions all of the residual LMM-binding material is confined to one localized area and is visualized in both channels (arrows). (e) Anti-desmin staining indicates the abundance of desmin in a TPA myosac. Note the circular nuclear arrangement in (f) and the numerous desmin-negative cells. (c-f: 300X).

In normal myotubes, 10^{-6} M Colcemid depolymerizes microtubules and induces the aggregation of vimentin and desmin into enormous cables that exclude all cytoplasmic organelles (438,445,448,449). It was of interest to determine whether these IFs would exhibit their characteristic response to Colcemid in the absence of myofibrils. As shown in Figure 48e, TPA myosacs recovered for 24 hours in Colcemid, assembled large tortuous cables of parallel-oriented IFs that were indistinguishable from those induced in normal myotubes. These cables bound both anti-vimentin and anti-desmin (434,450-452).

The effects of TPA on myogenic cultures were strikingly reversible. Recovery was rapid, with some striations being evident after only one day of recovery. Cultures allowed to recover in normal medium for 4 days displayed enormous numbers of typically striated myofibrils (Figure 48b). These myofibrils were distributed peripherally, forming a tube-like configuration in cross section, the center of which was occupied by a single row of nuclei. In most of these recovered myotubes, anti-vimentin and anti-desmin bound to longitudinally-oriented filaments of indefinite length. In some, the anti-desmin was bound not only to longitudinal filaments, but also localized in the I-Z band regions (Figure 48a). It should be noted that myotubes in cultures recovering from TPA were the result of both the recovery of myosacs, and the fusion of mononucleated postmitotic myoblasts into _de novo_ myotubes. Many fusion competent postmitotic myoblasts that were born in the presence of TPA but blocked from fusing by the drug, fused when returned to normal medium.

As shown in Figure 49a, day 5 control muscle cultures synthesized the major muscle-specific proteins including desmin, α-actin, α- and β-tropomyosins (α_1 and β_1) and their phosphorylated variants (α_2 and β_2), fast myosin light chains 1 and 2 ($LC1_f$ and $LC2_f$), the phosphorylated form of $LC2_f$ and troponin C. Vimentin, β-tubulin, β- and α-actins and nonmuscle light chains could also be identified. These proteins were identified by comigration with cold standards.

Two-dimensional electrophoresis of day 5 muscle cultures treated with TPA from days 3 to 5 in culture correlated well with immunofluorescence: in both cases the loss of muscle-specific proteins, with the exception of desmin, was evident. Figure 49b shows a typical fluorograph of a TPA-treated culture in which synthesis of most muscle-specific proteins has been lost or greatly reduced. The absence of $LC1_f$, $LC2_f$, and its phosphorylated

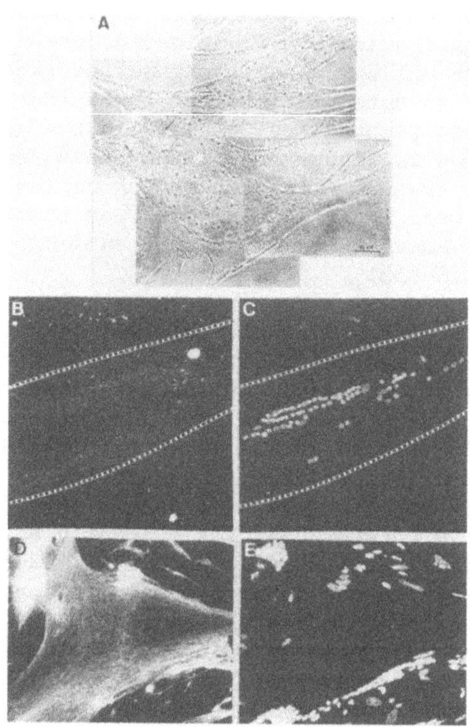

FIGURE 48: (a,b) TPA-treated cultures recovered in normal medium for 4 days. (a) Desmin localized to the I-Z band region in some myotubes, and (b) LMM resumes a normally striated pattern. (370X). (c,d) Identical fields of EMS-treated cultures recovered in normal medium for 5 days and stained with: (c) anti-desmin, and (d) anti-LMM. Note the longitudinally oriented desmin IFs, but the striated distribution of myosin. (370X). (e) TPA-treated cultures were allowed to recover in Colcemid for 24 hours and were stained with anti-desmin. The cabling of intermediate filaments is accentuated in these myosacs which contained no organized myofibrils. (600X).

variant are evident. When cold myosin carrier was comigrated with ^{35}S-Methionine-labeled TPA-treated samples and the light chain spots were subsequently excised, only background counts could be detected in such samples. Protein immune blots using anti-LMM showed a great reduction of muscle-specific myosin heavy chain accumulation in TPA-treated cultures. All of these data combined indicated an almost complete loss of thick filaments with TPA treatment.

The synthesis of thin filament proteins was differentially altered by TPA. Figure 49b shows a virtual absence of alpha-actin. Both two-dimensional electrophoresis and protein immune blot showed a great reduction, but not a complete absence of α-actin. However, the muscle-specific tropomyosins and their phosphorylated variants were completely lost. Spots seen in the tropomyosin region of this gel did not comigrate with the muscle-specific tropomyosins. Troponin C was also completely lost in TPA-treated cultures. Experiments are underway to determine if these changes are due to changes at the level of transcription or translation.

Although synthesis of thick and thin filament proteins was greatly reduced by TPA, that of desmin was not (Figure 49b). The presence of intermediate filament proteins was evident in immunofluorescence, two-dimensional electrophoresis and one-dimensional electrophoresis.

The majority of non-muscle proteins readily identified in these gels were unaffected by TPA-treatment. Synthesis of β- and α-actins, vimentin and β-tubulin is apparent in Figure 49b. Although $LC1_f$ and $LC2_f$ were not synthesized in TPA, the nonmuscle myosin light chains were synthesized. The synthesis of one protein which is common to muscle and fibroblast cultures and which has not been positively identified was substantially reduced by TPA (compare Figure 49a,b,c).

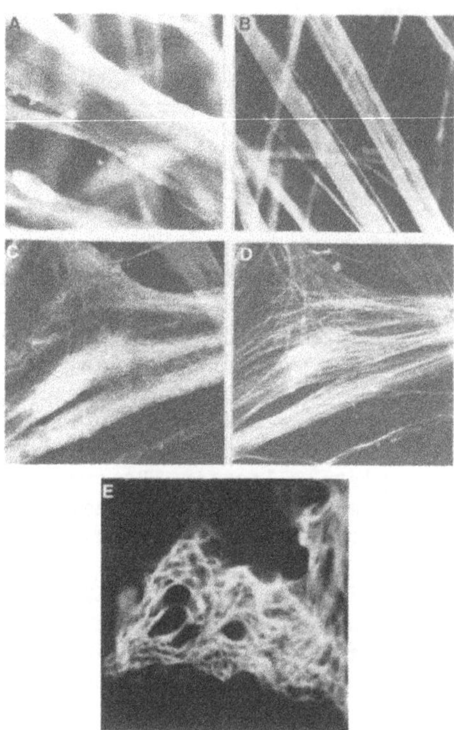

FIGURE 49: Fluorographs of two-dimensional polyacrylamide gels showing the synthetic patterns of: (a) day 5 control cultures; (b) day 5 cultures treated with TPA from days 3-5; and (c) TPA-treated cultures recovered in normal medium for 4 days. Note the loss of most muscle-specific proteins in (b) and their recovery in (c). D=desmin; α, β, γ = actin isoforms; TM=muscle-specific tropomyosins; ?=unidentified protein; $LC1_f$ and $LC2_f$ = fast myosin light chains; TN= troponin C. The arrows in (b) and (c) correspond to proteins labeled in (a).

Recovery of the synthesis of muscle-specific proteins after TPA-treatment was rapid. Cultures recovered in normal medium for 4 days synthesized all of the muscle-specific proteins (Figure 49c).

EMS and TPA affected myogenic cultures in some similar and some dissimilar ways. Unlike TPA, the carcinogen EMS is an alkylating agent, and is toxic to replicating presumptive myoblasts and fibroblasts. Consequently, day 4 myogenic cultures exposed to EMS from days 1-4 were grossly different in appearance from TPA-treated cultures. The total number of cells in day 4 EMS-treated cultures was less than 10% of that in TPA-treated or control cultures. All the rare surviving mononucleated cells were excessively flattened, fibroblastic and probably postmitotic. However, EMS did not block fusion as did TPA. Therefore, multinucleated structures formed in these treated cultures. As shown in Figure 50a, these multinucleated structures were immense and were inordinately flattened. For these reasons, they were distinguished from TPA-treated myosacs and were termed myosheets. EMS-induced myosheets often exhibited enormous areas of sarcoplasm that were devoid of nuclei (Figure 50e). Morphologically, they are somewhat reminiscent of the highly atypical myotubes that emerge in lines of immortalized L6 and L8 cells.

EMS-Treated Myogenic Cultures

EMS and TPA exhibited very similar effects at the cytoimmunochemical level. Figure 50b,c illustrate the total lack of binding of anti-LMM and the clustering of nuclei in the center of a single EMS-induced myosheet. Figure 50b,c of a triple-stained myosheet illustrate not only the total absence of binding of anti-LMM, but also the curious clustering of nuclei--this time to the periphery of the EMS-induced myosheet. Of particular interest in Figure 50d is the widespread, although uneven, distribution of desmin. In the absence of myofibrils, desmin ramified throughout the sarcoplasm, even into the fine processes that extend from the body of the myosheet. Within a single myosheet, there are considerable variations in fluorescence intensity following staining with anti-desmin and anti-vimentin. As yet we have not succeeded

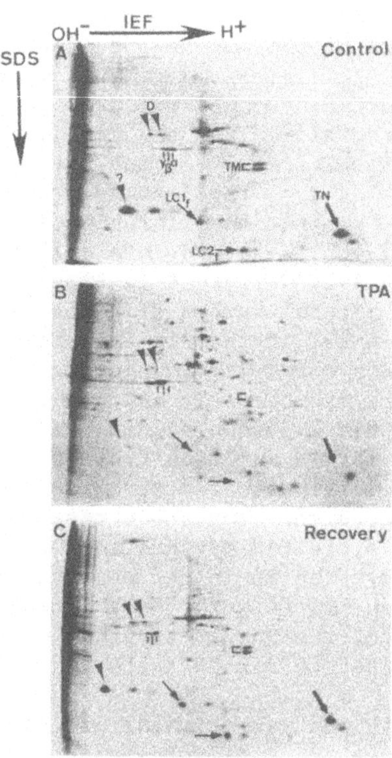

FIGURE 50: Day 4 muscle treated with EMS from days 1-4. (a) is a phase micrograph showing a very large, flat EMS myosheet (100X).
(b,c) Identical fields fluorescently labeled with: (e) anti-LMM, and (c) bisbenzimid. The dotted line indicates the myosheet border. (d,e) Identical fields triple-stained with: (d) anti-desmin, and (e) anti-LMM plus bisbenzimid. Note the widespread but irregular distribution of desmin, and the absence of nuclei in the central portion of the myosheet in (e). (b-e: 150X).

in correlating these fluorescent "hot spots" with other organelles.

Two interesting criteria distinguish EMS-induced myosheets from TPA-induced myosacs: (1) Myosacs did not display unusually prominent stress fibers when labeled with anti-nonmuscle myosin, anti- alpha-actin or rhodamine-phallodin. In contrast, EMS-induced myosheets stained with the same fluorescent reagents revealed exceedingly prominent arrays of very long, branching stress fibers; and (2) Antibody to α-actin that bound very weakly, or not at all, to the β- and α-actins of fibroblast microfilaments, bound strongly to the microfilaments in EMS-myosheets.

Recovery of EMS myosheets, as monitored with labeled antibodies, was much slower than recovery from TPA. Myosheets shifted to normal medium required 4 to 5 days to display numerous definitively striated myofibrils (Figure 49d). Because these myofibrils were long, narrow, and well-separated, they could be clearly visualized. The protracted period required for recovery, coupled with the unique flattened geometry of EMS myosheets, allowed studies on the topographical relationship between transitory microfilaments and the subsequent assembly of nascent myofibrils. It was observed that the earliest assembly of muscle-specific thick filaments occurred in proximity to the transitory microfilaments subtending the sarcolemma. The transitory microfilaments composed of β- and α-actins, etc. appeared to serve as a template for the longitudinal polymerization and for orientations of the muscle-specific myosins, α-actin, etc. These nascent myofibrils were subsequently displaced from their subsarcolemmal location into the body of the myotube. These data will be presented elsewhere. It will be interesting to determine whether the "striated" microfilaments themselves gradually transformed into the definitively striated myofibril, or whether they merely served as a temporary scaffold.

Biosynthetic studies on EMS-treated and recovered cultures confirmed cytoimmunofluorescent studies. Myosin heavy chains were not accumulated in myosheets reared in EMS for 3 days as determined by Western blots. The synthesis of MHC was readily detected after 4 or 5 days of recovery in normal medium. Two-dimensional SDS-PAGE of EMS-treated and recovered cultures revealed synthetic patterns similar to those of TPA-treated cultures

(Figure 50b,c): synthesis of myosin light chains, tropomyosins and troponin C was blocked by EMS. Like TPA, EMS did not affect the synthesis of desmin. However, EMS myosheets appeared to have modest amounts of α-actin.

Discussion

The differentiation program of newborn, definitive, unfused myoblasts is characterized by their unique option to coordinately accumulate and assemble myofibrillar isoforms, desmin, and those cell membrane molecules required for fusion into myotubes. It has been suggested that: (1) The acquisition and expression of this global program - so different from that of their mothers - is determined by the myoblast's mitotic history. It is not determined by exogenous molecules; and (2) The differentiation program of the definitive myoblast requires, and stems from, changes in chromosomal structure initiated as presumptive myoblasts undergo their terminal quantal cell cycle (434,435,437,450-452). In vivo, the developmentally regulated embryonic myofibrillar isoforms are replaced by regulated neonatal and adult isoforms. There is no evidence that the switch from embryonic to neonatal, to adult isoforms, requires DNA synthesis. From this we suggest that the genetic control of types and quantities of muscle-specific isoforms involves at least two distinct mechanisms. One establishes the "basic" myogenic options; the other modulates the quantitative changes in isoforms associated with maturation.

Definitive myoblasts are born with the option to transcribe all those genes whose proteins are, or will be, synthesized in either immature or mature muscle. Whether the option to transcribe a particular gene for one or another muscle-specific isoform is or is not expressed depends on exogenous conditions. It is to be stressed that these exogenous conditions, however, are not involved in initially establishing the myoblast's differentiation program. This dual genetic regulation which allows a modest choice among functionally coupled molecules with a broader, but strictly pre-determined, limited differentiation program has precedent in the differentiation and/or maturation of definitive autonomic neuro-blasts. These postmitotic autonomic neuroblasts are born with the option to express an adrenergic or cholinergic phenotype. No other cell type is born with these two options. Which transmitter is given immature autonomic neuroblast actually synthesizes, however, is determined by apparently "trivial" exogenous cues impinging on the maturing cell.

TPA- and EMS-treated myogenic cells are paradigms of how exogenous molecules, which have nothing to do with establishing any cell's differentiation program, differentially alter the expression of parts of that program. The entire inherited myogenic program need not be turned on or off as a coordinated block by these drugs.

TPA and EMS probably have different primary cell targets. TPA promptly blocks fusion while stimulating cell replication. EMS does not block fusion, but kills both replicating presumptive myoblasts and fibroblasts. Both agents reduce the total number of myotubes that form in day 5 cultures, but by different mechanisms. TPA inhibits the actual event of fusion by fusion-competent postmitotic myoblasts; it mimics the effect of EGTA, cytochalasin-B, etc. In contrast, EMS precludes the generation of fusion-competent myoblasts by depressing the replication of presumptive myoblasts: it mimics the effect of lacking a collagen substrate, lectins, transferrin, hyaluronate, etc.

By mechanisms currently unknown, both drugs reversibly block the synthesis of embryonic $LC1_f$, $LC2_f$, α- and β-tropomyosins and troponin C. TPA greatly reduces the synthesis of α-actin, whereas the synthesis of α-actin is less affected by EMS treatment. Additional experiments are required to quantify this inhibition of α-actin synthesis, but even in EMS this inhibition is greater than 50%. Translation of total mRNAs from EMS myosheets in a lysate system indicates the presence of mRNAs for α-actin and desmin (data not shown); similar experiments with mRNAs in TPA myosacs are in progress. Total protein synthesis is not grossly depressed by either drug. While both drugs differentially block the synthesis of many myofibrillar proteins, neither drug blocks the synthesis of desmin. This suggests a greater coupling between the synthesis of several myofibrillar proteins than between the myofibrillar proteins and desmin.

Because TPA and EMS alter myotubes morphologically as well as block the synthesis and cause the degradation of most myofibrillar proteins, they are excellent tools for studying myofibrillogenesis. EMS myosheets display unusually prominent stress fibers. These prove to be transitory structures, disappearing as striated myofibrils form during recovery. The earliest sites of assembly of the muscle-specific thick filaments occur in close association with these transitory subsarcolemmal microfilaments. This intimate topographical relationship between the contractile proteins comprising microfilaments and those comprising myofibrils leads to interesting speculations regarding the spatial interactions of contractile proteins in both nonmuscle and muscle cells.

The loss of myofibrillar proteins, but the retention of desmin in TPA- and EMS-treated cultures, focuses again on the intriguing, but largely unknown, role of desmin in myogenesis. In immature myotubes, TPA-myosacs, and EMS-myosheets, desmin is found associated with vimentin in longitudinally-aligned filaments of indefinitive length. Clearly, neither desmin nor vimentin play any role in the assembly of early definitively striated myofibrils, for A-, I- and Z-bands are well formed long before desmin secondarily associates with the I-Z band (443-446). It will be interesting to determine what function desmin serves that selects for its early synthesis and accumulation as longitudinal filaments in postmitotic myoblasts, and whether this function relates to its function at the I-Z region in more mature muscle.

CHAPTER 16: SYNTHESIS AND ACCUMULATION OF MYOSIN ISOZYMES IN TISSUE CULTURE

Robert G. Whalen*, Lawrence B. Bugaisky*, Gillian S. Butler-Browne*, Marion S. Ecob** and Christian Pinset*

*Departement de Biologie Moleculaire, Institute Pasteur
**Muscular Dystrophy Laboratories, New Castle General Hospital, Newcastle upon Tyne, Great Britain

Several questions can be asked concerning the synthesis and accumulation of myosin subunits and their isoforms in muscle cells grown in tissue culture. Do any of the transitions which characterize muscle development *in vivo* take place in tissue culture? Do myoblasts taken from animals of different ages, or from different muscle types synthesize the same myosin isozymes? Is morphological maturity of a muscle fiber in culture paralleled by accumulation of adult muscle myosins? We have examined each of these questions in three different tissue culture situations.

Myosin Light Chain Types in Rat Satellite Cell Cultures

We investigated the possibility that satellite cells taken from different muscle types (fast and slow) or from innervated versus denervated muscles might show differences in the myosin light chains that were ultimately synthesized by the myotubes formed from these cells in culture. We analyzed the light chains since the synthesis of these proteins can be directly examined using two-dimensional gel electrophoresis of radioactively labeled extracts of the myotube cultures (453). This approach allows us to analyze the embryonic, fast and slow light chain types (454).

Cultures were made from the gastrocnemius and soleus muscles of 3-4 week old rats; the gastrocnemius is composed of ca. Ninety percent fast fibers while the soleus contains about two-thirds slow fibers at this age. Comparisons were also made between the normal gastrocnemius muscle and the same muscle taken from rats that had been denervated at 7 days of age (214).

In all cultures examined, irrespective of the source of satellite cells, fast myosin light chains were the major forms being synthesized. In only 2 of the more than 20 cultures analyzed, faint spots in the region of slow light chains were detected in the electropherograms. We conclude that slow light chains, if they are synthesized at all, must only be minor components.

All cultures also synthesized the embryonic LC1 light chain. The ratio of synthesis of $LC1_{emb}$ compared to the adult fast LC1 was very high in these cultures. In the innervated or denervated gastrocnemius cultures, this ratio was as great as 10-15 to 1 in the early stages of myotube formation, and it decreased to 3-4 to 1 in older cultures. In the soleus cultures, the $LC1_{emb}/LC1_F$ ratio was nearly 20 to 1 in the early stages and 4-5 to 1 in the late stages. By way of comparison, primary cultures of fetal myoblasts synthesize nearly equal amounts of these two light chains at about one week after myotube formation (455).

These results suggest then that myotubes formed in culture from satellite cells express a qualitatively identical phenotype no matter what type of muscle the satellite cells are taken from. Quantitatively, differences in the ratio of embryonic and adult LC1 synthesis can be observed which seem to be correlated to the origin of the myotube precursors.

One limitation to the approach taken here to search for differences in phenotype is the possibility that there is a certain trauma experienced by the satellite cells in dissociating them from the muscle tissue. This trauma might influence the phenotype expressed in culture and overwhelm any intrinsic differences in the various satellite cell preparations.

Myosin Heavy Chain Transitions in Primary Cultures

In the myotubes formed from myoblasts dissociated from fetal or newborn muscle tissue, embryonic myosin accumulates as the major heavy chain isozyme. Even in avian cultures maintained for periods up to one month, the embryonic isozymes remain the predominant form (384,456). Since in our previous studies (55) we had isolated myosin from rat myotube cultures maintained for only about one week, we examined the myosin types present throughout the first two weeks after myotube formation.

Using antibodies specific to embryonic and neonatal myosins (175,457), we first used immunocytochemistry to determine the types of myosins present at different times after myotubes formed (Figure 51). Within the first week after fusion, all myotubes were stained with the embryonic antibody while the staining with the antibody to neonatal myosin was negative. During the second

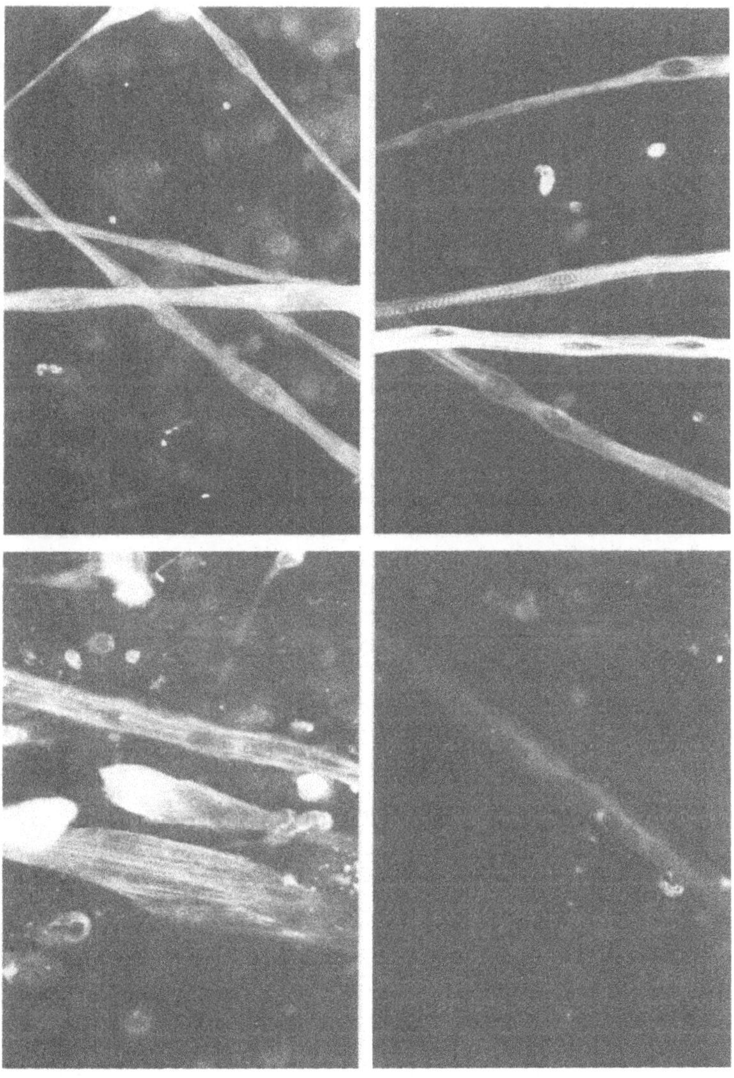

FIGURE 51: Immunofluorescent staining of primary cultures of rat myotubes. The cultures were examined at 5 and 13 days after myotube formation using antibodies to embryonic and neonatal myosins, as indicated.

week, however, many myotubes in the cultures stained strongly with neonatal antibody; furthermore, myotubes were seen in the cultures which stained only weakly with embryonic antibody.

These results suggested that neonatal myosin was appearing in these primary cultures of myotubes, and that the transition embryonic - neonatal was therefore taking place. To confirm presence of neonatal myosin, we prepared myosin from long term cultures and carried out polypeptide mapping as described previously (55,175). In these polypeptide maps, the pattern of embryonic myosin was still predominant when polypeptides were detected by standard Coomassie blue protein staining. However, if the polypeptide cleavage products were transferred to nitocellulose sheets and then reacted with the specific neonatal antibody, polypeptides were stained which corresponded to those found in control neonatal myosin treated in parallel. This approach to the identification of the neonatal myosin isozyme, which is present along with an excess of embryonic myosin, takes advantage of the specificity of the antibody used as well as the characteristic polypeptide cleavage pattern of the neonatal myosin.

The conclusion from these experiments is that the embryonic neonatal myosin transition is occurring in tissue culture myotubes. The transition seems to be nearly complete in some myotubes which have lost embryonic myosin, according to the immunocytochemical results. The factors controlling this transition are not known, but the fact that it occurs in aneural tissue culture strongly suggests that it is not strictly nerve-dependent.

Even though myotubes in tissue culture often become striated and contractile, this morphological and functional maturity is not accompanied by the accumulation of adult myosin isozymes, as discussed above. We have, therefore, investigated another, quite different system comprised of organotypic nerve-muscle cultures of fetal mouse spinal cord and mouse muscle.

Accumulation of Adult Myosin in Organotypic Nerve-Muscle Cultures

In this system, mouse muscle fibers develop as a result of regeneration, forming beneath the basal lamina of the parent fibers, and they become innervated and contractile, acquire cross-striations and can survive for many months (149,290). Although the amount of material is rather limited, the cultures are amenable to morphological examination, including histochemistry and immunocytochemistry.

In these experiments, the regenerated fibers were examined from cultures that had been maintained for a total of 20-34 days; the fibers had developed cross-striations after 10-17 days in vitro and had been contracting continually for 10-21 days (149). The bundles of regenerated muscles were composed mostly of large (8-15μ) and small (2-6μ) diameter fibers. When the regenerated fibers were excised from culture, frozen and sectioned, the large diameter fibers could be easily followed in serial sections. It was determined that these fibers showed a histochemical reaction typical of type IIB fibers (Figure 52): they were resistant to alkali incubation, sensitive to pH 4.3 acid preincubation, and they stained in an intermediate fashion after preincubation at pH 4.6 (458).

Serial sections were also reacted with antibodies to embryonic, neonatal and adult fast myosin. In the cultures examined, 39 out of 40 large diameter fibers reacted with the adult fast antibody but not with the embryonic or neonatal antibodies. In contrast, most of the small diameter fibers reacted with neonatal, some with embryonic, and only a few with adult fast antibody; the combinations of myosins present in a given fiber could not readily be determined, since it was difficult to recognize the same small fibers in different serial sections.

These results (149) demonstrating the presence of adult myosin in tissue culture, represent the first such system in which adult myosin has been found. The large diameter muscle fibers formed in these organotypic cultures are probably innervated, since accumulations of acetylcholine receptor and acetylcholinesterase are found on the muscle fibers, in the same regions where nerve axons are in apparent contact with the fibers (290).

It is, therefore, possible that the presence of adult myosin in this tissue culture system is due to innervation by the nerve cells present. This would be quite different from the in vivo situation where fast myosin can accumulate in a nerve-dependent fashion (214,459).

In spite of these possible differences, the organotypic culture system will allow further investigation into the factors controlling the appearance of adult myosin.

Conclusions

The various tissue culture systems used here have allowed us to investigate some questions concerning the expression of the muscle phenotype, particularly regarding the myosin subunits. We find no qualitative differences in the types of light chains synthesized by satellite cell cultures, compared to fetal myoblast cultures, even if the satellite cells are taken from fast or slow muscle, innervated or denervated muscle. Although these results do not rule out intrinsic differences among these different satellite cell populations, they provide no evidence in support of this idea for rat muscle. Some changes in phenotype can however be observed in tissue culture, in the case of the myosin heavy chain. Primary cultures will

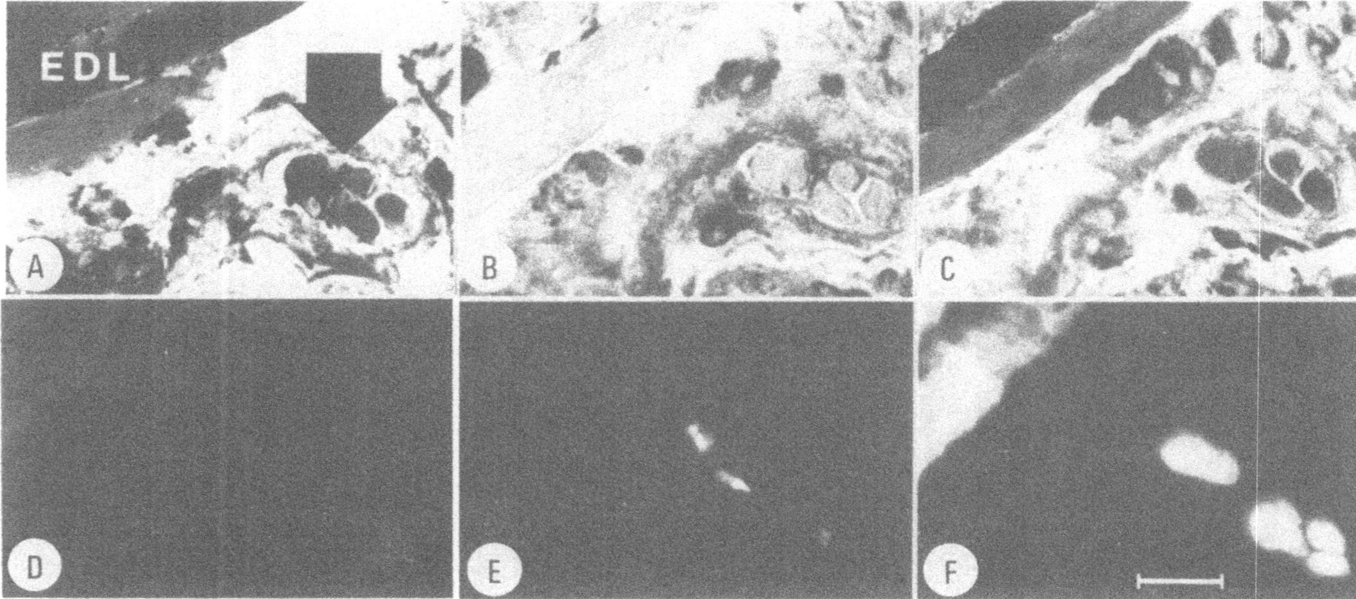

FIGURE 52: Histochemistry and immunofluorescent staining of organotypic cultures. The bundle of regenerated muscle fibers (large arrow in A) was sectioned along with a control mouse fast muscle (EDL: extensor digitorum longus). The results of histochemical reactions are shown for alkaline incubation (A), after pH 4.3 preincubation (B) and after pH 4.6 preincubation (C). The immunofluorescence was performed using antibodies to embryonic (D), neonatal (E) or adult fast (F) myosin. The scale bar in E equals 10 µm.
From Ecob et al, 1983.

undergo the embryonic - neonatal myosin transition, indicating therefore that this step of development is probably independent of the nerve. Finally, we have found a tissue culture system in which adult myosin is present, and these organotypic cultures can be further investigated and manipulated in an attempt to demonstrate what factors might control the appearance of this adult form.

PART IV

REGULATING EXPRESSION OF PROTEIN ISOFORMS

CHAPTER 17: OVERVIEW

Donald A. Fischman*, David Bader* and Takashi Obinata

*Department of Cell Biology and Anatomy
Cornell University Medical College
New York, NY

More than 75 years have passed since the pioneering studies of Harrison (460) in which methods for the tissue culture of frog muscle were first demonstrated. In the intervening years, hundreds, if not thousands, of studies have relied on *in vitro* systems for analyzing selected aspects of muscle differentiation. These studies have been essential in establishing:

1. the stability of the myodifferentiated state *in vitro*;

2. the sequence of morphogenetic steps which occur during myogenesis including mitosis, cessation of DNA synthesis, cytoplasmic fusion and myofibrillogenesis;

3. the postmitotic, diploid state of myotube and myofiber nuclei;

4. the concept of a coordinate expression of many "muscle-specific" genes during terminal differentiation;

5. the proof that regulation of coordinate gene expression is primarily at the level of mRNA transcription;

6. the existence and nature of intermediate filaments in myogenic and non-myogenic cells;

7. the parameters of acetylcholine receptor and acetylcholinesterase biosynthesis, distribution and turnover;

8. the biophysical properties of the myotube plasma membrane and their changes upon innervation;

9. methods for the clonal analysis of myogenic cells;

10. the isolation of permanent cell lines which offer the opportunity to genetically dissect many regulatory steps of myogenesis;

11. the nutritive requirements for muscle cell growth and differentiation.

Clearly, these are impressive achievements which have had an important bearing on the attractiveness and popularity of muscle as a developmental system for exploring a whole range of questions relevant not only to myogenesis and disease of muscle, but to the phenomena of cellular determination, oncogenesis, cell-cell recognition, synaptogenesis, cellular senescence and protein degradation.

However, as the sensitivity of our techniques has improved and the relevant questions been more precisely defined, it has become apparent that current in vitro models do not reproduce several important features of myodifferentiation. It is the aim of this introduction to highlight some of these deficiencies in the hope that they might be addressed and corrected in the ensuing decade.

Based on the recent experiments employing chick-quail transplantation (461), it is now fairly certain that most, if not all, muscle cells of the limbs arise from myotome-derived precursors (462,463) whose determination may be established in early, epithelial stages of the somites. As emphasized by several investigators (464-466), the concept that there exist in the limb bud pluripotent stem cells which are capable of both cartilage and muscle differentiation must now be seriously questioned. Clonal cell cultures of the early chick or limb (443) form cartilage or muscle but not both. Furthermore, the studies of Hauschka and colleagues (293) would suggest the existence of several myogenic cell types in embryonic limbs at different stages of embryogenesis. None of these studies have yet addressed a central question in this field. Are there multiple cell lineages in presumptive skeletal muscle? Are the

Muscle Cell Lineages

myogenic cells which derive from the early somite analogous to early neuroblasts which migrate away from the central canal of the neural tube? If these are separate muscle cell lineages, do they relate to subsequent fiber type diversity in adult muscle?

Recently, a series of manuscripts have appeared from the laboratory of Marcus Jacobson in which the clonal derivatives of peroxidase-marked blastomeres have been followed in Xenopus embryos (467). These studies have demonstrated the feasibility of tracking cell lineages from blastomeres through neurula stages of development and, most importantly, have provided suggestive evidence that primary motor axons display a preferred association with clonally related myotubes of the ventral myotome (468). In other words, motor nerves and myotubes derived from the same parent blastomere may form preferential neuromuscular associations. These observations are especially significant in light of the experiments of Lance-Jones and Landmesser (469,470) in which segmental specificity of neuromuscular connections was demonstrated during chick embryogenesis. With few exceptions (471), experimentors in this field have treated myoblasts as a relatively homogeneous population differing only in their stage of progression through the mitotic cycle. Yet, it is well-recognized that skeletal muscles of both vertebrates and invertebrates differ in growth characteristics, morphology, speeds of contraction and relaxation, resistance to fatigue, sensitivity to oxygen debt or lactic acid accumulation and, perhaps most significantly, as the target for specific myopathic disorders. Clearly, the phenotype of a muscle can be modified by its innervation and work history (472). What is less certain is the extent of genetic vs. epigenetic influences on muscle gene expression during embryonic and postnatal stages of life. Do myoblasts respond equivalently to extracellular cues? Recent studies by Stockdale and colleagues (473) suggest that different muscles of the chick embryo contain myogenic cells which express fast and slow-type myosin light chains _in vitro_, and do so in the absence of innervation. Were these cells epigenetically imprinted to synthesize tissue specific myosin isoforms, or were they of differing clonal lineages of restricted phenotypic potential? Techniques at hand can now resolve this question.

A related question concerns the homology of myonuclei within single myofibers. Do all myonuclei within a common sarcoplasm transcribe identical mRNAs? Do all myonuclei respond identically to the same cytoplasmic regulatory factors? Recent studies by Blau et al (474) and Wright (475) suggest that positive regulation of muscle-specific gene expression can cross both species and tissue barriers. With cDNA probes specific for muscle proteins of different species, and improved _in situ_ hybridization techniques, it will now be feasible to explore gene expression at the cytological level and probe the phylogenetic conservation of myonuclear regulation in chimeric myotubes.

Muscle Gene Expression *In Vivo* & *In Vitro*

Although the concept of coordinate gene expression has dominated models of terminal myodifferentiation over the past decade, recent evidence that many contractile proteins exhibit isoform transitions during late stages of muscle development (476) has necessitated a reevaluation of gene regulation in the post-differentiated myofiber.

It is to this latter topic that I shall address my remarks. Recent studies from our laboratory (477-480), using a variety of monoclonal antibodies (McAbs) specific for the myosin heavy chain (MHC), C-protein and myosin light chain 2 (LC_2) have been used to analyze gene expression during chick muscle development *in vivo* and *in vitro*. It is apparent from these studies that isoform transitions in the cultured myotubes exhibit significant differences from those observed *in vivo*.

Three McAbs (MF20, MF30 and MF14), which are all specific for the rod domain of the MHC of adult pectoralis muscle (PM) exhibit differential reactivity with myosin extracted from PM of 12 day-old embryos (Figures 53-54). McAb MF20 binds equivalently to PM myosin from embryonic, post-hatch and adult stages of development. In contrast, MF30 does not bind to myosin from 12 day-old embryos but does so to myosin from late stage embryos and older birds. A third stage in myosin antigenicity can be detected with MF14 which only binds to PM myosin after the first week post-hatching. Thus, three McAbs are at hand which discriminate three immunochemical changes in the MHC, one between the mid and late embryonic stages of development, a second between late embryonic and post-hatch stages of growth and, finally, between post-hatch and adult stages of development.

Using these 3 McAbs, we next examined the question of whether these immunochemical changes in the MHC occur in muscle cell culture. To this effect, 11 day-old chick PM was trypsin dispersed and plated in monolayer and then tested for reactivity with McAbs MF 20, 30 and 14 by immunoblot and solid phase radioimmunoassay (RIA). The results were quite dramatic; little or no reactivity of the myosin in cultured cells could be detected even if the cultures were maintained for 28 days (Figures 55-56). Thus, some regulatory factor or factors are missing from the cell culture system which are apparently required for the expression of MHC isoforms which react with McAbs MF30 and 14. The obvious candidates are: a) input from the nervous system; b) hormones or unknown

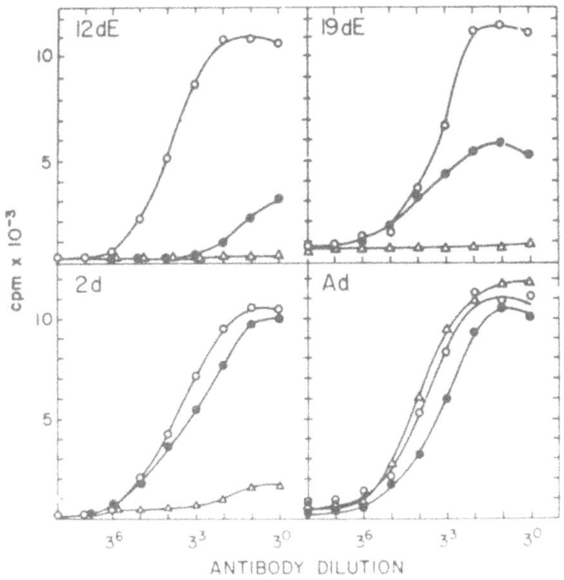

FIGURE 53: RIA analysis of myosin with MF20, MF30, and MF14. 1 μg of myosin from 12 and 19-d embryonic, 2-d posthatching and adult pectoralis muscles was reacted with McAbs in 1:3 dilutions of the hybridoma supernatants. All points represent the average of two analyses. MF20 (O); MF30 (●), and MF14 (Δ).

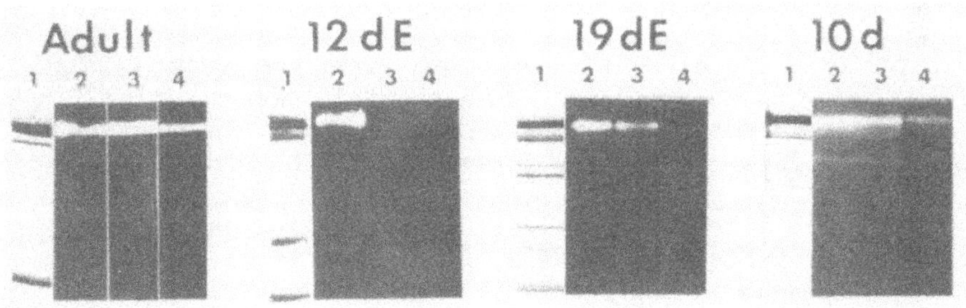

FIGURE 54: Immunoautoradiography of myosin from adult, 12 and 19-d embryonic 10-d posthatching chicken pectoralis muscles. Immunoblots with MF20 (2), MF30 (3) and MF14 (4) were performed as described. The amount of protein added to each gel was adjusted so that equivalent amounts of MHC (12%) was present.

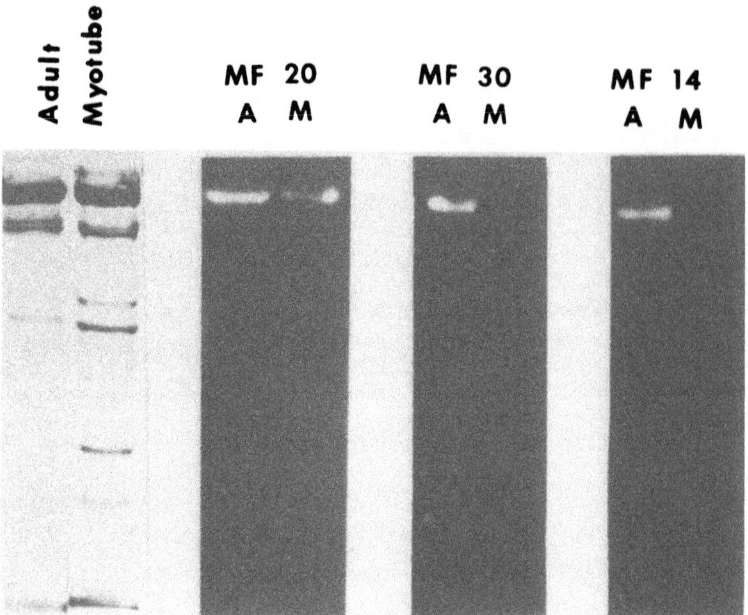

FIGURE 55: Immunoautoradiography of myosin from adult chicken pectoralis muscle and muscle cell cultures 10-d after plating with MF20, MF30, and MF14. The gel lanes at the left are crude myosin preparations of adult muscle and myotube cultures stained with Coomassie Brilliant Blue. The same myosin samples were used for the accompanying immunoblots.

growth factors; and c) absent components from the extracellular matrix. Using these sensitive immunochemical assays, it will now be feasible to identify and hopefully to isolate the putative regulatory factors in the near future.

A separate line of investigation has focused on another thick filament protein, C-protein, first identified by G. Offer and his colleagues in England (481). We have now prepared another set of McAbs which bind to this protein and are capable of discriminating isoforms which we term fast and slow type because of their distribution in fast-twitch PM (MF1 and MF21) and slow-tonic ALD (ALD66) muscles of the chicken (478,479).

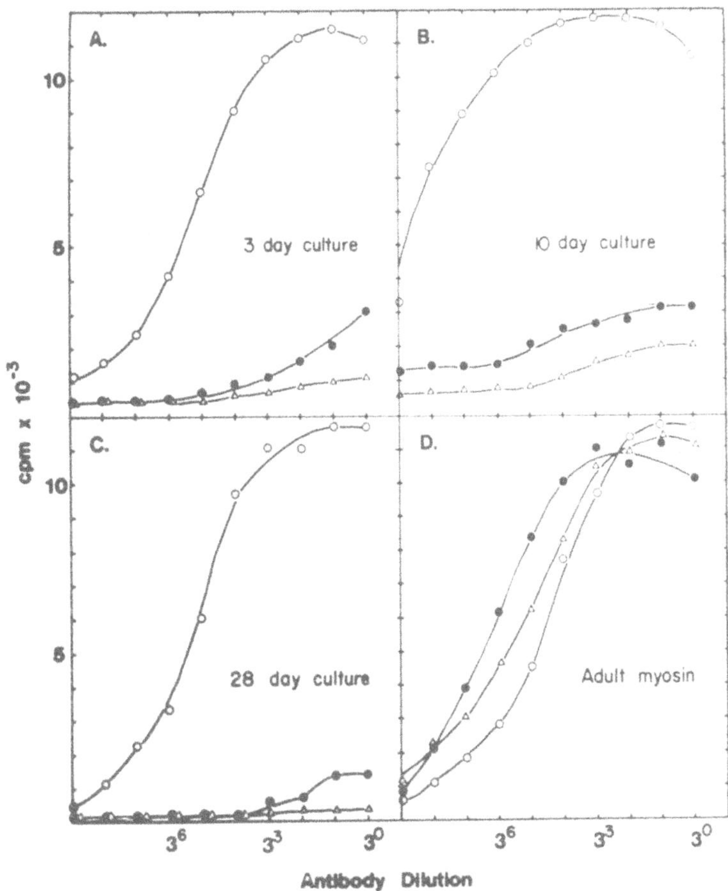

FIGURE 56: RIA analysis of myosin from cell cultures at 3, 10, and 28-d after plating with MF20, MF30, and MF14. 1 µg of myosin from cell cultures and adult pectoralis muscle was reacted with MF20 (O), MF30 (●), and MF14 (Δ) in 1:3 dilutions of mybridoma supernatants.

Recently, we have begun to analyze the expression of these C-protein isoforms during development to see if the transitions in MHC expression occur in parallel with C-protein changes (480). Is there a coordinate remodeling of all thick filament components?

As with the McAbs to MHC, we tested the C-protein antibodies by immunoblot, RIA and immunofluorescence. All of these experiments gave the same result: during the course of PM development in vivo there is the appearance of a C-protein isoform reactive with ALD66 (slow type isoform) about the 15th day of egg incubation (Figures 57-58). At this stage, the PM is unreactive with McAb MF1 which reacts with fast type C-protein. However, by the 17th day of embryonic development, both fast and slow type isoforms are clearly expressed in the muscle, although not all myofibers contain equivalent amounts of both proteins. By one day post-hatching, almost every myofiber, every myofibril and every sarcomere contains both fast and slow type C-protein isoforms. This situation is a developmental analogue of the adult PLD muscle in which 2 C-protein isoforms have been detected and localized by electron immunocytochemistry in all A bands of this muscle. During the first week post-hatching, however, there is a shut-down in expression of the slow type C-protein in the PM. By 14 days post-hatch, no binding of ALD66 can be detected by immunofluorescence (Figure 58) or RIA (results not shown; see 480). As discussed in a recent publication, the timetables for MHC, C-protein and myosin light chain isoform transitions during chick embryogenesis do not appear to be coordinate. Admittedly, the data are not complete but, nevertheless, they do suggest that the myosin heavy and light chains change independently during PM development. The same also appears to be true of C-protein.

Recently, Dr. Obinata while working at Chiba University, Japan, has observed the antibodies specific for cardiac C-protein react with embryonic PM at earlier stages of development than McAb ALD66. His work now suggests that the earliest form of C-protein which is expressed in PM may either be a cardiac isoform or a unique embryonic isoform with shared epitopes common to the adult cardiac protein. Assuming that the embryonic pectoralis muscle expresses an adult cardiac form of C-protein, then this would be one additional contractile protein encoded by a cardiac gene in early stages of skeletal muscle differentiation (482-487).

Preliminary studies have been performed on the expression of C-protein in monolayer cultures of PM. Using a McAb (MF21) which is specific for C-protein from fast-twitch muscle (i.e., it does not bind to cardiac C-protein) we have found that cross-striated myotubes are completely unreactive with MF21 (Figure 59) even though C-protein is evident on SDS acrylamide gels of crude myosin extracts. At these same stages of culture, a McAb specific for cardiac C-protein stains the myofibrils in a typical C-protein pattern (Figure 60). Thus, as in vivo, the first C-protein detectable in muscle cultures of 11 day-old PM appears to be the cardiac isoform. Further work is in progress to assess the C-protein isoform transitions in culture. In contrast to MHC, in which an arrest of isoform switching was observed in monolayer

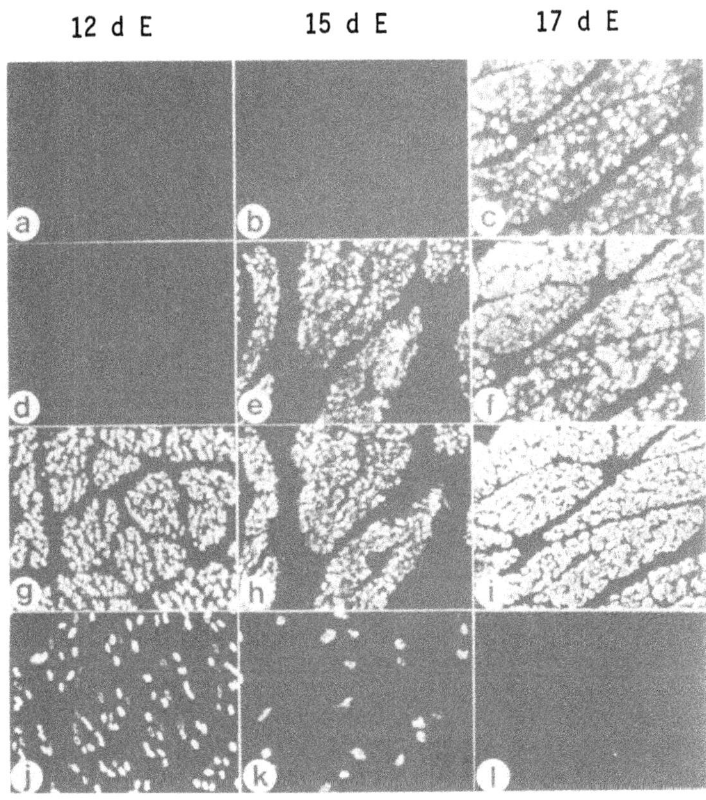

FIGURE 57: The reactivity of embryonic PM to antibodies against fast C-protein (MF-1), slow C-protein (ALD-66), fast myosin light chain (FLC1), and cardiac myosin light chain (CLC1). Frozen serial sections of PM from 12-day-old embryos (a,d,g, and j), 15-day-old embryos (b,e,h, and k), and 17-day-old embryos (c,f,i, and l) were reacted with MF-1 (a-c(, ALD-66 (d-f), anti-FLC1 (g-i) or anti-CLC1 (j-l). Serial sections were photographed under indirect immunofluorescence.

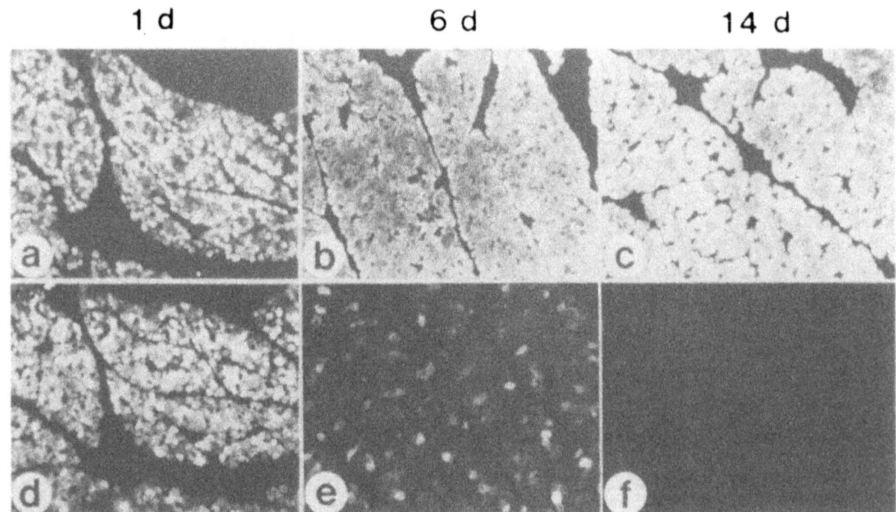

FIGURE 58: The reactivity of post hatched chicken PM to McAbs against fast C-protein (MF-1) and slow C-protein (ALD-66). Frozen serial sections of 1-day (a and d), 6-day (c and f) PM. Photographs of the sections were taken with indirect immunofluorescence.

culture, preliminary studies by Dr. Obinata indicate that C-protein transitions do take place in vitro.

Taken together, these experiments indicate a rather complicated set of regulatory steps which operate in the post-differentiated myotubes and myofibers of skeletal muscle. Some of these regulatory steps appear to be operative in monolayer culture (e.g., the C-protein conversions, while others are absent (e.g. the MHC isoform switches)). More questions than answers arise from our studies. First, it is currently a complete mystery why these isoform conversions take place at all. Possibly, the myosin isoforms possess different self-assembly characteristics (341,488) but improved assays for thick filament assembly will probably be necessary to prove that rigorously.

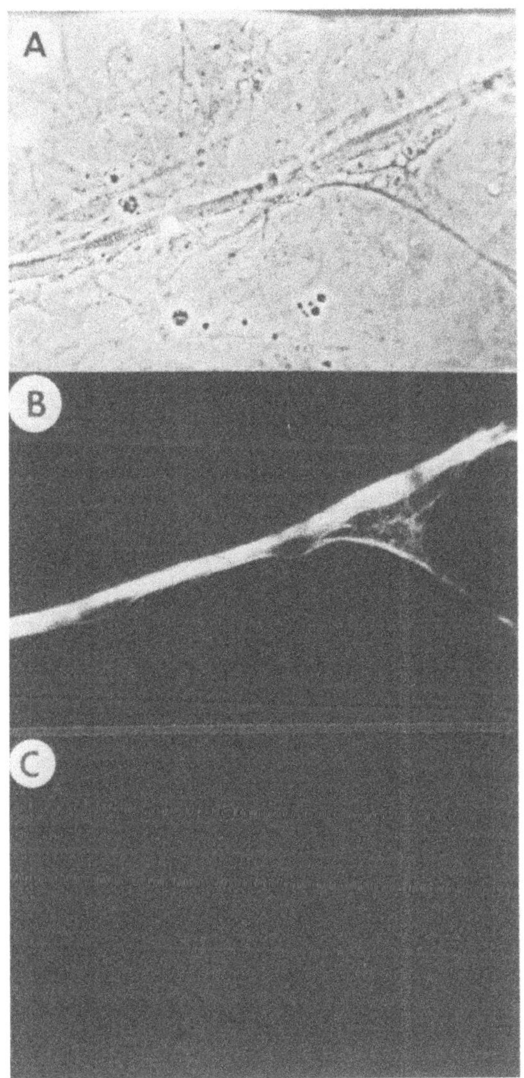

FIGURE 59: Direct immunofluorescence staining of cultures with MF20 and MF21. Primary muscle cultures were prepared for 11-day pectoralis muscles, grown for 14 days *in vitro* and processed for immunofluorescence. A. Phase contrast. B. TRITC-MF20. C. FITC-MF21.

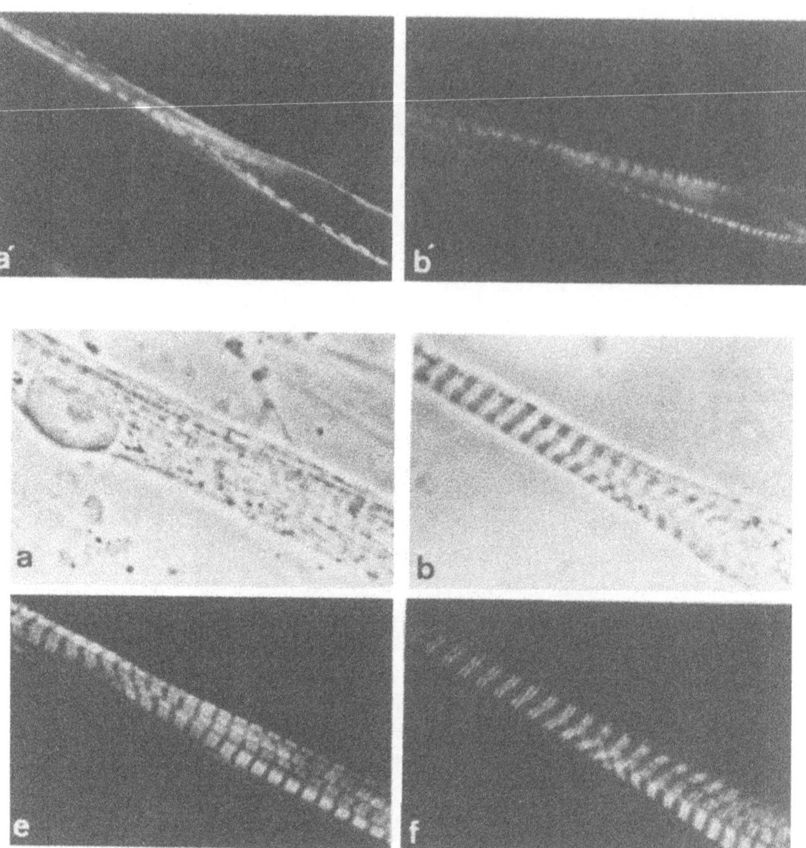

FIGURE 60: Immunofluorescent analysis of myosin LC and cardiac C-protein in embryonic chick pectoralis muscle cell cultures. In 2 day-old cultures (a' and b') myofibrils stain positively for both LC (a') and cardiac C-protein (b'). At 7 days of culture (a-f) myofibrils continue to synthesize both LC_1 (e) and cardiac C-protein (f). Corresponding contrast photomicrographs are shown in Figures a and b.

It is tempting to speculate that these isoform conversions of the contractile proteins may only represent the "tip of an iceberg." Transitions of other proteins, perhaps enzymes involved in regulating the full maturation of skeletal muscle must now be considered seriously in any discussion of those myopathies which become manifest at predictable stages of development. Is Duchenne dystrophy the result of a defective isoform conversion?

CHAPTER 18: MYOSINS A & B IN THE ORGANIZATION OF MYOFILAMENTS

Henry F. Epstein

Jerry Lewis Neuromuscular Research Center
Baylor College of Medicine
Houston, TX

I will discuss the question of two myosin isoforms in the same muscle from a genetical, as well as biochemical, viewpoint. For an overview, I will begin by reviewing the sliding-filament model for the molecular mechanims of muscle contraction by Huxley (489).

Figure 61 shows the interaction of actin and myosin to produce muscle contraction. The thin filaments are assembled from actin; the thick filaments from myosin. Today's undergraduate students of cell biology would not see the interaction of actin and myosin as a uniquely skeletal muscle phenomenon, but as a rather broad general scheme of a process that can occur in any eukaryotic cell. We now recognize that proteins, are indeed universal building blocks of eukaryotic cells. Morevoer, there is a great deal of homology at the protein level, and more recently, recombinant DNA methods have shown that there is homology between the genes that code for the proteins expressed in different cell types. When we refer to muscle specific gene expression, we are dealing with the expression of certain proteins to form a highly specific physiological entity, the skeletal muscle fiber in distinction to very similar proteins that are forming structures and performing rather diverse functions in non-muscle cells. These phenomena can also be analyzed phylogenetically.

Figure 62 shows the sequential branching appearance of life forms: viruses, bacteria, plants and on up the ladder of the metazoa. Proteins such as actin and myosin, as well as many other

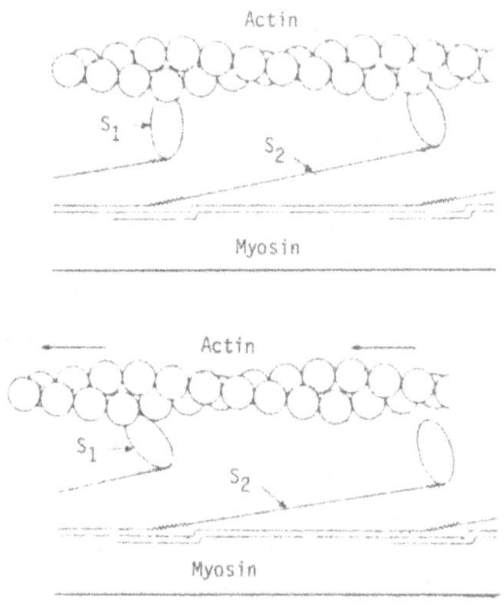

FIGURE 61

proteins discovered originally in skeletal muscle appear throughout eukaryotic phylogeny with a high degree of homology. The adaptive and specialized forces that operated to produce these diverse species have led to very different structures being formed from these homologous proteins.

Recombinant DNA has permitted analysis of myosin heavy chains from nematode, insect, avian and mammalian species including human. The technique has shown that there is a great deal of homology, for example, between the rod region of the major nematode myosin heavy chain and the homologous region in rabbit skeletal muscle myosin (490). There is about 32% identity of the derived amino acid sequences. In the DNA sequence encoding the myosin head, the so-called subfragment-1 region, the identity is about 47%. Recombinant DNA is a powerful tool for comparing the structures of genes through a vast array of organisms.

Throughout the histological and phylogenetic diversity, there persists a common basic structure of myosin. Each molecule contains two heavy chains and usually two copies of each of two kinds of light chains.

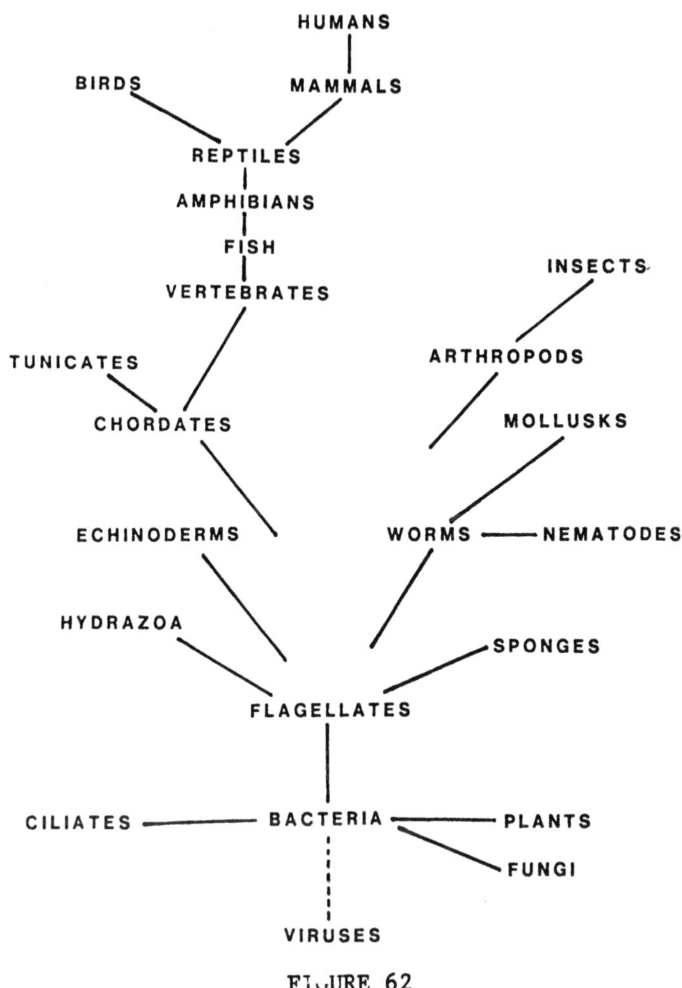

FIGURE 62

Only one exception has been found to this basic myosin structure, the so-called myosin type 1 of Acanthamoeba which seems not to have two copies of the heavy chain (491). It is more like a one-half molecule of myosin, and perhaps this protein is a pre-myosin. Even in Acanthamoeba there is a Type 11 myosin which more closely resembles the more general myosin structure that prevails from Dictyostelium (slime mold) all the way up to humans in a vast variety of cell types, including muscle, nerve, fibroblast, etc.

One very critical issue is how are such diverse structures derived from actins which have 95% amino acid sequence homology from Acanthamoeba to rabbit skeletal muscle and myosin heavy chains which also have a high degree of homology from nematodes to rabbits. Part of the explanation may lie in the isoform differences we have been discussing. Another major part of the explanation may be that actin and myosin molecules exist in a milieu of interacting proteins that may differ from cell to cell and from species to species leading to characteristic structures.

Table 10 is a listing of some of the different kinds of protein that are known to interact with myosin. F-actin was discovered as the activator of myosin ATP-induced viscosity change (492). In addition, there are myosin light chain kinases that markedly influence the enzymatic activity in certain non-muscle and smooth muscle systems.

From this viewpoint, myosin light chains may be considered accessory proteins which interact with the basic myosin structure within the dimer of heavy chains, thereby modulating enzymatic and other properties. Myosin light chain kinase has been shown to regulate smooth muscle turkey gizzard myosin and also certain non-muscle myosins in vitro. Phosphorylation in myosin heavy chain as an effect in Dictyostelium opposite to that of the light chain phosphorylation in other systems. There are proteins in muscle that clearly interact stoichiometrically with myosin. A classic example is paramyosin. Vertebrates are one sub-phylum of metazoa where paramyosin has not been demonstrated in muscle.

Dr. Fischman has discussed C proteins which have a specific stoichiometry to myosin in many vertebrate skeletal muscle thick filaments. There are several so-called M band proteins that cross-link myosin filaments in vertebrate skeletal muscles. The array of thick filaments in the muscles certainly requires the intrinsic properties of myosin and actin, but additional proteins must interact for the organization at the filament and lattice level.

Our work has been on the nematode, Caenorhabditis elegans. It is a simple organism 1.5 mm long and 100 µm wide with a well-defined set of cells. Mutants affecting muscle can be analyzed and assigned to specific loci upon the organism's six chromosome pairs. Many of these issues about isoforms have to deal with stages of different muscles and between different types of muscles.

With respect to myosin heavy chain isoforms in this system, we have evidence that the two isoforms form only homodimeric myosin molecules (493). Previous immunochemical studies with polyclonal antibodies indicated all body muscle cells and probably all sarcomeres seem to contain both isoforms (494).

TABLE 10

Proteins that Interact with Myosin

Proteins that influence ATPase activity _in vitro_:

F-actin

myosin light chains

myosin light chain kinase

Proteins regulating myosin polymerization _in vitro_:

myosin light chain kinase

myosin heavy chain kinase

myosin heavy chain phosphatase

Proteins interacting stoichiometrically with myosin in filaments:

paramyosin

C protein

H protein

Z protein

end filament protein

core proteins

myosin light chains

Proteins linking myosin filaments:

M band proteins

myomesin

creatine kinase MM isoform

Using the monoclonal antibodies, we have verified that indeed not only do all body wall muscle cells and their sarcomeres contain these two isoforms, but the two isoforms appear specifically localized within the sarcomeres.

When monoclonal antibody 28-2 is incubated with immunoblots of a mixture of proteins, we find only material at the uppermost myosin heavy chain band is reacted. This material is specifically the B myosin heavy chain within the band, verified by the fact that only the specifically mutant band of the E675 strain reacts with the monoclonal antibody (Figure 63). No protein reacts when there is no chemically detectable B isoform as in the E190 mutant. In contrast, the monoclonal antibody 5-6 reacts with only the upper band representing A myosin heavy chain in all three of these situations (495).

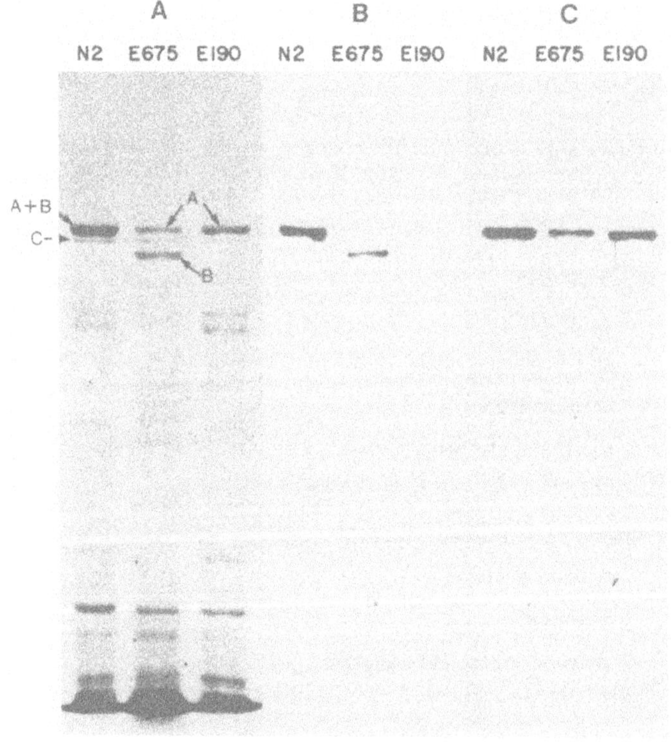

FIGURE 63

As an example, the same cell has been reacted with the two monoclonal antibodies (Figure 64). In the first instance, it was reacted with monoclonal antibody 28-2. The outer edges of A bands are reacted, but there is a fine gap at the center of the A band. The monoclonal antibody 5-6 reacts with that central region only (495).

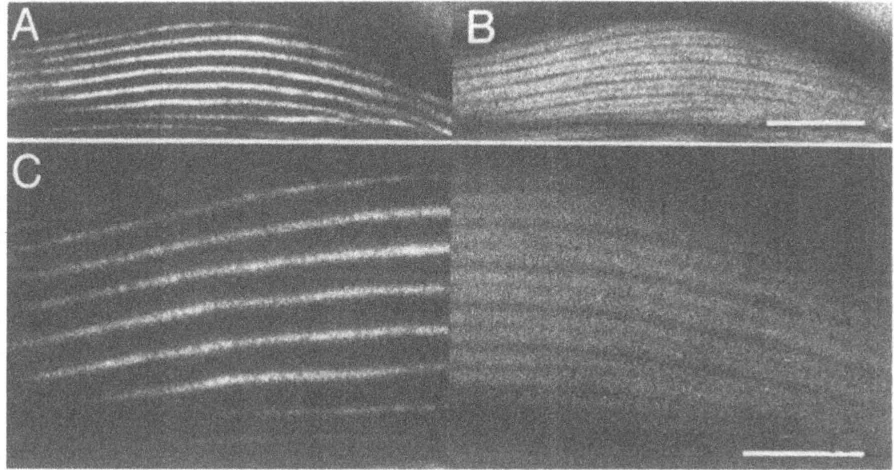

FIGURE 64

These results are verified at the electron microscopic level with isolated thick filaments. The antimyosin B antibody reacts with the polar 4.4 μm segments of each thick filament whereas the anti- A myosin reacts only with the central 1.8 μm of each filament.

One interpretation of these localization results is that indeed the isoforms are within all the same filaments but in different places on these filaments. As pointed out by Dr. Fischman, an alternative explanation could be that there are different packing arrangements of each myosin along the filament zones; therefore, zones of differential reactivity would represent regions of differential accessibility because of changes in packing. We have verified that we can isolate from the mutant E190 filaments that contain only myosin A; the antimyosin A monoclonal antibody reacts along the entire length of these filaments. There does not seem to be any necessary inaccessibility in one part of the filament or another of myosin A to this antibody.

In salt dissociation experiments, we can solubilize 80% of the myosin and 90% of the paramyosin leaving a central stub that reacts only with the myosin A. In addition to the myosins and paramyosin, some material forms a core structure that emanates from the central stub all the way to the end, about 4 μm in either direction. This material does not react with any of our antibodies to myosin or paramyosin and seems to be composed of presently unidentified protein. This new structure and paramyosin appear necessary for the regulated assembly of myosin into very long filaments. (Figure 65).

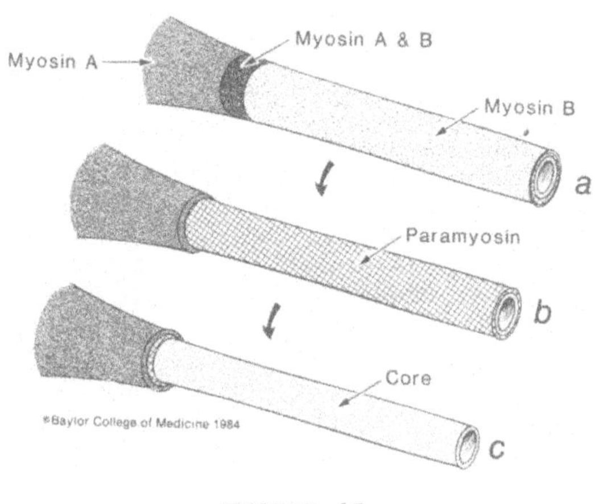

FIGURE 65

We are now examining various other mutants including mutants that are not in the unc-54 structural gene for myosin heavy chain B which lies on chromosome 1 but affect unc-52, an apparent regulatory gene, on chromosome II. These mutations depress the amount of myosin B produced. The result seems to be to block the aggregation of myosin into organized filament arrays within sarcomeres (496).

We plan to test the hypothesis that both myosin isoforms are necessary for the normal structure of thick filaments and, once assembled, for these filaments to be organized into the regular arrays of developing sarcomeres.

CHAPTER 19: A SET OF ACTIN-FILAMENT ASSOCIATED PROTEINS CHARACTERIZED BY QUANTITATIVE TWO-DIMENSIONAL GEL ELECTROPHORESIS

James I. Garrels, Shigeko Yamashiro-Matsumura,
Jim J.-C. Lin and Fumio Matsumura

Cold Spring Harbor Laboratory
Cold Spring Harbor, New York

Our laboratories have been using two-dimensional gel electrophoresis and monoclonal antibody techniques for the study of contractile and structural proteins. The resolving power of the two-dimensional gels, combined with computer methods for quantitation and pattern matching, have been used in previous studies to analyze the proteins of cultured L6 muscle cells as they differentiate from myoblasts to myotubes (453,497,498). Highly specific monoclonal antibodies have made possible the identification and biochemical characterization of major and minor structural proteins. Matsumura et al (1983) have used the monoclonal antibodies to tropomyosins to identify 5 isoforms that are present in several rat cell lines (499). These results confirm and extend the earlier identification of tropomyosin isoforms in L6 myoblasts (453). Matsumura et al (1983) have further shown that actin-filament assemblies can be purified from non-muscle and muscle cells as ordered bundles cross-linked in a highly regular fashion by monoclonal antibodies to tropomyosin. (500). This report combines the data obtained by computer-analyzed two-dimensional electrophoresis of differentiating L6 muscle cells with the identification of minor actin-binding proteins revealed by the monoclonal antibody technique. An interesting and previously undescribed set of phosphorylated, myotube-specific actin-filament associated proteins have been identified.

In Figure 66 the acidic proteins (having isoelectric points lower than 6.0) of L6 cells are shown at three stages of differentiation. These cells have been allowed to incorporate [^{35}S]-methionine over a 2 hour interval before harvest for 2D gel analysis. The skeletal muscle alpha- and beta-tropomyosins,

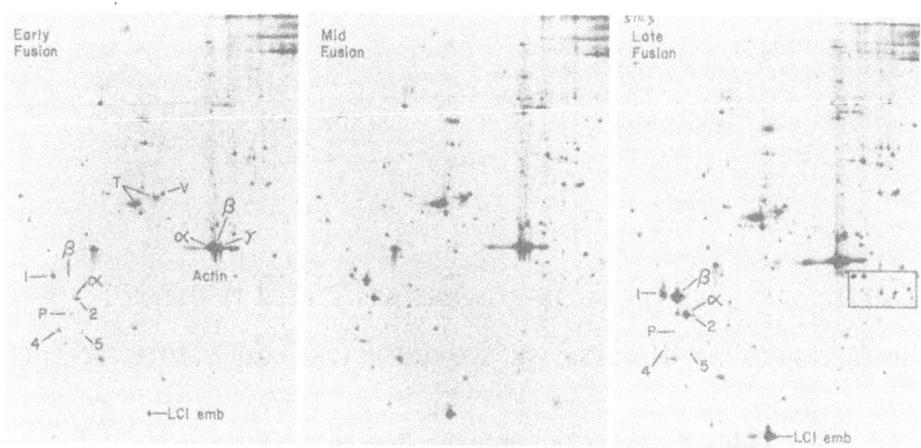

FIGURE 66: Protein changes during differentiation. Cultured L6 cells were labelled with [^{35}S]-methionine for 2 hr at 4.5, 7.5, and 11.5 days after plating. The proteins were resolved on two-dimensional gels containing pH 5-7 ampholytes in the first dimension. The identified proteins are actins (alpha, beta and gamma), tubulins (T), vimentin (V), PCNA (P), embryonic myosin light chain (LC1emb), and the tropomyosin cluster containing the skeletal muscle forms, alpha and beta, and the myoblast forms (TM-1 through TM-5. Acidic proteins are on the left.

and the 5 non-muscle forms are indicated at the left of each panel. The actins, tubulins, vimentin, and one myosin light chain are also visible on the gels shown. The protein PCNA, labeled "P", is a recently identified proliferation- and transformation-sensitive protein (501-503). The increase of muscle-specific proteins and the decrease of the non-muscle tropomyosins and PCNA are readily apparent during fusion.

In the region just below and more basic than actin (see box in Figure 66) is a group of proteins induced during L6 myogenesis. The 6 major induced proteins in this region are indicated by arrows in Figure 67b. It can be seen that the 6 spots occur as 3 pairs, suggesting that one member of each pair has been altered by a post-translational modification. Further information was provided by phosphate-labeling, using the isotope [^{33}P) which provides sharper spots than 32P (Figure 67c). Phosphate incor-

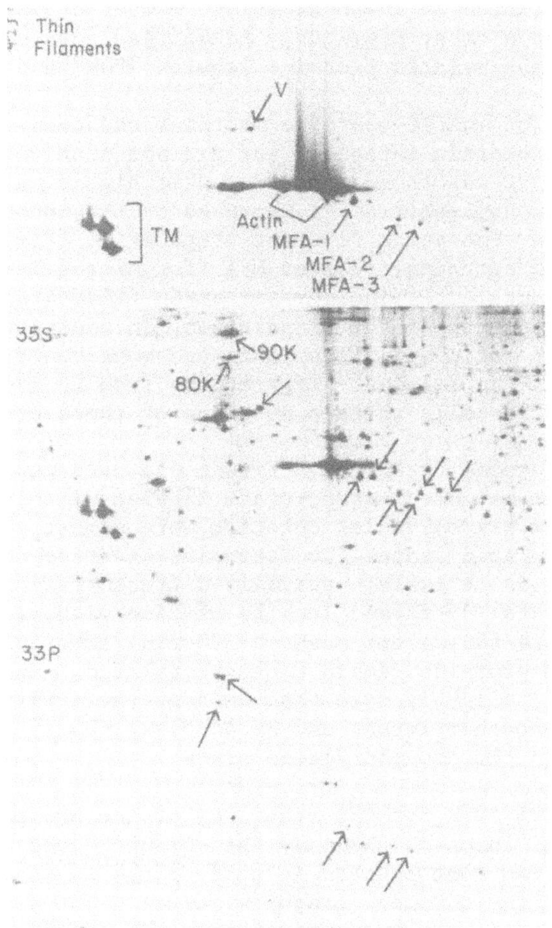

FIGURE 67: A group of myotube-specific proteins is phosphorylated and associated with actin-filaments. Proteins of purified thin filament preparations (top) are aligned with the pattern of total cellular proteins at mid-fusion (middle). Each of the MFA proteins (upward arrows) is accompanied by a more basic spot (downward arrows). Labeling with [^{33}P]-phosphate reveals that only the acid number of each MFA pair contains phosphate (bottom panel). L6 myotube proteins were labeled for 16 hr before actin-filament purification as described (500), proteins resolved in the middle panel were radio-labeled for 2 hr, and [^{33}P]-phosphate labeling was carried out for 24 hr in reduced-phosphate medium.

poration was detected in the most acidic member of each pair, as well as in some other previously identified phosphoproteins, such as the stress-related proteins labeled "80K" and "90K".

This group of muscle-specific proteins had been entered as part of our rat protein database, but did not receive any special attention until it was found that they were highly enriched in actin filaments prepared from L6 myotubes by the monoclonal antibody method. The actin filament preparation (Figure 67a) shows that these proteins, labeled MFA (for microfilament-associated, using non-muscle terminology for actin filaments), are significant components of the preparation, in addition to large amounts of actin and tropomyosin and some contaminating vimentin (V). Actin filament preparations from L6 myoblasts or from non-muscle cells reveals no trace of these components.

The MFA proteins detected in Figure 67a were purified from L6 myotubes that had been steady-state labeled with [^{35}S]-methionine. The MFA molecules detected were almost entirely in the phosphorylated state. To determine the time-course of phosphorylation in L6 cells, partially-differentiated cells were labeled for several different lengths of time with [^{35}S]-methionine. As seen in Figure 68a, after a short (30 min) labeling period, most of the MFA proteins remain unphosphorylated. During a 2 hour labeling period, slightly more than half of the newly synthesized molecules are phosphorylated, and by 4 hours, nearly all labeled molecules are in the phosphorylated state.

Quantitative data for the stability of the phosphorylated and unphosphorylated forms is shown by the computer-generated graphs in Figure 69. The spot pattern is part of the L6 standard map, as displayed on the computer graphics screen. The user selects any experiment that has been entered into the protein database and can select any spots visible on the screen. The computer reports the radioactivity of the spot as a fraction of the total TCA-precipitable radioactivity in the applied sample. For short labeling periods, the value reported is proportional to rate of synthesis; for long labeling periods, it is proportional to steady-state abundance of the protein. Each graph represents the radioactivity in one spot, plotted for each sample prepared as part of the selected experiment. (The graphs are plotted so

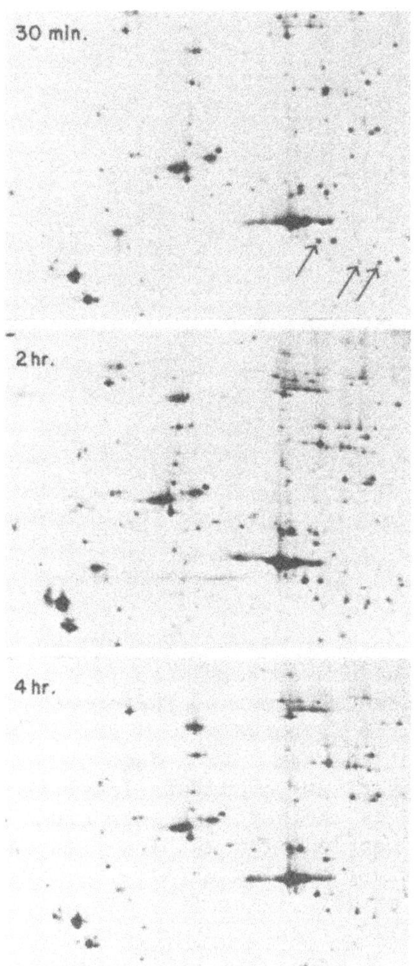

FIGURE 68: Unphosphorylated MFA proteins do not accumulate in L6 cells. Mid-fusion cells were labeled for the times indicated, and the proteins were resolved on pH 5-7 gels. The phosphorylated MFA forms (arrows) are under-represented at 30 min relative to longer labeling periods. The unphosphorylated forms contain less radioactivity, relative to surrounding spots, in the longer labelings.

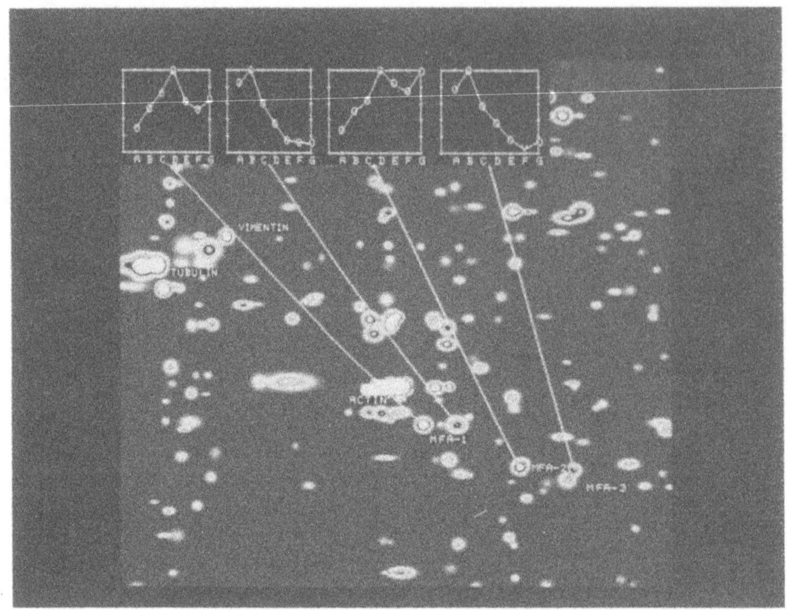

FIGURE 69: Quantitation of the MFA proteins. Phosphorylated and unphosphorylated forms of MFA-1 and MFA-2 have been selected on the computer graphics screen, and the database values are displayed as the graphs at the top. Each data point represents the disintegrations per minute (dpm) in the one spot divided by the total protein radioactivity in the applied sample. The samples plotted represent labeling periods of 30 min (A), 1 hr (B), 2 hr (C), 4 hr (D), 8 hr (E), 16 hr (F), and 24 hr (G). Each graph is scaled to put the highest data point at full scale. At 1 hr, the radioactive incorporation in the 4 indicated MFA forms (in parts per million of total protein radioactivity) was: MFA-1 phosphorylated, 706, MFA-1 unphosphorylated, 788; MFA-2 phosphorylated, 293; MFA-2 unphosphorylated, 365.

that the highest point on each graph is at full scale, but the numerical values of each data point are simultaneously reported on a terminal). The data plotted in Figure 69 indicates that the phosphorylated forms of MFA-1 and MFA-2 are accumulating, relative to total protein, for a period of about 4 hours after synthesis, after which their relative levels are reasonably steady. The unphosphorylated forms represent a much higher fraction of radioactivity in a short (30 min) labeling period than in a longer (2-24 hr) labeling period, indicating that they do not accumulate. These data suggest that the unphosphorylated forms are being converted to phosphorylated forms. A pulse-chase experiment (not shown) has confirmed that [^{35}S]-methionine incorporated into the unphosphorylated forms during a short pulse can be detected in the phosphorylated forms after a "chase" in (non-radioactive) media.

The newly-identified actin-filament associated proteins do not appear to correspond to any previously-described contractile proteins. We have not yet surveyed other muscle lines or tissues for their presence, but they have not been detected in several rat (non-muscle) cell types. It will be of interest to determine the time of phosphorylation relative to the assembly of newly-synthesized molecules onto actin filaments. Possibly the phosphorylation is involved in the mechanism of assembly, but it might also be essential for the functional regulation of the molecules. The highly phosphorylated state of the MFA proteins argues against their role as dynamic regulators of function, but it is possible that in immature L6 myotubes the mechanism which regulates the state of phosphorylation is not yet developed. Further quantitative electrophoresis work can reveal more about the regulation of synthesis, modification, and turnover of these molecules, and further biochemical work can begin to clarify their functional role in the contractile apparatus of muscle cells.

DR. BLAU: I am a little concerned that the relative change, even relating a protein to total incorporation, may not be very good. We know for instance in myogenesis, protein synthesis changes so you may be getting changes in the amount of total protein.

DR. GARRELS: I am not saying anything about the absolute amount of proteins in the cell. We can only say that the incorporation into a particular protein is going up or going down relative to the incorporation into all of the protein of the cell.

DR. KEDES: You are talking about relative changes in specific proteins. Thus some proteins may be dropping although their relative percentage may be increasing.

DR. GARRELS: If total protein synthesis increases dramatically at some point, then it is possible that the absolute rate of synthesis per cell goes up for a protein, even though our graphs show a decline in relative synthesis.

DR. BUCKINGHAM: I have a question about the tropomyosins in the L6 cell line. Do I understand that the one tropomyosin spot is the one that you think is from the smooth muscle?

DR. GARRELS: Yes. The tropomyosin-1 form co-migrates under a variety of conditions with tropomyosin from smooth muscle.

DR. WOOD: Have you attempted to use this for studies on normal human muscle or dystrophic muscle?

DR. GARRELS: No. So far our studies have been mostly concentrated on rat as we are becoming familiar with the system and the changes during the differentiation.

DR. WOOD: Do you see this technique as being useful at some specific point in studying human muscle?

DR. GARRELS: Yes, definitely. If you have pure populations of cells, dystrophic vs. normal, I think there is a good chance that you will see differences. There may be more differences than you expect so you may not know which are the primary ones.

DR. FISCHMAN: I gather there is still a discrepancy between a known number of mRNAs predicted from hybridization and the number of spots detected on the gels. I was wondering how close you are coming now to correlating the known number of unique messengers and the known number of spots?

DR. GARRELS: I'm not sure there is really a discrepancy. We have not fully catalogued all of the spots from our gels. We will have over 3000 spots in our standard map pretty soon. By fractionating cells, we can see many more proteins. There may be 5,000 to 10,000 possible spots from these cell fractions, although some represent modified forms of other proteins.

DR. HAUSCHKA: Using your critera for non-change how many proteins did change?

DR. GARRELS: Many of the proteins in any cell line we studied change from 2 to 4 fold, but you don't see many changes greater than 10-fold. About 5% of the proteins appear when the muscle cells fuse and about the same number will disappear in the myotube relative to the myoblast.

CHAPTER 20: MUSCLE GENE EXPRESSION IN HETEROKARYONS

Helen M. Blau, Choy-Pik Chiu, Grace K. Pavlath and Cecelia Webster

Department of Pharmacology
Stanford University School of Medicine
Stanford, CA

One approach to the study of how gene regulation occurs during muscle differentiation and development is to put a non-muscle cell into an environment where it is reprogrammed to synthesize muscle proteins, which it would never normally express. One way to do this is to fuse two cells together. In this talk I will show you how this kind of fusion system can be used to ascertain the requirements for gene expression and to address certain questions about the determination and differentiation.

Determination describes the transition from a stem cell with multiple options to a cell type which is restricted to a specific differentiation pathway. In the case of muscle, the determined cell is a myoblast which is restricted to the myogenic lineage. Under appropriate conditions, the myoblast undergoes a second transition, commitment, following which it differentiates to become a myotube and expresses muscle functions.

The most common product of cell fusion is the hybrid. Figure 70A shows the result usually obtained when a non-muscle cell and a myoblast are fused together using polyethylene glycol. First a binucleated cell is produced, which upon cell division yields a mononucleated cell called a synkaryon. This familiar type of hybrid has been particularly useful in the mapping of genes to specific chromosomes. However, there are two major problems in studying gene regulation with such hybrids:

Cell Hybrids

1. Extensive chromosome loss is common during the propagation of hybrids, especially when they are

formed between the cells of two different species. This unstable situation complicates studies of regulating the expression of a structural function or the gene coding for the structural function itself.

2. The earliest steps involved in gene activation cannot be analyzed. This is because hybrids are obtained following numerous cell divisions in a selective medium.

As an alternative approach we have taken advantage of the fact that in the course of differentiation myoblasts normally fuse to form multi-nucleated cells, or myotubes, in which there is no nuclear division. When a non-muscle cell, in this case an amniotic fibroblast, is fused with a myotube, a stable heterokaryon is obtained (Figure 70B). This multinucleated cell can exist in

Production of Heterokaryons

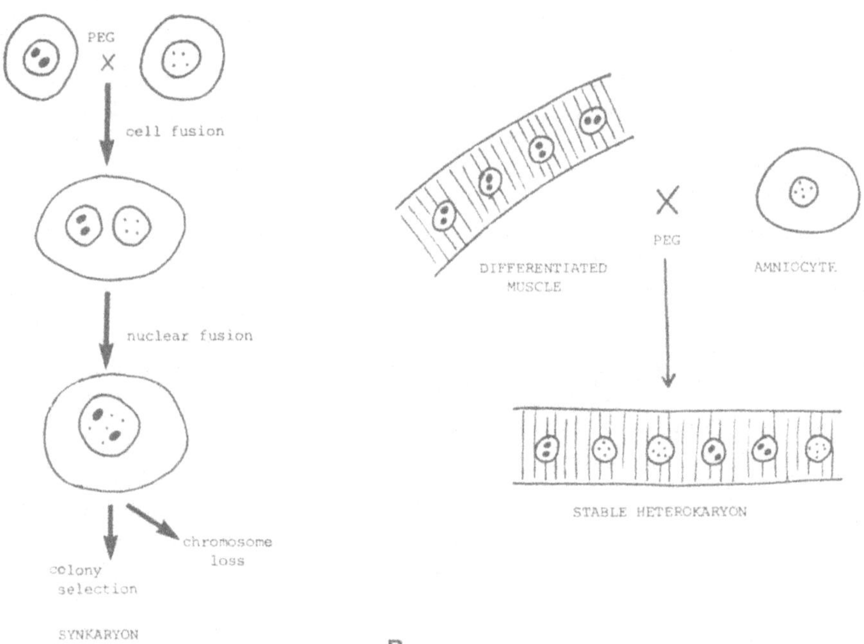

FIGURE 70: Formation of Synkaryons (A) and Heterokaryons (B) from Muscle Cells and Non-Muscle Cells.

culture for up to two weeks and will often actively contract. The advantages of a heterokaryon over a synkaryon are that one can analyze gene expression immediately after fusion, and that since there is no cell division, there is no chromosome loss. The result is a fusion product in which both the nuclear and cytoplasmic components of both cell types remain present.

We produce these heterokaryons by fusing the C2 line of mouse muscle cells isolated by Dr. Yaffe, with human amniotic fluid fibroblasts using polyethylene glycol (Figure 71). Selective agents, ouabain and cytosine arabinoside, are then added to eliminate the unfused parental cell types (474). The species difference between mouse and human nuclei enables us to confirm that the myotube is a heterokaryon composed of nuclei of the two cell types (Figure 72). The mouse muscle nuclei contain satellite DNA which has AT-rich sequences; consequently, when stained with Hoechst 33258, the mouse nuclei exhibit punctate fluorescence while the human nuclei appear uniformly stained. As a result, we can readily determine the precise number of mouse and human nuclei present in each heterokaryon. The frequency with which we get these heterokaryons in culture is 75 ± 2%. In other words, a very high proportion of the myotubes in the culture contain nuclei of both cell types, making possible studies of gene regulation in mass cultures.

In order to study the potential activation of human muscle genes in the non-muscle cell following fusion, species-specific markers were required. The first one we identified was creatine kinase (CK). Figure 73A shows a native polyacrylamide gel on which whole cell extracts from monolayer cultures were electrophoresed. We were able to visualize the CK isozymes using a coupled enzyme reaction with NADPH as its end-product. Since the enzyme is composed of two subunits, three isozymes are possible: BB is characteristic of non-muscle cells and undifferentiated myoblasts, MB of early differentiating myotubes, and MM of fully matured muscle. Amniocytes do not synthesize M subunits (lanes 1 and 2), and the mouse (lane 3) and human (lane 4) MM-CK bands have different mobilities and are readily distinguished by this assay.

CK Expression in Hybrids and Heterokaryons

Figure 73B shows the results of a fusion experiment. As a reference, the isozymes in an extract of cultured mouse and human muscle cells mixed in vitro is shown (lane 1); the MB and MM isozymes of the two species are distinct. Lane 2 shows a co-culture in which mouse myotubes and human fibroblasts were plated together but were not treated with polyethylene glycol. In the absence of fusion no activation of the human muscle CK occurs and

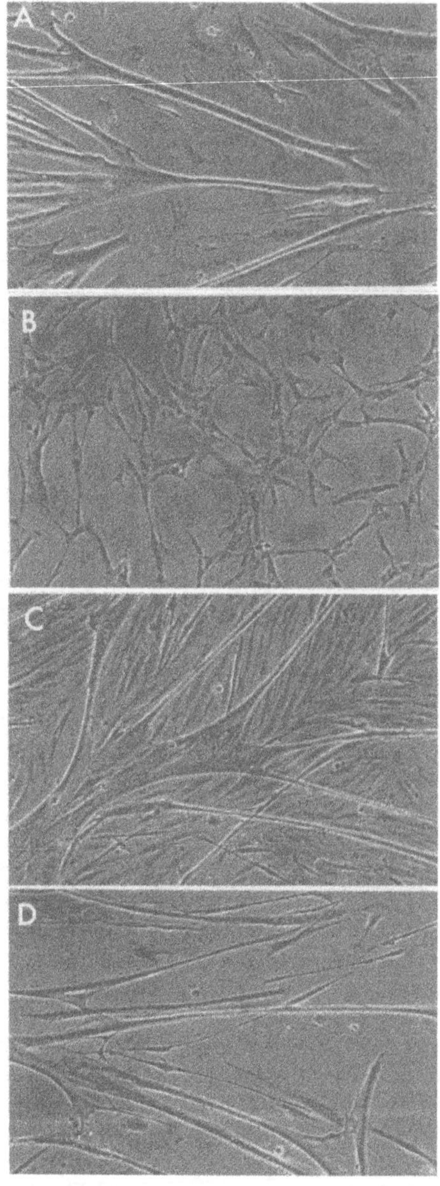

FIGURE 71: Formation of heterokaryons by fusion of mouse muscle cells and human amniocytes with PEG. Phase contrast micrographs of cells in vivo. Mouse myotubes (A), human amniocytes (B), confluent co-culture of myotubes and amniocytes just prior to PEG treatment (C), and the same culture six days after fusion with PEG and treatment with selective agents (D). (Mag X 500).

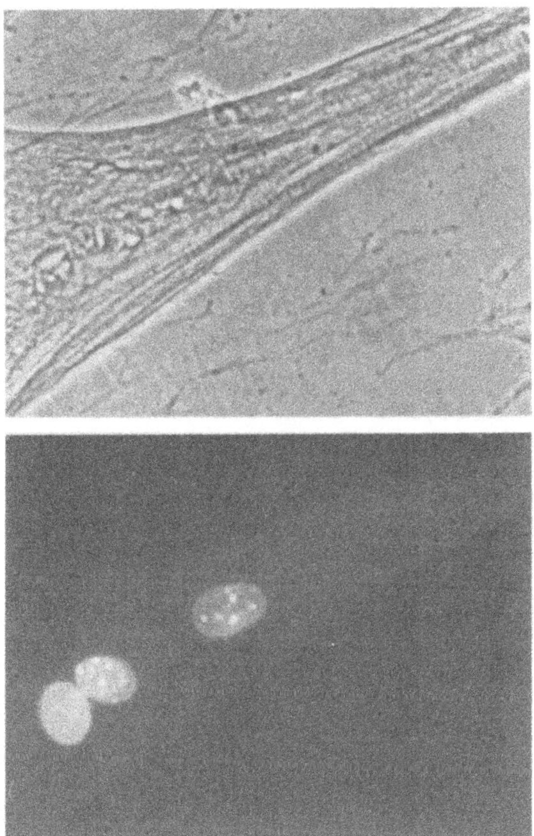

FIGURE 72: Mouse-Human Heterokaryons Stained with Hoechst 33258. Multinucleated myotubes are shown in phase contrast (bottom) and by fluorescence (top). Punctate mouse and uniformily stained human nuclei are clearly distinguished using the Hoechst stain (Mag X 70).

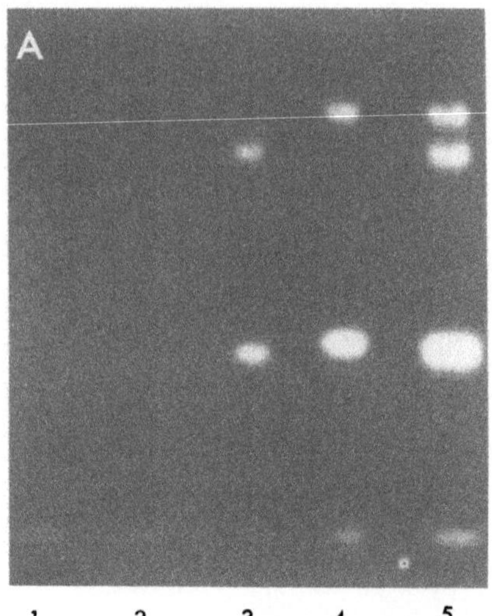

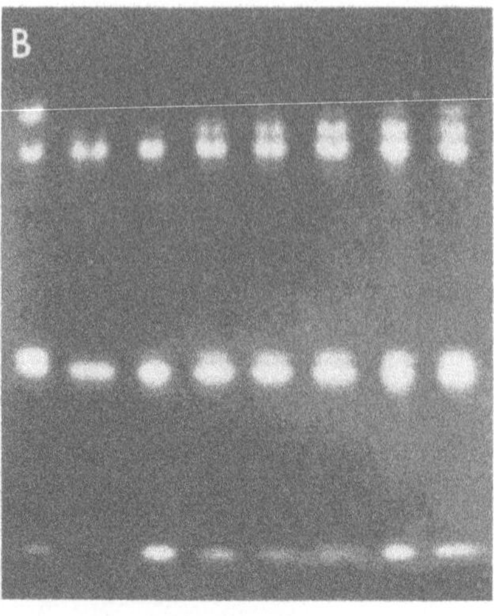

FIGURE 73: Expression of Human M-CK in Mouse-Human Heterokaryons. Whole cell extracts were subjected to electrophoresis on non-denaturing polyacrylamide gels for 4 hr (A) and 7 hr (B). CK isozymes (BB, MB, and MM) were detected with U.V. illumination using a coupled enzyme reaction with NADPH as its end product. A. Isozymes from amniocytes alone (lane 1), amniocytes + PEG (lane 2), cultured mouse muscle (lane 3), cultured human muscles (lane 4), and cultured mouse and human muscle extracts mixed in vitro (lane 5). B. Isozymes from cultured mouse muscle and human muscle mixed in vitro (lane 1); co-culture of mouse muscle and human amniocytes after six days without PEG (lane 2); heterokaryons of mouse muscle and human amniocytes at time intervals after PEG fusion: one day (lane 3), three days (lane 4), four days (lane 5), five days (lane 6); six days (lane 7); heterokaryons of mouse muscle and human muscle formed spontaneously (lane 8). Arrows indicate CK isozymes containing human subunits.

only the mouse isozymes are visible. Activation is not induced when the cells are merely present in the same culture dish; apparently there is no "activating factor" that is transmitted from one cell type to the other via the medium. The CK isozyme present in extracts from heterokaryons on different days after fusion are shown in lanes 3-6. One day following fusion a trace of the human MB isozyme is apparent and it progressively increases in amount on days 2 through 6. In addition, a novel isozyme in the MM region of the gel is evident and increases in amount with time after fusion. Finally, by day 6 there is a trace of the pure human MM isozyme. We reasoned that the novel isozyme with a mobility intermediate between the human and mouse MM-CK might be composed of M subunits of both species. In order to test this possibility we grew mouse muscle cells and human muscle cells in the same dish and found that the muscle cells recognized each other and spontaneously fused. The isozymes in these spontaneous heterokaryons included pure human, the hybrid, and pure mouse MM-CK. Thus, the novel isozyme is a hybrid enzyme composed of mouse and human subunits and it is a functional enzyme, since the assay is based on enzyme activity. From this type of experiment we concluded that by fusing human fibroblasts into the mouse muscle myotubes, the gene coding for the human M-CK subunit was activated.

We then studied the expression of structural proteins of the contractile apparatus which could be distinguished for the two species. Figure 74A shows immunoblots (504) of two-dimensional gels of the proteins produced by muscle cultures from human, mouse, and mixed extracts of the cultured muscle cells of both species. The electrophoretically transferred proteins were reacted with a monoclonal antibody, generously provided to us by Dr. Frank Stockdale, which recognizes the myosin light chains of both species. Using this antibody it is possible to distinguish the human and mouse isoforms of four distinct myosin light chains: one slow, two fast and a fetal myosin light chain (70) that differ in their electrophoretic mobility. These differences provide a means for determining whether the human genes coding for myosin light chains have been activated in heterokaryons.

Myosin Light Chain Expression

Figure 74B shows the myosin light chains synthesized in heterokaryons. Autoradiograms of ^{35}S-methionine labeled proteins are compared for cultures of the human aminocyte and mouse muscle parental cell types and for heterokaryons formed between the two. As indicated, in the heterokaryons, but not in the parental cells, human myosin light chains Ls, 2f, fetal and trace of 2s were synthesized. Thus, we have evidence that genes coding for four distinct human muscle myosin proteins are activated in the heterokaryon.

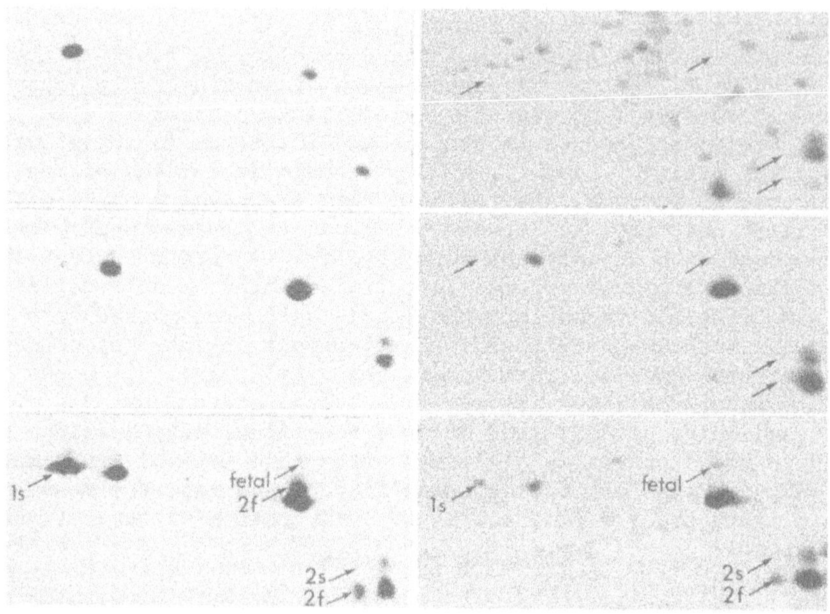

FIGURE 74: Expression of human myosin light chains in mouse-human heterokaryons. Left: Identification of myosin light chains on immunoblots. Contractile proteins were partially purified from cultured human muscle (top), cultured mouse muscle (middle), and cultured mouse and human muscle mixed in vitro (bottom) and electrophoresed on two-dimensional gels. Myosin light chains of human and mouse species were identified on Western blots using a monoclonal antibody to myosin light chains and a second antibody coupled to horse radish peroxidase. Right: Myosin light chain synthesis in heterokaryons. Human amniocytes + PEG (top); mouse muscle cells + PEG (middle); heterokaryons four days after fusion with PEG (bottom). Cultured cells were labeled with ^{35}S-methionine, the contractile proteins partially purified, fractionated on two-dimensional gels, and processed for autoradiography. Proteins were identified by co-migration with unlabeled contractile protein standards. Amniocyte proteins were coextracted with unlabeled mouse muscle proteins to ensure precipitation of contractile proteins. Mouse muscle cells and heterokaryons were grown in the presence of ouabain and cytosine arabinoside. Electrophoresis of gels in A and in B was performed at separate times. The positions of the human myosin light chains are indicated by arrows. Myosin light chains 1s, 2f and fetal are clearly induced in heterokaryons; a trace of 2s is also evident.

From these results we can draw a number of conclusions. We estimate from the ratios of mouse to human CK isozymes and the average ratios of the nuclei of the two species that almost every human nucleus incorporated into a heterokaryon is activated to express human muscle functions. Since the nuclei of the heterokaryon remain separate and distinct, activation occurs via the cytoplasm. Moreover, the presence of the activator in muscle cells which have already differentiated suggests that it may be important not only for the initiation of myogenesis, but als for the continued expression of the muscle phenotype. Activation occurs across species; the mouse muscle activator is capable of gaining access to a foreign nucleus of a different cell type and of a different species, suggesting that the molecule(s) is highly conserved. Activation involves reporgramming cells not normally destined to be muscle. The human amniotic fibroblast would never normally express muscle functions and yet it has been programmed to do so in response to the mouse muscle cytoplasm. In summary, we conclude that muscle cytoplasmic components are capable of dramatically altering the function of the nucleus and inducing the expression of a number of different proteins and that the nucleus is highly responsive to such cytoplasmic cues.

We have taken advantage of the heterokaryon system to ask certain questions about the requirements for cell determination. In particular, we have asked whether specific changes in the genome that require DNA synthesis accompany the transition from "stem" cell to determined myoblast. The experiments described thus far emphasize the importance of the cytoplasm. In the experiments described below, we are exploring the role of the nucleus in gene expression. Specifically, we are asking whether the nucleus must undergo a sequence of changes associated with one or more rounds of DNA replication in order to express muscle functions. Is there a requirement for the amniotic fluid fibroblasts to replicate their DNA in order to activate and express muscle genes?

To address this question we examined what happens to gene expression in heterokaryons when DNA synthesis is inhibited. Amniotic fibroblasts were fused with mouse muscle cells and the heterokaryons were labeled with tritiated thymidine immediately following fusion. We were able to identify the nuclei contributed by each species by their fluorescent staining pattern and to monitor DNA synthetic activity in these nuclei by their autoradiographic labeling pattern (Figure 75). With our conditions for autoradiography, a cell which as undergone only one-fifth of a round of replication can be detected (505). Three different experiments were carried out in which amniocytes were exposed to an inhibitor of DNA synthesis, cytosine arabinoside (ara-c), 24 hr prior to and continuously after fusion with mouse myotubes. Control cultures were not treated with ara-c until 24 hrs after fusion. Heterokaryons were labeled with 3H-thymidine for the first 24 hours after fusion, cultured for a total of 4 or 6 days, fixed, processed for autoradiography, and scored for the percent of labeled amniocytes they contained. In the presence of ara-c, DNA synthesis, as determined by the incorporation of isotope into TCA precipitable counts, was reduced to 1% of control levels (505). The expression of CK isozymes in these heterokaryons was compared and found to be equivalent whether or not DNA synthesis was inhibited (Figure 76).

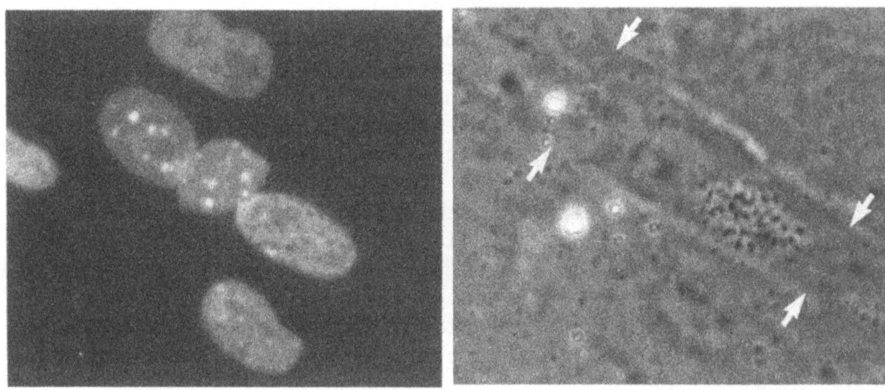

FIGURE 75: Detection of DNA Synthesis in Mouse-Human Heterokaryons. Heterokaryons were labeled with ^{3}H-thymidine for 1 hr and immediately fixed, processed for autoradiography and stained with Hoechst 33258. A multinucleated heterokaryon containing two punctate mouse nuclei and one uniformly stained human nucleus is shown by fluorescence microscopy (left). The same heterokaryon (outlined by arrows) viewed with phase contrast optics reveals the presence of silver grains over the human nucleus indicating that it synthesized DNA during the labeling period (right).

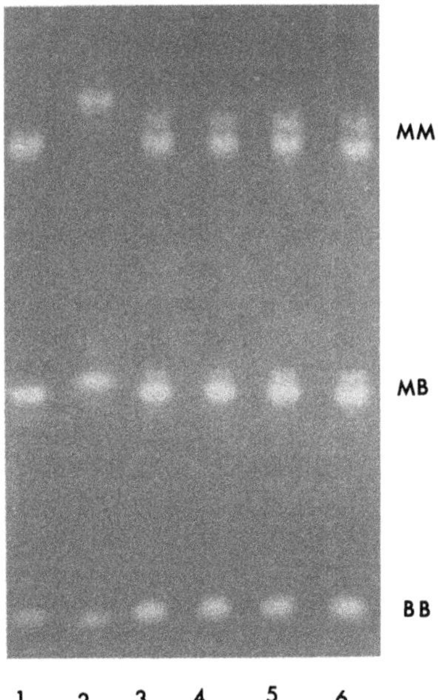

FIGURE 76: Expression of Human M-CK Gene in the Absence of DNA Synthesis. CK isozymes were analyzed as described in Figure 73, and equal enzyme activity was loaded (Lanes 1 and 2) standard CK isozymes from cultured mouse and human muscle respectively. (Lanes 3 and 5) ara-c treated heterokaryons 4 and 6 days after fusion (Lanes 4 and 6) control heterokaryons 4 and 6 days after fusion.

From these results we conclude that DNA replication is not required for a non-muscle cell such as an amniotic fibroblast to make muscle proteins. In other words, changes in the chromatin structure of the genes which depend on DNA synthesis, such as methylation (506), need not occur.

We then developed methods for examining gene expression at the single cell level in individual heterokaryons. This permitted us to determine definitively whether DNA replication is required for gene activation. In these studies we fused a different strain of human fibroblast, the MRC-5 from fetal lung, with the mouse myotubes. We assayed the expression of a human muscle cell surface antigen, 5.1H11 using a monoclonal antibody generously provided to us by Dr. Frank Walsh (507). Figure 77 shows that the antibody reacts with human myotubes, but not with either of the parental cell types used in the heterokaryons. It is therefore a good marker for the activation of a human muscle specific gene.

As shown in Figure 78, the human cell surface antigen is expressed in heterokaryons. We studied the activation of 5.1H11 in individual heterokaryons in four separate series of experiments (Table 11). Gene activation occurred at high frequency; in fact, greater than 93% of the heterokaryons in each experiment expressed 5.1H11. Yet, only a very small proportion (<20%) of these heterokaryons contained labeled nuclei. Clearly, gene activation was a very frequent phenomenon when a human fibroblast nucleus was contained in a muscle cell, and DNA synthesis was not required.

The analysis of individual heterokaryons has resulted in some particularly interesting and unexpected findings. First, as shown in Figure 78A, heterokaryons can contain more fibroblast than muscle nuclei and still exhibit human muscle gene activation. In fact, activation has been observed at every conceivable nuclear ratio; all that is required is that human non-muscle and mouse muscle nuclei share the same cytoplasm. Second, activation of the human muscle gene for the 5.1H11 antigen can occur in a nucleus which as undergone a round of DNA replication, evident from the intensity of ^{3}H-thymidine labeling revealed by autoradiography (505). Figure 78B shows a heterokaryon in which gene activation occurred when only one human nucleus was present and that nucleus was heavily labeled. Since no mitotic figures have been observed in heterokaryons, this nucleus must have been in either the S or G2 phases of the cell cycle.

In conclusion, it is evident from these experiments that DNA synthesis is not required for novel gene expression in heterokaryons. This raises questions about mechanisms of gene activation during differentiation that are thought to require DNA synthesis, such as changes in methylation. It also raises questions about many long-held assumptions regarding changes in chromatin conformation in the course of stem cell determination. Finally, contrary to several reports (49,508) we find that novel muscle gene expression can occur in phases of the cell cycle other than G1.

DR. KUNKEL: I have a question related to the definition of activation. I think it could be re-defined a little bit since there still may be mRNA in those amniotic fibroblast cells. I noticed that the pictures you showed had more human than mouse nuclei. You could be putting in a fair amount of mRNA from amniocytes, although I am not saying you are. Have you looked with direct DNA probes, to see if those mRNAs are present in the cells before fusion?

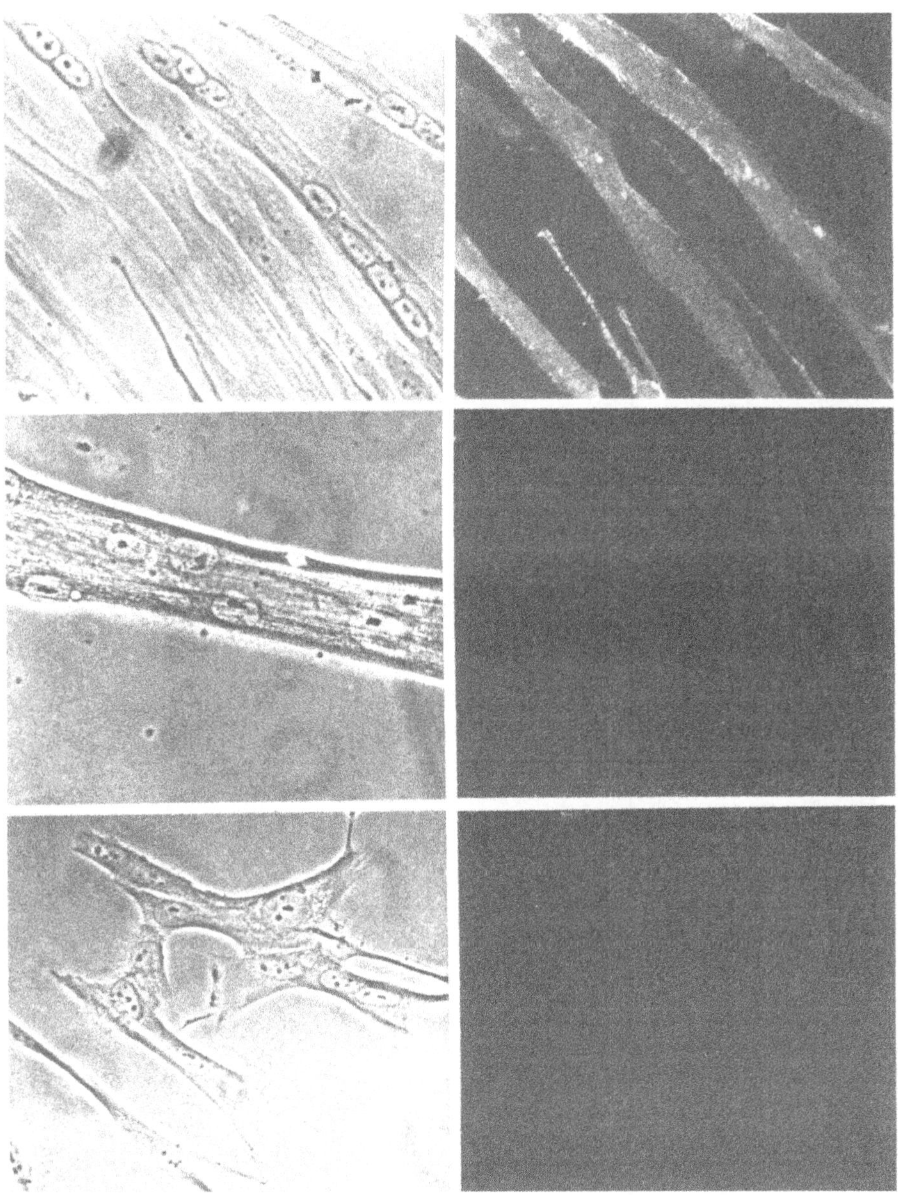

FIGURE 77: Specificity of 5.1H11 for Human Muscle Cells. Cells were incubated with the monoclonal antibody, 5.1H11, and stained with a rhodamine-conjugated second antibody. Cultured human muscle (top), cultured mouse muscle (middle), and MRC-5, human fetal lung fibroblasts (bottom) are shown in phase contrast (left) and fluorescence (right).

TABLE 11

DNA Synthesis and Human 5.1H11 Activation

Expt.[a]	Ara-c[b]	Heterokaryons Scored (n)[c]	Nuclei Scored[d]		% Heterokaryons[e]	Nuclear Ratio (M:H)[f]	% Hetero-karyons with labeled Nuclei[g]	% Hetero-karyons Expressing 5.1H11[h]
			M	H				
1 (A)	-	43	138	134	96	2:1	19	93
(B)	+	64	348	195	83	2:1	5	97
2 (A)	-	43	203	123	83	2:1	16	95
(B)	+	52	196	153	87	2:1	4	94

[a]Heterokaryons were produced by fusing mouse muscle cells with human fetal lung fibroblasts (MRC-5). Cells were labeled ^3H-thymidine for the first 48 hr following fusion. Heterokaryons were processed for autoradiography and assayed for 5.1H11 expression 4 days later.

[b](-) Heterokaryons were not exposed to ara-c until 24 hr after fusion. (+) Heterokaryons were exposed to ara-c prior to fusion for 1 hr (Expt.1) or 24 hr (Expts. 2-4) and continuously thereafter.

[c]Total number of heterokaryons scored (n). [d]Total number of mouse (M) and human (H) nuclei scored in all the heterokaryons. [e]Percent of total myotubes which were heterokaryons. [f]The ratio of mouse (M) to human (H) nuclei was determined for each heterokaryon and the mean ratio for each experiment is shown. [g]Percent of total heterokaryons which contained at least one labeled human nucleus. Nuclei with 10 or more grains, or 3-fold above background, were scored as labeled. [h]Percent of total heterokaryons which were positive for 5.1H11 by immunofluorescence.

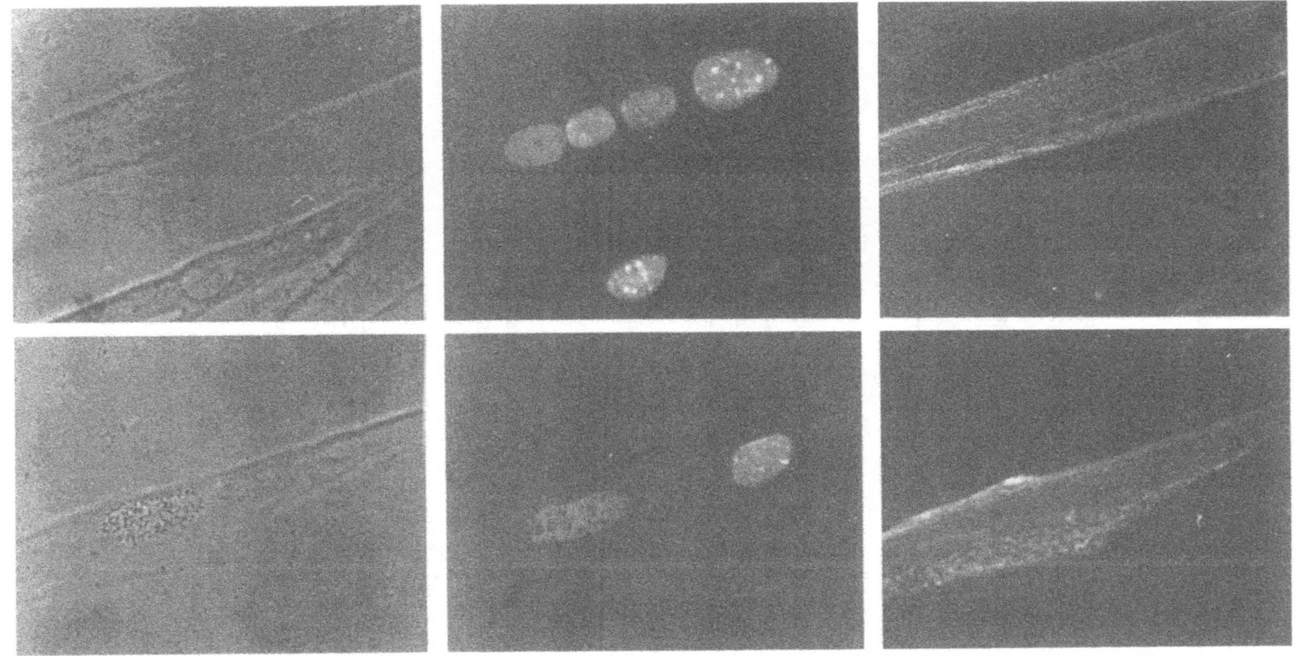

FIGURE 78: Activation of 5.1H11 (A) in the Absence of DNA Synthesis and (B) in Cell Cycle Phase other than G_1. Heterokaryons of mouse muscle and human fetal lung fibroblasts were labeled for 48 hr with ^{3}H-thymidine and assayed 4 days later for 5.1H11 by immunofluorescence and for DNA synthesis by autoradiography. Heterokaryons are shown with phase contrast optics (left), Hoechst fluorescence (middle) and rhodamine fluorescence (right). (A) Heterokaryon containing 1 mouse and 3 human nuclei (middle), of which none was autoradiographically labeled with silver grains (left), yet the heterokaryon expressed 5.1H11 (right). Note that the pure mouse myotube in the bottom of the field was not expressing 5.1H11. (B) Heterokaryon with 1 mouse and 1 human nucleus (middle), with >50 silver grains over the human nucleus (left), and expression of 5.1H11 was evident (right).

DR. BLAU: I understand your point. What you are questioning is the level of regulation, that is, whether it is transcriptional or post-transcriptional. I think activation is definitely occurring and that we are looking at the synthesis of novel gene products. However, soon we will be able to address that question directly using isotype and species-specific probes developed in Dr. Kedes' lab.

DR. KUNKEL: Are you really looking at activation of a specific gene or genes in the DNA of that cell? Is it necessary to use so many human cells to get high efficiency of fusion as well as any expression? If you use 1/10 the number of human cells in your fusion experiments, would you get the same results?

DR. BLAU: As I showed you in the final slide, gene activation is detected in single cells of widely differing nuclear ratios. In fact, we have observed human muscle gene expression in heterokaryons in which the muscle:non-muscle ratio was 25:1.

DR. KEDES: In regard to Dr. Kunkel's question about messages, I remember that Dr. Blau once pointed out to me regions on the 2-D gels of heterokaryons where non-muscle related human proteins characteristic of amniocytes did not appear. So it would seem highly coincidental or else would require a whole new mechanism of messenger leakage and specific messenger activation in muscle in order that human muscle proteins appear but human non-muscle proteins not show up on a 2D gel. The only ones that seem to show up are muscle-specific.

DR. BLAU: There is another point. Most of the evidence for stored mRNAs which are later activated is in oocytes. I don't think that there is much evidence that stored mRNAs exist in differentiated somatic cells.

DR. KUNKEL: I actually wasn't referring to stored RNAs in large quantities. I was referring to only trace quantities, 3 to 4 messengers per cell of the human origin for those particular genes that wouldn't be translated into protein in a normal cell. I was referring to the ratios of cells that went in.

DR. BLAU: Even when there is only one human nucleus in a heterokaryon we still see human muscle gene expression.

DR. EPSTEIN: You don't really know per heterokaryon what is actually being expressed, you only know that in a mass sort of way.

DR. BLAU: No, that isn't so. The data presented in the last part of my talk was all based on single cell assays and gene expression in individual heterokaryons.

DR. HOLTZER: Why the one-way differentiation if indeed you have intervention? Why aren't the muscle nuclei now switched into an amniocyte?

DR. BLAU: We do not know that. As yet, we have no markers for amniocyte functions. With such markers it would be possible to determine whether coexpression of two phenotypes can occur and whether with excess non-muscle nuclei the muscle cell can also be reprogrammed.

DR. HOLTZER: We don't find very many striations in our heterokaryons. Do you find striations?

DR. BLAU: We observe very nice striations and active contractions as well. This is probably because our heterokaryon cells last for up to 12 days in culture.

DR. MAURO: How do you control the ratio of nuclei, just by fooling around with PEG and time exposure, etc?

DR. BLAU: No, the PEG protocol is constant and is not easily varied because it is highly toxic. We vary the ratio of cells on the dish prior to PEG treatment.

DR. FISCHMAN: Several people a number of years ago thought that instead of cloning the genes coding for hormones in bacteria that it would be possible to use hybridoma technology to make hormones. For example, one could fuse a myeloma cell with a pancreatic beta cell from an embryo, and get a system that would crank out insulin and be immortal. A number of people have tried those experiments and failed. It turns out you don't get insulin synthesis in that combination. People have done it with the hepatocyte too. When you fuse a hepatocyte with a myeloma cell, for example, you don't get liver specific gene expression. It is very puzzling.

DR. BLAU: Actually gene activation has been seen by some other people in hybrids, i.e. synkarons (509,510). Darlington has shown that if you fuse a mouse hepatoma cell with a human fibroblast, you can turn on the liver specific functions of the other species (510). However, I believe that our results constitute the first example of novel gene activation in a heterokaryon.

CHAPTER 21: MYOSIN ISOZYME TRANSITIONS IN DEVELOPING AND REGENERATING RAT MUSCLE

Robert G. Whalen*, Gillian S. Butler-Browne**, Lawrence B. Bugaisky*, John B. Harris** and Danielle Herliocoviez***

*Departement de Biologie Moleculaire, Institut Pasteur, Paris; **Muscular Dystrophy Laboratories, Newcastle General Hospital, Great Britain; ***Laboratoire de Neuropathologie, Chu Cote de Nacre, Caen, France

During the fetal and post-natal development of rat muscles, certain myosin isozymes are present which are distinct from the adult forms (380,381). The embryonic and neonatal myosins appear and disappear in an apparently sequential fashion, and, in the case of developing fast muscles, they are replaced by adult fast myosin (381). In order to study the metabolism of these proteins at the cellular level, we have prepared polyclonal antibodies to each of the developmental and adult forms and have used them in immunochemistry (214,511). Biochemical analyses have also been carried out, in many cases on the same muscles used for immunocytochemistry, to confirm the presence of those myosins detected by the antibodies. For these analyses, electrophoresis of native myosin (402,512) is particularly well suited, since it can be performed on unfractionated muscle extracts from relatively small amounts of tissue.

It is important to define the context of known myosin isozymes that are used to establish the specificity of the antibodies; this consideration is relevant whether one uses polyclonal or monoclonal antibodies. Our previous biochemical and immunochemical results established the existence of an embryonic myosin heavy chain, present in fetal muscle as well as in myotubes in cell culture, and a neonatal heavy chain found in muscle tissue beginning in late gestation and persisting into the third week after birth (380,381). We have thus prepared antibodies specific to these two forms. Our data do not exclude the possibility that each of these rat isozymes might be micro-heterogeneous, but currently no evidence suggests that they are. We have also obtained antibodies specific to adult fast and slow myosin. Protein sequence chemical data (514,515) have provided strong evidence for at least two fast heavy chain forms, which may correlate to the two histochemical types of fast fibers revealed by ATPase staining and referred to as type IIA and IIB (458). Our antibodies to adult fast myosin do in fact seem to react preferentially with certain adult fast fibers (511).

Development of Fast Myosin-Containing Fibers

We have used the antibodies against neonatal and adult fast myosin to examine the fiber distribution of these two myosins in the post-natal period when the transition between the two isozymes is occurring. Figures 79A,B show the immunocytochemical results obtained with the gastrocnemius muscle of a 22-day-old rat in a region composed of fibers destined to become the fast type. Approximately half of the fibers react with both antibodies, while about 25% react with only anti-neonatal and another 25% with only anti-fast (214). The presence of the doubly stained fibers strongly suggests that the neonatal - fast transition occurs within individual fibers, as opposed to the existence of two fiber populations each containing only one myosin type and which change their relative abundance during development. These results also illustrate that the neonatal - adult fast transition occurs asynchronously; that is in a small region of a single muscle some fibers already possess only fast myosin and others only neonatal myosin, while many contain both. The results of Figure 79 could therefore be interpreted as showing that the transition is initiated in different fibers at different times.

We have investigated the role of innervation in the neonatal to adult fast transition. Hind limb muscles of 7-day-old rats were denervated by cutting the sciatic nerve, and myosin types were analyzed by immunocytochemistry and electrophoresis of native myosin between 3 and 5 weeks of age. We find that denervation does not block this transition: adult fast myosin appears with approximately the same time course as in the innervated muscles, as judged by electrophoretic analysis (214). The neonatal myosin content also decreases although possibly less rapidly or less completely than with innervated muscles. Figures 79C,D illustrate that at 22 days after birth (about 2 weeks after denervation) nearly all the fibers in this region of the gastrocnemius muscle are stained by the neonatal and the fast myosin antibodies. This dual staining of all fibers at this time is a clear difference compared to the innervated muscles (Figures 79A,B). Within the next 2 weeks (by 35 days after birth), neonatal staining decreases in most fibers while fast staining is retained (214).

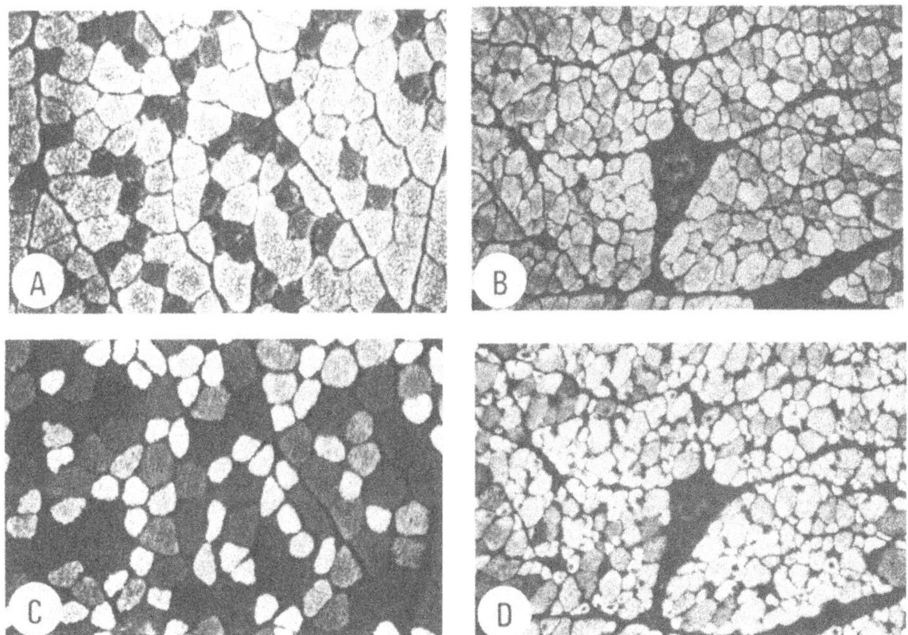

FIGURE 79: Immunofluorescent staining of serial section of innervated (A,BO or denervated (C,D) gastrocnemius muscles from 22-day-old rats. The antibodies used were directed against adult fast myosin (A,C) and neonatal myosin (B,D). The staining of the individual fibers can be evaluated by comparing the photos of the two antibodies for a given muscle. From Butler-Browne, et al, 1982

These results show that <u>continued</u> innervation of the muscle is not required for the neonatal - adult fast transition. We cannot exclude a possible influence of the nerve on the developing muscles prior to experimental denervation. However, our experiments on denervated regenerating muscle suggest that fast myosin can appear even if the muscle fibers have never been innervated.

One factor which seems to have an important influence on this myosin transition is the thyroid status of the animal. Newborn rats can be rendered hypothyroid during the first 3-4 weeks of life if their mothers are treated with anti-thyroid drugs such as methylthiouracil from mid-gestation onward. In these animals, neonatal myosin is a major component of the gastrocnemius muscle up to at least 28 days after birth, as determined from the analysis of native myosin isozymes shown in Figure 80, and by immunocytochemistry (516).

Although these results suggest that thyroid hormone levels are important, they do not allow the conclusion that the effect is the result of a direct action on the muscle fiber. The endocrinological status of the rat is changing rapidly in the several weeks after birth, and other hormones may be dependent on thyroid hormone levels. For example, post-natal increase in growth hormone levels is also diminished in hypothyroid rats (517). If growth hormone were involved in the control of myosin transitions, then the effect could be via the somatomedins which are the natural mediators of classical growth hormone action. Thus, the effect of hypothyroid may not necessarily be due to a direct effect of thyroid hormone on the muscle fibers.

Development of Slow Myosin-Containing Fibers

The soleus muscle in adult rats (greater than 6 months of age) is composed of 80-90% slow contracting fibers (518), and it is frequently chosen for the study of development of slow myosin-containing fibers. However, the soleus is not composed of a uniform type in the young rat. Rather it is composed of two phenotypically different fiber populations: one population (about half the total fiber number) contains neonatal but not slow myosin, while the other contains slow myosin but not the neonatal isozyme (511). These results are shown in Figure 81A-B. Using the antibodies to the four myosin isozymes (embryonic, neonatal, fast and slow), we

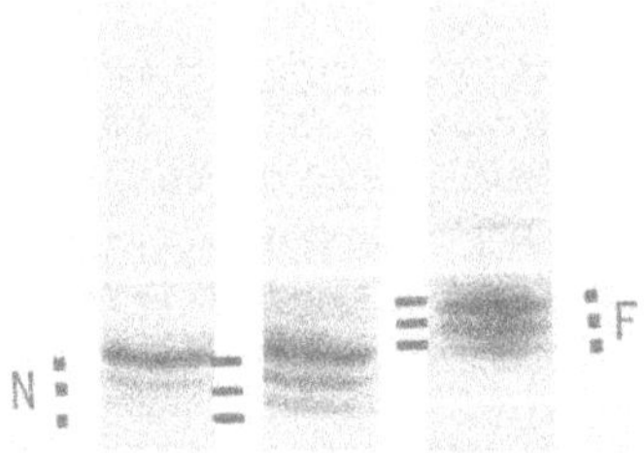

FIGURE 80: Electrophoretic analysis of native myosin isozymes in extracts of gastrocnemius muscles. The three samples analyzed are taken from: normal 7-day-old rats (N-7d), a 28-day-old hypothyroid rat (H-28d), and a 28-day-old normal rat (N-28d). The three bands marked N correspond to neonatal myosin, and those marked F correspond to adult fast myosin.

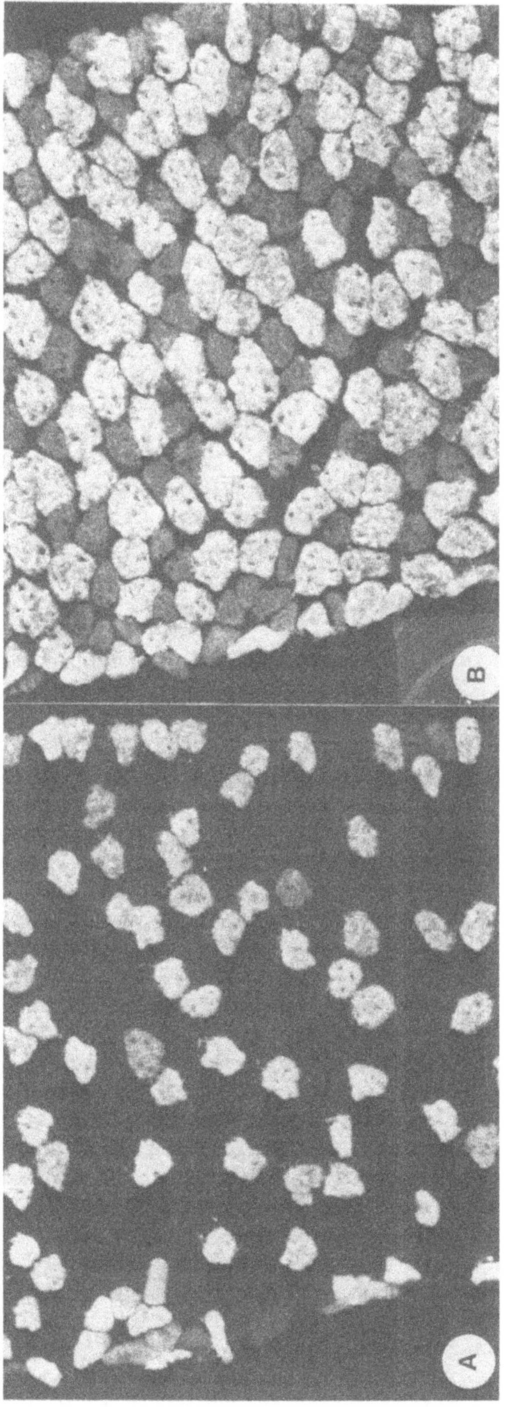

FIGURE 81: Immunofluorescent staining of the soleus muscle taken from a 14-day-old rat using antibodies to neonatal (A) and slow (B) myosin.

have followed the evolution of the myosin phenotype in the soleus muscle between 1 and 6 weeks after birth.

The results of this study (511) have been interpreted in the following manner. One population of fibers undergoes an embryonic - slow transition, without accumulating either neonatal or fast myosins. The other population first undergoes an embryonic-neonatal transition and subsequently either acquires slow myosin directly or acquires fast myosin. These fast myosin-containing fibers can be converted to slow fibers over a period of several months, as described by Kugelberg (519). These transitions are illustrated schematically in Figure 82.

Another experimental model for studying the formation of slow myosin-containing fibers is regeneration of the soleus muscle of young adult rats (519). Regeneration can be induced by injection of a snake toxin, motexin, which provokes complete degeneration of the soleus muscle fibers while leaving the basement membrane substantially intact. Fibers then re-generate in a scaffold of basement membrane which leads to good fiber orientation and probably contributes to the rather complete regeneration attained in this model.

We have used this regeneration system to demonstrate the nerve-dependence of slow myosin appearance. Figure 83A shows the results of native myosin analysis, demonstrating that slow myosin is accumulated as the major species in a 4 week regenerated muscle. However, if the sciatic nerve is cut at the time that toxin is injected, then fibers regenerate in the complete absence of innervation. Although the fibers are quite atrophic by four weeks after toxin injection, immunocytochemistry (Figure 83B) shows quite clearly that they accumulate fast myosin. In the innervated muscles, staining with fast antibody is weak and is only seen for a short period, but never at 4 weeks of regeneration.

All of the myosin isozyme transitions seen in the various situations that we have studied are included in the diagram of Figure 82 . The conclusion implicit in this diagram is that fast and slow muscle fiber development can be reconciled into a single context by the following proposition. There exists a series of myosin transitions (embryonic - neonatal - fast) that will occur in a "pre-programmed" fashion; the basis for this conclusion is the results of the denervation studies on developing and regenerating muscles. At any time during these transitions, slow myosin can be induced and the other isozymes are repressed. The induction of slow myosin in a fast myosin-containing fiber (i.e. the fast to slow fiber transformation in the adult) is apparently due to innervation by a "slow type" motor unit, or more precisely a certain activity pattern imposed by the nerve (192,193). This transformation seems to occur directly from fast to slow myosin, since no neonatal myosin is detected during the

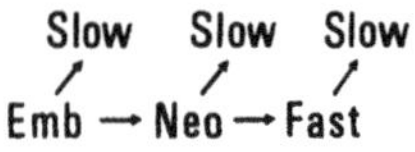

Slow Slow Slow
↗ ↗ ↗
Emb → Neo → Fast

FIGURE 82: Schematic illustration of the myosin isozyme transitions observed in the developing rat soleus muscle. From Butler-Browne and Whalen, 1984.

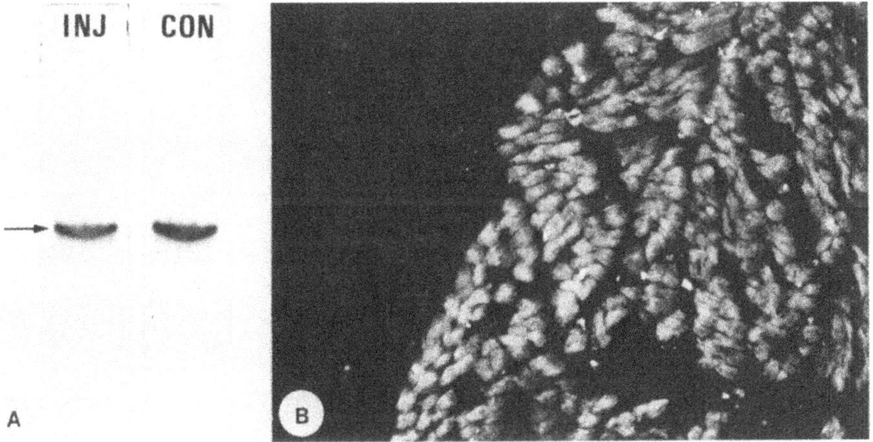

FIGURE 83: Myosin isozymes found in the innervated and denervated regenerated rat soleus muscle. In part A are shown the electrophoretic analyses of the myosin present in an innervated regenerated muscle, 28 days after motexin injection (Inj), and the contralateral control muscle taken from the same animal. The arrow indicates the slow myosin band. Part B shows the immunofluorescent staining of a denervated 28-day regenerate using an antibody to adult fast myosin. The regenerated muscle, stained positively by the antibody, is seen in the right of the photo; part of a control soleus muscle, negative with the antibody, is in the upper left of the photo.

conversion (515). Whether this same signal would be responsible for the presence of the slow myosin seen in neonatal (or even fetal) muscle is unclear. A precise description of the myosin types in fetal muscle fibers is not yet available, and more experiments are required to shed some light on what mechanisms might control the appearance of those myosins.

DR. HOH: Are you implying the nerve is dependent on muscle activity?

DR. WHALEN: If the muscle activity is that which is imposed by the nerve, then I would call it nerve-dependent. Specific patterns of nerve-muscle activity could be imposed by slow motor neurons which might be the cause of the induction of certain muscle proteins.

DR. WOOD: Do tissue culture cells utilize thyroid hormones?

DR. WHALEN: we have not yet observed any effect of thyroid hormone on myotubes in culture. As I mentioned, it is not certain that thyroid hormone acts directly on the muscle cell.

DR. FISCHMAN: I wanted to call to your attention the recent paper in Cell that suggests activity cannot be the whole explanation in the sense that the conversion of the troponin can be programmed by nerve extracts under conditions that make it unlikely that activity levels are changling in culture (484).

DR. STROHMAN: I get the suggestion from one of Joseph Hoh's slides that the denervation process may have some impact on the ability of the muscle to repress for example the denervated muscle. I got the impression that fetal chains were there more than they usually are and it could be interpreted as a failure of the denervated muscle to repress fetal light chains. Matsuda at Berkeley last year showed the same effect occurs *in vivo*. The breast muscle normally represses beta tropomyosin but very quickly after you denervate the breast the beta tropomyosin comes right back up. It is the removal of the nerve that releases an ongoing repression. The same thing is true for leg type component T which is absnet in the breast; when you denervate the leg type components T comes back up, so the denervated muscles seems to not repress what it normally represses.

The same thing is true in the chick, if you denervate neo-neonatally and then look several weeks later the adult myosin heavy chain is there so that the nerve is not important in the chick breast for the expression of the adult myosin. In the same muscle the failure of repression shows up. It is simply an example of a degree to which all of a variety of different peptides are regulated independently of one another. If this shows us anything, it shows the independence of expression of one of these proteins.

DR. SCHULTZ: What effect does toxin have on the nerve? In your regeneration experiments how much of the muscle was degenerated?

DR. WHALEN: The effect of the toxin on the nerve is slight. However, degeneration of the muscle is nearly complete when we have used young, that is 4-5 week old rats. This is seen histologically and also from the biochemical results where we have seen only small amounts of persisting slow myosin during the first week of regeneration.

DR. SCHULTZ: I would suspect that the toxin would not spare the satellite cells.

DR. WHALEN: The fact that the satellite cells dc seem not to be destroyed by the toxin might just be an effect of the relative target sizes of the muscle fibers versus the satellite cells.

CHAPTER 22: MYOSIN EXPRESSION DURING REGENERATION AND IN DENERVATED SKELETAL MUSCLE

Richard C. Strohman and Ryoichi Matsuda

Department of Zoology
University of California
Berkeley, CA

Myosin and Tropomyosin Expression in Regenerating Muscle

During skeletal muscle regeneration new fibers are built from the population of satellite cells that is normally associated with each fiber (72). As the adult fiber is injured the indwelling satellite cells are stimulated (somehow) to divide. At the same time invading macrophages clear out the degraded products of the old fiber and the new population of satellite cells, now myoblasts, are able to fuse within the space of the old basal lamina to produce the new muscle fiber (363,520). The questions we have focused upon are the following: When the new fiber differentiates in the old adult fiber space, what is the sequence of gene expression for the various muscle proteins? Does the regenerating fiber take its cues from the adult environment and express adult forms of muscle proteins? Or does the regenerating fiber in the adult recapitulate embryological development? If the latter case is true then we should be able to detect a sequence of myosin expression in which the new fiber first synthesizes embryonic myosin heavy chains (MHCs) followed by neonatal followed by adult MHCs (56). Figure 84 summarizes the possibilities for programmed growth during muscle fiber regeneration.

We have followed regeneration in a cold-injured skeletal muscle preparation in the chicken. Adult pectoralis major (PM), a fast muscle and anterior latissimus dorsi (ALD), a slow muscle are cold injured and allowed to recover. At various times after muscle injury we inject the regeneration site directly with ^{35}S methione and remove the muscle for analysis of type of muscle protein being synthesized. The results are clear. During the

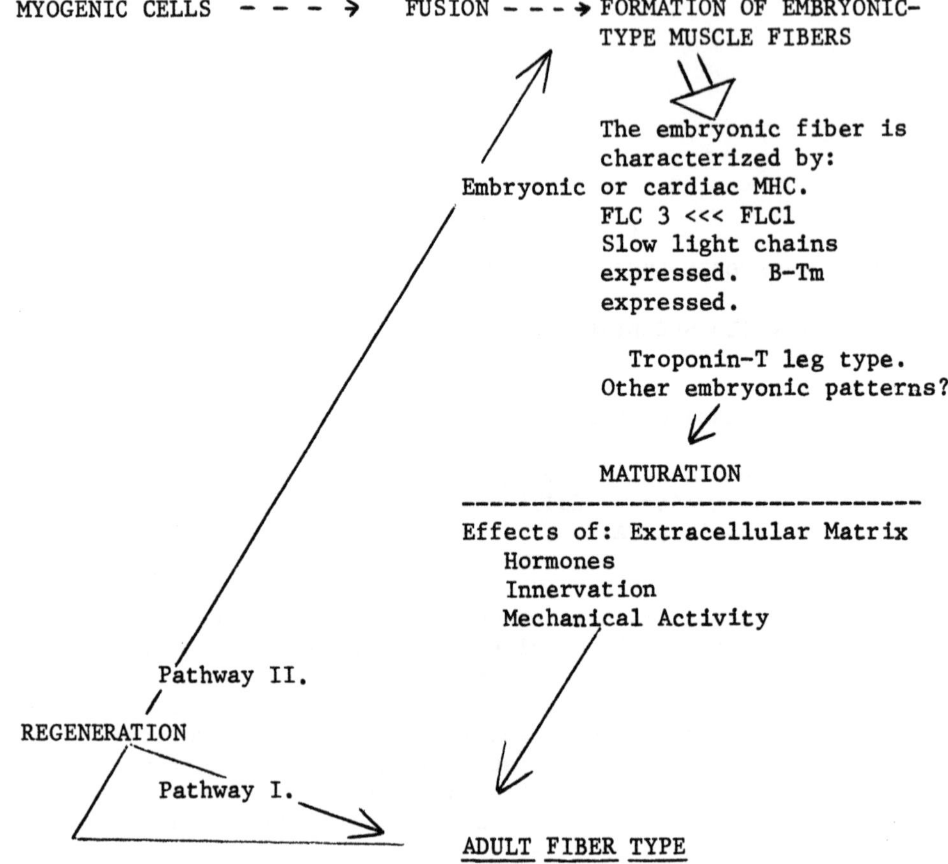

FIGURE 84: Possible Pathways for Gene Expression during Regeneration in Chicken Pectoralis Major Muscle.

Regenerating fibers might be expected to immediately reexpress the adult fiber phenotype (Pathway I.). Alternatively, the regenerating fiber may need to run through a program in which it essentially recapitulates embryological development (Pathway II). As we point out in this paper (61) pathway II is followed in regenerating chicken PM muscle.

first week of regeneration the PM muscle synthesizes an embryonic myosin heavy chain and a pattern of myosin light chains that is characteristic of embryonic muscle. In addition, the regenerating PM synthesizes an embryonic pattern of tropomyosins (521). That is, normally the adult PM synthesizes only α-fast tropomyosin and represses β-tropomyosin sometime during late embryonic development. Regenerating muscle reexpresses β-tropomyosin together with α-fast.

Finally, while the adult, uninjured muscle synthesizes myosin light chains in a normal pattern (FLC1=FLC3), the regenerating muscle shows a reduced synthesis of FLC3. Reduced amounts of FLC3 are characteristic of embryonic skeletal muscle (522). The results for myosin heavy chains, light chains and tropomyosin are summarized in Table 12 (61). Regenerating muscle therefore displays a recapitulation of embryonic development in terms of its synthesis of myosin and tropomyosin. By 3-4 weeks post-injury the recapitulation was complete and only adult type isoform patterns were seen (61).

TABLE 12: ^{35}S-methonine incorporation into proteins of regenerating muscle in vivo and into myotubes of satellite cells in vitro.

Regeneration in PM Muscle for:	Percent Incorporation					
	B-Tm	FLC1	FLC2	FLC3	SLC1	SLC2
1 week	27.2	39.3	36.8	16.5	1.8	5.3
control	2.0	10.9	54.5	32.7	nil	nil
4 weeks	4.5	12.9	52.9	33.8	nil	nil
control	1.5	12.8	57.1	29.8	nil	nil
Satellite Cell Cultures						
PM Muscle	31.2	47.0	36.7	4.6	3.9	7.8
ALD Muscle	23.7	40.1	23.0	0.5	20.1	16.3

Values for alpha slow and alpha fast Tm are not shown.

The satellite cell cultures from each muscle type were allowed to grow for 7 days in culture during which time well-developed myotubes were formed.

Similar results were obtained when we cold-injured the chicken adult ALD. The regenerating ALD in vivo reverted to an embryonic pattern of myosin and tropomyosin expression which was transient and gave way to an adult pattern within 3-4 weeks post-injury (61).

We were anxious to know if satellite cells cultured from adult fast and slow muscle would generate muscle fibers characteristic of their originating fiber type.

Satellite Cells of Fast and Slow Muscle: Programs of Gene Expression in Cell Culture

We established cultures of satellite cells from PM and ALD muscles respectively. After 7 days of culture these cells fused to produce muscle fibers that were indistinguishable from those produced by embryonic myoblasts of either PM or ALD muscle. By biochemical analysis however the myotube/myofiber populations generated from the two types of satellite cells were distinctly different. The myotubes from PM satellite cells synthesized only or predominantly myosin fast light chains while myotubes from ALD satellite cells synthesized both fast and slow myosin light chains. In addition, the ALD myotubes synthesized the embryonic MHC equivalent to that found in PM cultured myotubes but synthesized as well a MHC that comigrated on 5% SDS-PAGE with the SM2 MHC of slow muscle. Since SM2 and cardiac MHC comigrate on these gels it is possible that ALD myotubes synthesize a cardiac MHC but we are not clear about this at the moment. What is clear is that the satellite cell of the ALD and PM adult muscle express quantitatively and qualitatively different programs of myosin heavy and light chains under identical culture conditions (61).

Since nerve cross-innervation experiments have demonstrated the ability of the nerve to reprogram the muscle (66,67,523) we were interested in determining whether or not and to what extent there was a coordinated shift in gene expression in several muscle proteins following denervation.

Denervated Skeletal Muscle Shows Discoordinate Regulation for Muscle Protein Synthesis

We denervated the PM muscle just after hatching at which time the muscle was synthesizing a neonatal MHC but was synthesizing adult patterns of tropomyosin (α-tropomyosin only), myosin fast light chains (FLC1=FLC3), and troponin-T (breast type troponin-T). We waited 7 months at which time the muscle was found to have remained uninnervated and had a mass of less than 50% of the control muscle (contralateral side). The results of this experiment are summarized in Table 13 (524).

The denervated PM muscle had made the transition from expression of neonatal to adult MHC so it was apparent that continuous input from the motor neuron was not a necessary part of this regulatory shift (214). The nerve was necessary, however, for the appropriate expression of tropomyosin, myosin light chains and troponin-T. The denervated muscle no longer repressed β-tropomyosin or leg type troponin-T and these were coexpressed together with α-fast tromyosin and breast type troponin-T. In addition, the denervated muscle showed depressed levels of expression of myosin FLC3.

TABLE 13: ^{35}S-methionine incorporation into muscle proteins in regenerating and control PM muscle.

Time after Denervation	Tropomyosins α-fast	Tropomyosins Beta	Myosin Light Chains FLC1	FLC2	FLC3	SLC1	SLC2
7 months*	76.5	22.7	26.6	53	20	0.2	0.1
control	97	2.2	13.2	62	24	0	0.5
*the above experimental muscle was denervated neonatally.							
6 weeks*	64	34	52	31	15	0	1.0
control	96	2.5	13	51	33	1.1	0.7
*the above muscle was denervated at an adult stage.							

The denervated muscle always showed, in addition to the above patterns of myosin light chain and tropomyosin synthesis, a significant expression of leg type troponin T and adult type myosin heavy chain. At the time of neonatal denervation the MHC being synthesized was the neonatal type and there was no expression of either β-tropomyosin or leg type troponin-T.

Finally, Bruce Paterson (69) has found that chicken PM muscle expresses cardiac α-actin throughout embryological development. Cardiac α-actin is replaced by α-skeletal actin at about day 18 in the embryo. RNA from our denervated PM muscle was probed with cDNAs that distinguish between both of these actins. The denervated muscle was identical to the control muscle; both expressed α-skeletal actin. Thus, the denervated muscle does not regress to embryonic patterns for the major structural proteins actin and myosin heavy chain. For the muscle regulatory proteins, however, it appears that the nerve exerts an important influence in controlling gene expression. It is interesting to speculate that in the nerve cross-reinnervation experiments cited above, the muscle may use a switching mechanism that works first through changing gene expression for proteins regulating cross-bridge interaction.

CHAPTER 23: PARVALBUMIN REDUCTION IN RELATION TO POSSIBLE PERTURBATIONS OF CA^{2+}-HOMEOSTASIS IN MUSCULAR DYSTROPHY

Dirk Pette, Gary Klug and Heinz Reichmann

Faculty of Biology
University of Konstanz
D-7750 Konstanz, West Germany

It has been suggested that muscle wasting in muscular dystrophy is causally related to a perturbation of Ca^{2+}-homeostasis in the muscle fiber (8,525-530) due to an increased permeability of the sarcolemmal membrane. An elevated sarcoplasmic Ca^{2+} concentration would result from an increased Ca^{2+}-influx and would thus lead to an activation of Ca^{2+}-dependent proteases. Ca^{2+} has also been shown to play an important role in the regulation of glucose-1,6-biphosphate (531,532) a powerful effector of several enzymes in glucose metabolism (533). This modulator has been shown to be significantly reduced in muscles of dystrophic mice (534,535).

The sarcoplasmic free Ca^{2+}-concentration results from influx, various Ca^{2+}-pumping activities (sarcolemma, mitochondria, sarcoplasmic reticulum) and from the concentrations of several Ca^{2+}-binding proteins. Among the latter parvalbumin represents a major component in fast-twitch mammalian muscles (536). It appeared of interest therefore to study whether or not the disturbed Ca^{2+}-homeostasis in dystrophic muscle is accompanied by changes in the content of this major Ca^{2+}-binding protein in the sarcoplasmic compartment.

Results of parvalbumin determinations in different hindlimb muscles of normal and dystrophic mice by the method of Blum et al. (537) as described elsewhere (538) are presented in Table 14. As compared to the muscles of normal C57 BL/6J of the same age, the dystrophic muscles are characterized by a significant decrease in their parvalbumin content. In the average, parvalbumin is reduced to 60% of its level in normal muscle. Assuming a molecular weight of 12,000, the reduction of parvalbumin of 40% would correspond in these muscles to a reduction from a mean value of 450 μmol/kg

TABLE 14

Parvalbumin Content in Hindlimb Muscles of 15 Wk Old Normal (C57 Bl/6J) and 15 Wk Old Dystrophic Mice (C57 Bl/6J dy^{2J}/dy^{2J})

Muscle	Parvalbumin Content (mg/g w.wt.)	
	Normal	Dystrophic
m. quadriceps femor.	5.82 ± 0.31 (5)	3.44 ± 0.31 (5)*
m. gastrocnemius	5.53 ± 0.27 (5)	2.98 ± 0.40 (5)*
m. tibialis ant.	4.86 ± 0.32 (5)	3.24 ± 0.40 (5)*

*$P < 0.001$

of muscle. Referred to the two Ca^{2+} -binding sites, this results in a decreased Ca^{2+} -binding capacity of 360 µmol/kg of muscle. This remarkable decrease in sarcoplasmic Ca^{2+} -binding capacity would add to the increased Ca^{2+} -influx and therefore represent another factor responsible of an increase in sarcoplasmic free Ca^{2+}. Although no data are available on the effective increase in free Ca^{2+} in the dystrophic muscle, recent measurements of Nylen and Wrogemann (539) provide independent evidence in support of this suggestion. These authors observed Ca^{2+} -overloading of mitochondria in skeletal muscle of dystrophic mice. This observation points to a compensatory mitochondrial Ca^{2+} -uptake in consequence of an elevated sarcoplasmic Ca^{2+} -concentration.

It has been shown that the concentration of glucose-1,6-biphosphate (Glc-1,6-P_2) is decreased in skeletal muscle and in myotube cultures under conditions which are suggested to result in an increase of sarcoplasmic free Ca^{2+} (531,532,540). A decrease in Glc-1,6-P_2 has also been reported in skeletal muscles of dystrophic mice of the strain 129 ReJ (534,535). Since determinations of parvalbumin in this study were performed on mice of the strain C57 BL/6J dy^{2J}/dy^{2J} it was decided to investigate Glc-1,6-P_2 in the same muscles.

Table 15 compares Glc-1,6-P_2 levels between three hindlimb muscles of normal and dystrophic mice of strain C57 Bl/6Jdy^{2J}/dy^{2J}. There is a 60-75% decrease in the Glc-1,6-P_2 concentration in the dystrophic muscles which fully confirms the results of Beitner et al. (534,535). This decrease in Glc-1,6-P_2 may be explained not only by an increased activity of glucose-1,6-bisphosphatase in dystrophic muscle (541) but also by the discussed increase in sarcoplasmic free Ca^{2+}. There is evidence that glucose-1,6-bisphosphatase in muscle is activated by Ca^{2+} -calmodulin (542).

TABLE 15

Glucose-1,6-Bisphosphate Levels in Hindlimb Muscles of Normal (C57 Bl/6J) and of Dystrophic Mice (C57 BL/6J dy^{2J}/dy^{2J})

	Glucose-1,6-Bisphosphate (nmol/g/ w.wt.).	
Muscle	Normal	Dystrophic
m. quadriceps femor.	43.7 ± 9.5 (5)	13.1 ± 5.5 (6)*
m. gastrocnemius	65.5 ± 16.4 (5)	15.0 ± 3.3 (6)*
m. tibialis ant.	70.6 ± 27.0 (6)	24.9 ± 7.3 (5)*

[1] 2 months old; [2] 4 months old
* $P < 0.005$

It has also been shown that Glc-1,6-P_2 increases in muscle under the influence of the calmodulin antagonist trifluoperazine (543).

The decrease of Glc-1,6-P_2 is thus in accordance with the suggested increase in sarcoplasmic free Ca^{2+}. The observed reduction of parvalbumin might at least partially be related with this perturbation of intracellular Ca^{2+} -homeostasis. However, parvalbumin and Glc-1,6-P_2 levels might also be reduced in an unrelated manner and merely reflect an altered phenotypic expression of the dystrophic muscle fibers. It has been observed that the parvalbumin content of fast-twitch muscles responds rapidly to experimentally induced fiber type transformation. Thus, fast to slow fiber type transition as elicited by chronic nerve stimulation (538,544,545) or by high intensity endurance training (546), results in pronounced reductions of the parvalbumin content. Since muscle fibers undergoing the dystrophic process are different with regard to several properties from normal fiber types (e.g. 547-550), it is also conceivable that the relatively low parvalbumin content of dystrophic muscle is not causally related to the dystrophic process but represents another symptom of an abnormal phenotypic expression.

CHAPTER 24: MYOSIN ISOZYMES IN DEVELOPING CHICKEN MUSCLES

Susan Lowey

Rosentiel Basic Medical Sciences Research Center
Brandeis University
Waltham, MA

There is now general agreement among several laboratories that a minimum of three classes of myosin isozymes appear sequentially during the course of muscle development (56,381,386, 551). These classes include embryonic, neonatal and adult myosin. Even though the primary structure of these myosins is different (552,553), their overall size and shape remains unchanged (Figure 85B). A more difficult, and largely unresolved problem is the functional significance of this polymorphism. It is widely assumed that myosin isozymes have different enzymatic properties which can be related to the speed of shortening of the muscle from which the myosin is derived (554). Here it will be shown that this correlation does not necessarily apply to developing muscles, and that alternative explanations for myosin diversity need to be found.

Enzymatic Activity of Myosin Isozymes

With the exception of adult rabbit skeletal myosin, few detailed kinetic studies exist in the literature. In fact, most of the analyses are not even performed with myosin, but instead use the proteolytic subfragment, S1 (Figure 86 for nomenclature), which contains the nucleotide and actin-binding sites. Most investigators choose to determine the actin-activated Mg^{2+} ATPase activity of soluble subfragments rather than native myosin. Myosin and actin interact strongly only at low salt concentrations, where both myosin and actin are in the form of heterogeneous, high molecular weight polymers. At the actin concentrations needed to reach the maximum velocity of the reaction, V_{max}, the actomyosin suspension becomes sufficiently viscous to make such measurements unreliable (555).

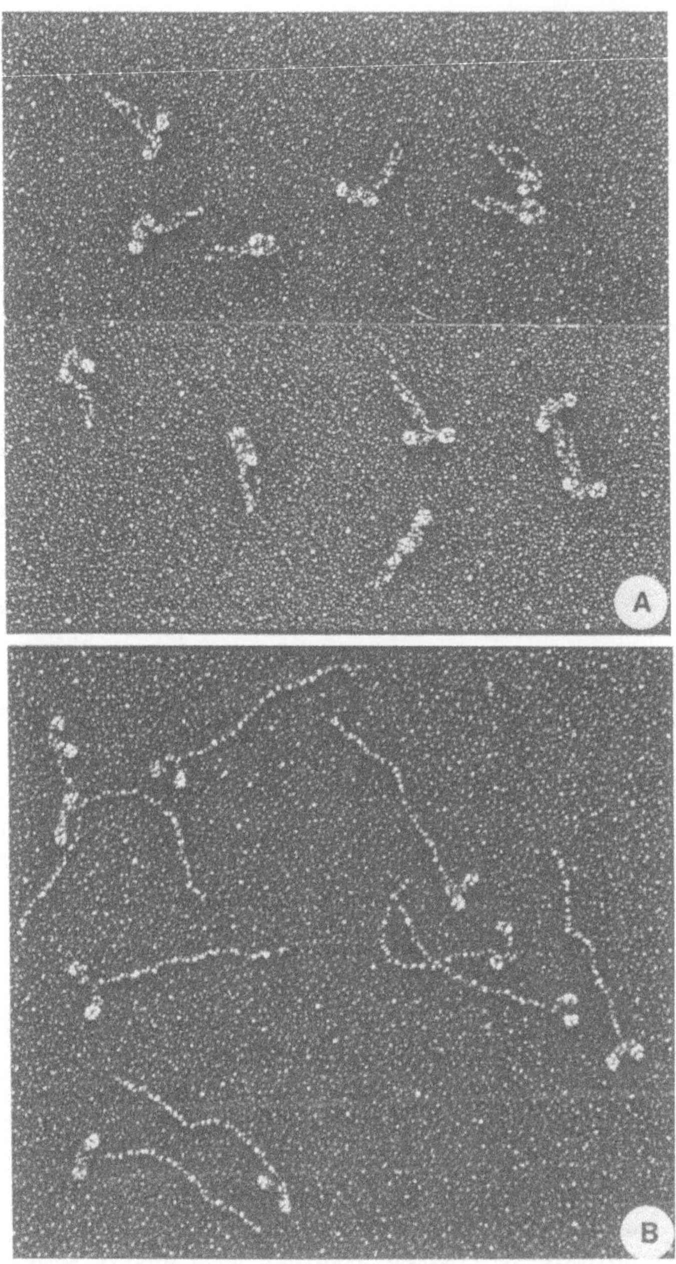

FIGURE 85: Electron micrographs of rotary-shadowed smooth muscle myosin molecules in the (a) folded and (b) extended conformations. (Courtesy of K.M. Trybus).

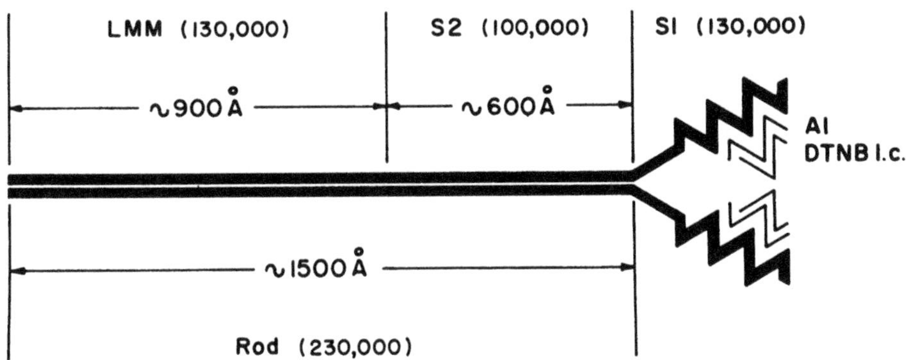

FIGURE 86: Schematic representation of the vertebrate skeletal muscle myosin molecule.

A significant improvement in kinetic studies was brought about by the introduction of myosin "minifilaments" (556). These minifilaments are formed by dialyzing myosin into a citrate-Tris buffer of low ionic strength. Instead of the conventional synthetic filaments comprised of several hundred myosin molecules, the "minifilaments" consist of only 16-18 myosin molecules assembled into a small bipolar aggregate (Figure 87). An unusual feature of the

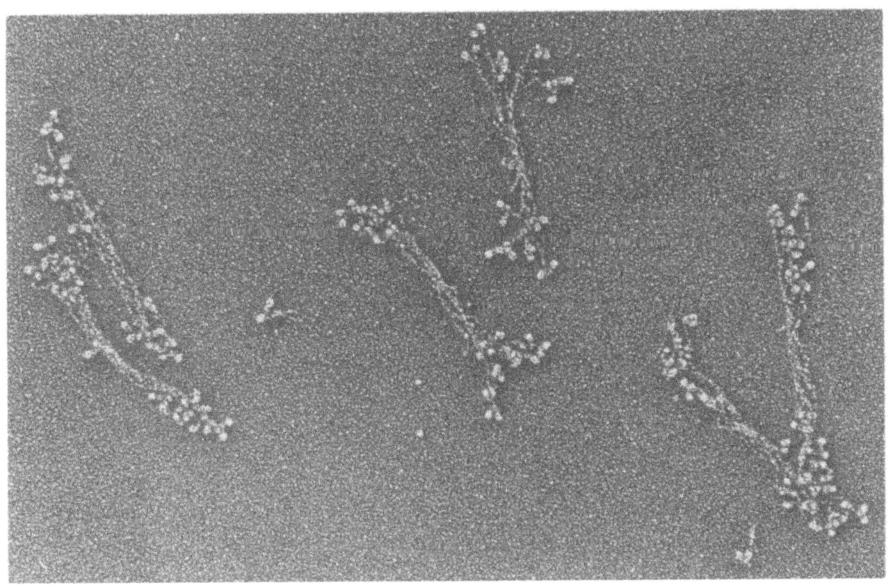

FIGURE 87: Electron micrograph of a field of rotary-shadowed smooth muscle myosin minifilaments. (Courtesy of K.M. Trybus). Skeletal muscle myosin minifilaments look similar in appearance.

minifilaments is their remarkable homogeneity compared to synthetic filaments; any heterogeneity seen in the electron microscope is probably introduced by fixation methods, and is not an inherent property of the minifilaments. When ATPase measurements are carried out with minifilaments and actin, the quality of the data is greatly improved, and the rates approach those obtained with the soluble subfragments (557,558).

In our initial kinetic experiments with 11-day embryonic myosin, we used synthetic myosin filaments in the assay medium (559). Preparation of subfragment-1 was not feasible due to the small amounts of protein present in these developing muscles. When we compared the actin-activated Mg^{2+} ATPase of 10-11-day embryonic chicken pectoralis myosin with that of adult chicken pectoralis myosin, the values were identical within experimental error (559).

More recently we have measured the kinetic properties for 18-day embryonic myosin and 12-day posthatch myosin, and again we find no significant differences among these isozymes (Table 16) The absolute values for the actin-activated Mg^{2+} ATPases are 3-fold higher than the rates obtained previously, but this increase in ATPase activity can be ascribed, in part, to the use of mini-

TABLE 16
Kinetic Constants of Chicken Myosin Isozymes*

Myosin		K^+(EDTA)ATPase (s^{-1})	Actin-activated Mg^{2+} ATPase V_{max}(s^{-1})	Actin-activated Mg^{2+} ATPase K_{app}(μM)
Pectoralis	adult	11	9	<23
PLD	adult	12	9	< 4
ALD	adult	7	1	<25
Pectoralis (18-d embryo)		12	10	< 3
Pectoralis (12-d posthatch)		13	10	<14
Pectoralis (11-d embryo)†		11.0	3.1	23
Pectoralis (adult)†		10.8	2.8	31

*The data given here represent a range of values from several experiments; a detailed analysis will be presented elsewhere (Lowey & Waller, in preparation); the activity is expressed in (mole P_i) (mole protein active sites)$^{-1}$ (s)$^{-1}$. Conditions for the K^+ATPase were 0.6M KCl, 2 mM EDTA, 50 mM Tris (pH 8.2), 2.5 mM ATP, 25°C. Assays in the presence of actin and minifilaments were in 5 mM KCl, 5 mM citric acid, 28 mM Tris (pH 8.2, 25°C), 3.75 mM $MgCl_2$, 2.5 mM ATP.

†Data reproduced from Lowey et al. (1983). The myosin is in the form of synthetic filaments, and the assay medium contained actin, 50 mM KCl, 2.5 mM ATP, 3.75 mM $MgCl_2$, pH 8.0, 25°C.

filaments in the assay (557). These results emphasize how dependent the ATPase activity is on the exact ionic conditions and the experimental procedures. For comparison, we have included the kinetic parameters of ALD (anterior latissimus dorsi) myosin. The almost 10-fold differences in V_{max} between ALD myosin and pectoralis or PLD (posterior latissimus dorsi) myosin is consistent with the well-known difference in the speed of shortening between the slow-tonic ALD muscle and the fast-twitch PLD muscle (560).

In conclusion, the kinetic properties of several myosin isozymes have been determined, and the results suggest no major differences in enzymatic activity for myosins isolated from muscles at different stages of development. There is, therefore, no experimental basis for ascribing the slow speed of contraction of embryonic muscles to the enzymatic activity of their constituent myosins.

Since the enzymatic function of myosin does not appear to be appreciably affected by polymorphism, we looked next at the structural basis for this diversity.

Structure of Myosin Isozymes

In the course of cellular differentiation, conformational changes within the myosin molecule and interactions between myosin molecules in the filament may have an important role in the maturation of the muscle cell. Peptide mapping first demonstrated that the primary structure of myosin changes during development (380,561), but the identification and location of these sequence alterations in the three-dimensional structure of myosin required a specific probe, such as monoclonal antibodies. Here I shall describe the properties of three such antibodies used in a topographical study of myosin (562).

An antibody specific for the amino-terminal 25 kD region of chicken myosin was shown to bind to the myosin head at a distance of about 140 Å from the head-rod junction (Figure 88). This portion of the head presumably contains the nucleotide-binding site (563). An unusual feature of this anti-S1 antibody is its strong reactivity with 18-day embryonic pectoralis myosin, but lack of reactivity with post-hatch myosin. This property provided a means for following the disappearance of embryonic myosin and the emergence of adult myosin (Figure 89). It also confirmed the existence of a post-hatch isozyme, previously deduced from peptide mapping (381,559,562), and non-denaturing gel electrophoresis (381). Similar conclusions were reached by the studies of Bader et al (386), using monoclonal antibodies against the LMM and S2 regions of myosin.

A second monoclonal antibody specific for the carboxyl terminus of the myosin rod (Figure 90) showed no reaction with

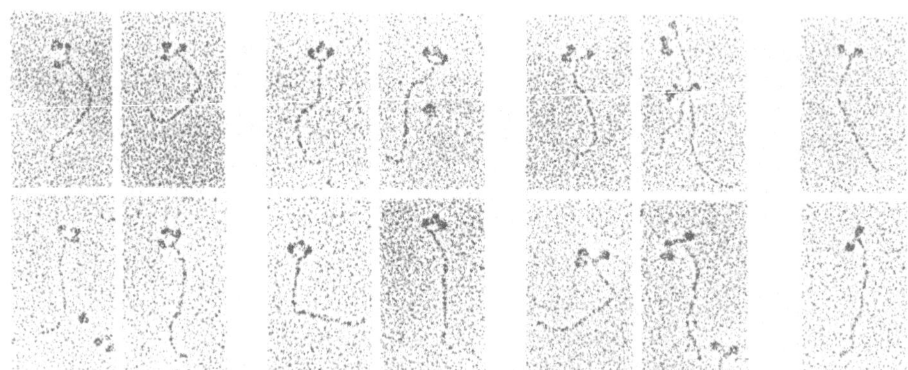

FIGURE 88: Gallery of rotary-shadowed skeletal muscle myosin molecules labeled with anti-S1 antibody. Antibody is seen bound to one head or bound symmetrically between the two heads. Unlabeled control myosin is shown on the extreme right for comparison. (Reprinted from Winkelmann et al., 1983).

adult isozyme. This anti-LMM antibody could therefore be used to detect the appearance of adult myosin, and confirm the time course obtained with anti-S1 (Figure 89). A third monoclonal antibody was mapped by immune electron microscopy to the so-called neck region of mysoin where the head joins the tail (Figure 91). This antibody, whose specificity is for the amino-terminal region of the LC2 light chain (otherwise known as DTNB light chain), reacts equally well with all the developmental myosin isozymes. This result is consistent with electrophoretic analyses which show no change in the size or charge of the light chains during avian muscle development (564).

What conclusions can be drawn from these limited structural studies of the myosin isozymes? It appears that sequence changes in myosin during development can occur in widely separated regions of the molecule, anywhere from the N-terminus in the myosin head to the C-terminus in the rod. These changes do not appear to influence the steady-state ATPase activity, but they may affect the assembly of myosin into a filamentous form. Aggregation of myosin is largely dependent on rod interactions, and it seems that the rod shows far greater sequence divergence than the head region (553,565).

It has recently been discovered that certain myosins, such as smooth muscle and non-muscle myosin can form unusual structures. Instead of assembling into filaments at low salt concentrations (∿0.1M), these myosins adopt a folded monomeric conformation upon

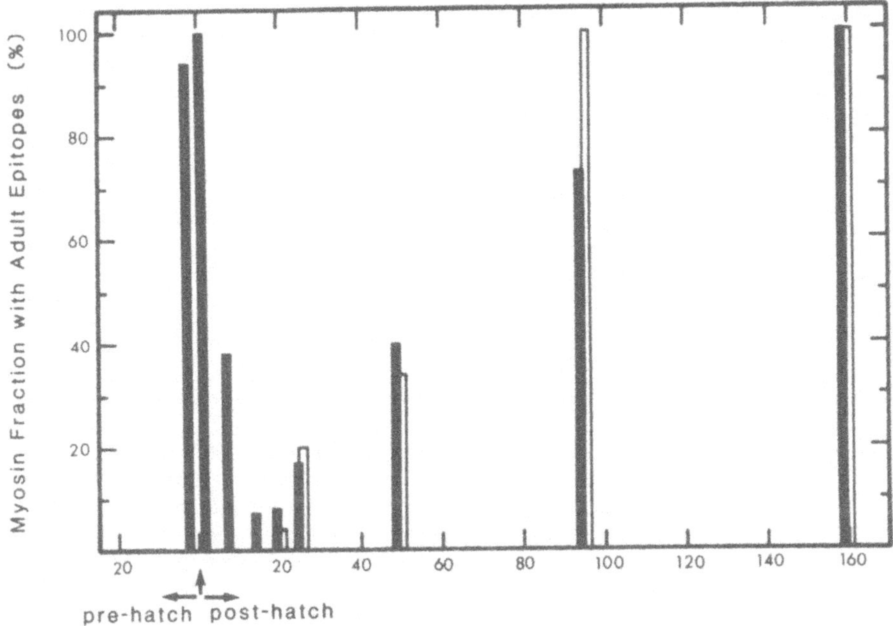

FIGURE 89: Histogram relating the myosin fraction having the LMM determinant (open bars) and the S1 determinant (shaded bars) to the age of the animals from which the myosin samples were isolated. (Reprinted from Winkelmann et al., 1983).

the binding of MgATP (566-569) (Figure 85A). Phosphorylation of the light chain, or raising the salt concentration to above 0.3 M, converts these myosins back to the extended form typical of skeletal muscle myosin (Figure 85B) (570). I am not suggesting that embryonic skeletal myosin assumes a folded conformation in the myotube (although this conformation may conceivably exist in a myoblast), but I do wish to emphasize the implications of this new structure. Smooth muscle myosin does not differ from skeletal muscle myosin in size and shape (Figure 85B), and the rod alone, after cleavage of the S1 region, forms only filaments at low ionic strength. The differences between smooth and skeletal muscle myosin arise predominantly from alterations in the head region (571). The message to be drawn from these studies is that small charge effects can lead to profound structural changes, and that the sequence alterations we have encountered in the embryonic and post-hatch isozymes may influence the assembly of myosin (381) and/or the organization of the filaments into the hexagonal lattice of the myofibril.

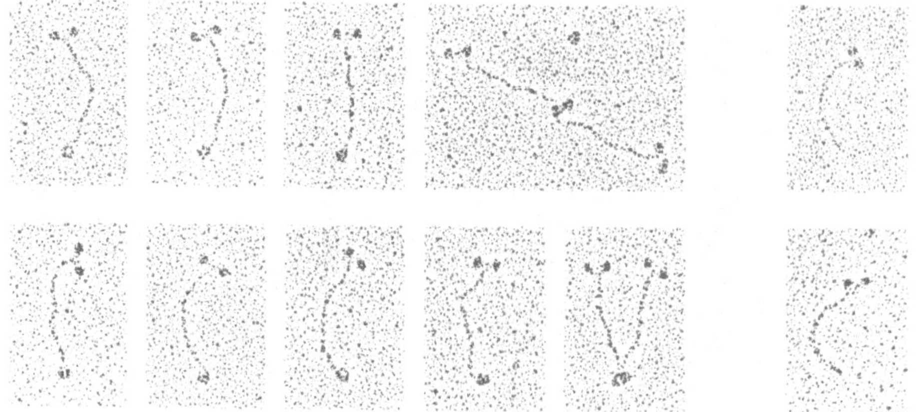

FIGURE 90: Gallery of rotary-shadowed myosin molecules labeled with anti-LMM antibody. The antibody is bound at the extreme end of the myosin rod. Unlabeled myosin is shown on the right for comparison. (Reprinted from Winkelmann, et al., 1983).

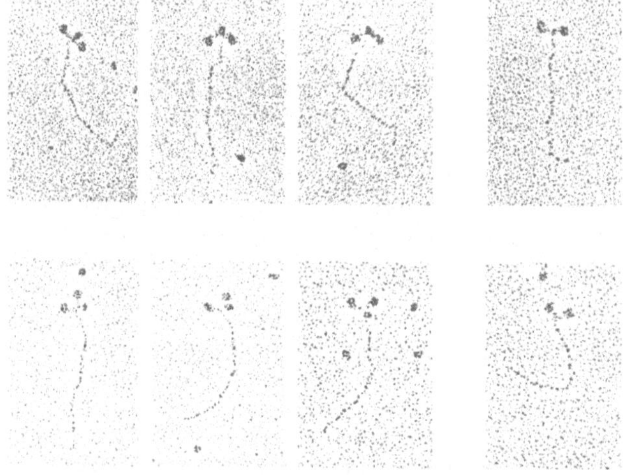

FIGURE 91: Gallery of myosin molecules labeled with an Fab fragment of anti-LC2 antibody. The antibody is bound near the head-rod junction. Unlabeled myosin is shown on the right for comparison. (Reprinted from Winkelmann, et al., 1983).

In the discussion so far, I have spoken of "embryonic" myosin as if it constituted a single unique species of myosin. The concept of embryonic myosin has undergone its own evolution: At first, some investigators believed that an intrinsic program in the muscle cell called for adult fast myosin, and that slow muscle myosin required extrinsic influences, such as innervation (379). Others reported that embryonic muscles reacted with antisera to fast and slow muscle myosin, which led to the hypothesis that both myosin types were present in the earliest stages of muscle development (50,572). The current concept of myosin in embryonic muscles favors a distinct embryonic heavy chain (380). I wish to modify this picture by reviewing data in support of several myosin isozymes appearing in the course of embryonic development prior to hatching.

Multiple Embryonic Isozymes

Immunocytochemistry can provide information regarding cross-reactive determinants between embryonic and adult myosins, but direct isolation and analysis of embryonic myosin was necessary in order to define its composition (573). By preparing an immunoadsorbent specific for slow (ALD) myosin, it was possible to fractionate 11-day embryonic myosin into a minor "slow" component, retained by the column, and a major "fast" component which subsequently bound to an anti-fast (pectoralis) myosin column (Figure 92). Gel electrophoresis showed that "slow"

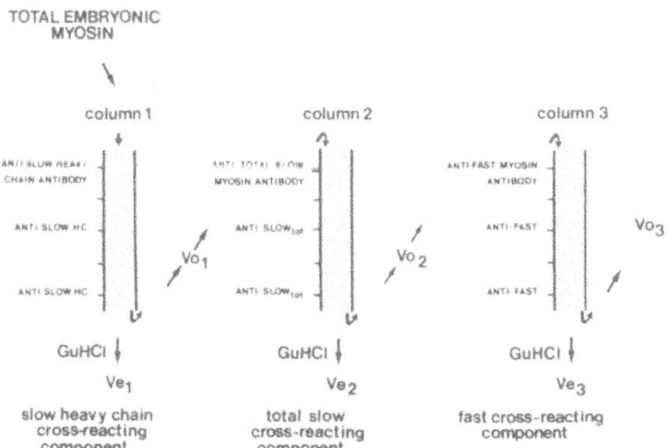

FIGURE 92: Procedure used to fractionate embryonic pectoralis myosin using antibody-affinity chromatography. Fractions bound to each column are denoted Ve, and the unbound fraction (Vo) is then passed through the next column in the series. Bound fractions (Ve) were eluted from each column using 4M guanidine hydrochloride (GuHCl). (Reprinted from Benfield, et al., 1983).

embryonic myosin was enriched in slow light chains (Figure 93), and peptide mapping of the heavy chain showed that the slow component (Ve_1) was distinct from both the fast component (Ve_3) and adult ALD myosin (Figure 94) (573).

Immunofluorescence results have indicated that the amount of slow embryonic myosin in the pectoralis declines by 18 days _in ovo_ (574), a time course consistent with the detection of slow light chains by monoclonal antibodies (52). It appears that changes in light chain expression may be linked to changes in

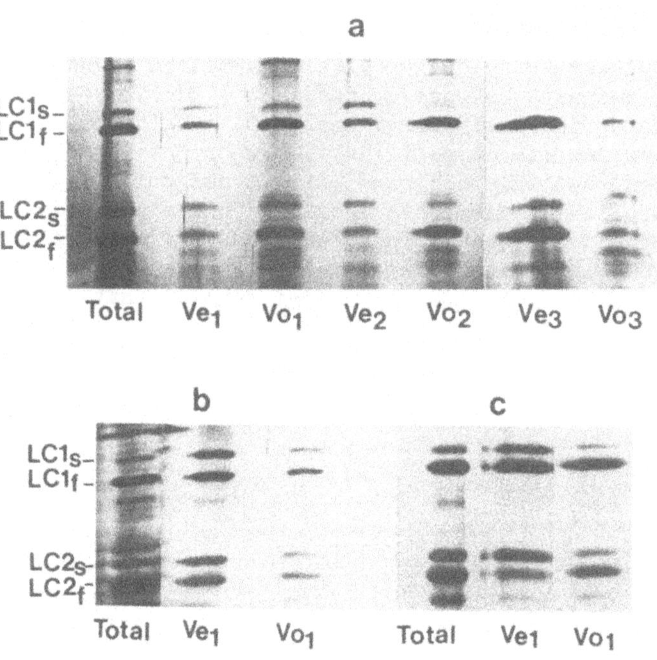

FIGURE 93: One-dimensional SDS-polyacrylamide gel electrophoresis of components of embryonic chicken pectoralis myosin fractionated by the procedure outline in Figure 92. (a), (b) and (c) represent fractionations of three different embryonic myosin preparations. (Reprinted from Benfield, et al., 1983).

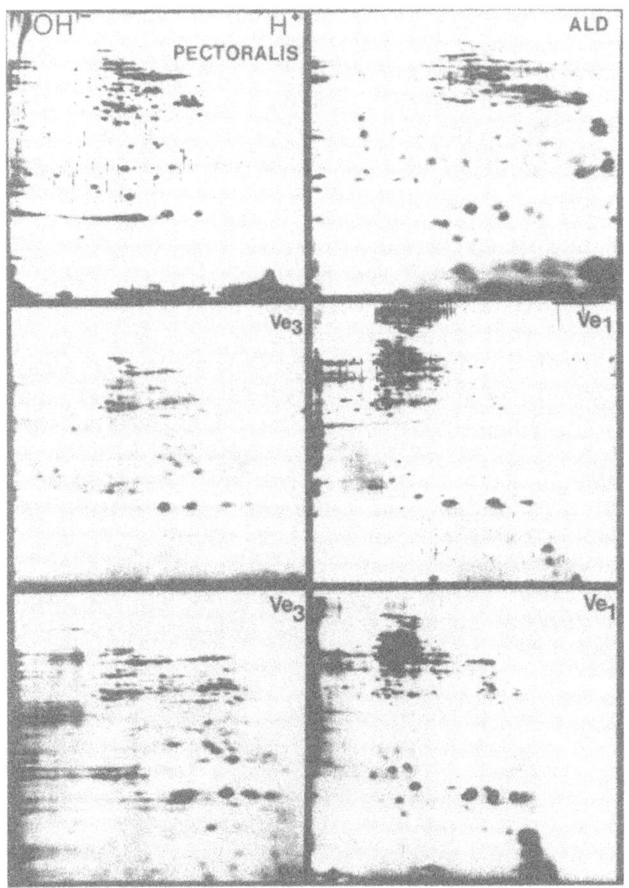

FIGURE 94: Two-dimensional SDS-polyacrylamide gel electrophoresis of partial chymotryptic digests of adult pectoralis and ALD myosins, together with embryonic pectoralis myosins fractionated as described in Figure 92. (Reprinted from Benfield, et al., 1983).

heavy chain expression, and that a "slow" embryonic myosin isozyme exists transiently during development, whose light chains (LC1S and LC2D) are associated with a unique slow heavy chain.

A third myosin isozyme has recently been demonstrated in the earliest stages of muscle development, before the myotome forms separate muscle masses. Monoclonal antibodies to cardiac ventricular myosin heavy chain reacted with the somitic myotome as early as day 2 *in ovo*, at a time when no visible reaction with antibodies against the adult skeletal myosins occurred (575). Low levels of reactivity with anti-PLD and anti-ALD myosin were observed by days 5 and 6, respectively. The cross-reactivity with the cardiac antibodies declined by day 20, and the muscle stained primarily with the homologous antibodies (575).

The combined experiments described here lead to the conclusion that at least three myosin isozymes are expressed in the embryo: first a cardiac-type, followed by a slow- and fast-type myosin. Only the fast-type embryonic myosin persists into the post-hatching period, where it is subsequently replaced by a post-hatch myosin. Adult myosin appears relatively late in development, not until 2-3 weeks after hatching, suggesting that the nervous system has a more pronounced influence in the terminal stages of muscle differentiation. As discussed above, the functional significance of this extensive myosin polymorphism during myogenesis remains unknown, but considering how little is understood about the development of form and function in any cell, it should come as no surprise that more than one developmental myosin isozyme is necessary to build a muscle cell.

PART V

RECOMBINANT DNA APPROACHES IN THE INVESTIGATION OF MUSCLE GENE EXPRESSION

CHAPTER 25: INTRODUCTION

Henry F. Epstein

Jerry Lewis Neuromuscular Research Center
Baylor College of Medicine
Houston, TX

Don Fischman made a very important point in regard to the use of antibodies, both polyclonal and monoclonal, in the detection of antigens. Very few of us, if any, know the value of the dissociation equilibrium constant for the binding of our antibody or antibodies to our antigen of interest, in this case myosin.

Over the years we might obtain such information, but it would probably require forming small soluble peptides and measuring them with proper physical chemical methods. The important thing is you have to think of what possible values those might be. Let us for the moment assume that the value of the equilibrium constant for the primary antigen and antibody is 10^{-8} M (576). The actual antibody concentrations used will be of that order of magnitude. Thus, in many experiments, only a small percentage of the antigen may be bound to antibody.

What we mean by specificity even in a monoclonal antibody is probably relative; that is the equilibrium dissociation constant is much lower for an epitope on one kind of myosin compared to another. In considering homologous proteins, the most likely explanation is that there are amino acid substitutions in the sequences composing the local protein structures represented as epitopes. Such differences are consistent with factors of about 1000 between equilibrium constants. Exclusive binding to a unique myosin may rarely arise if there is substantial modification or deletion of the epitope in other isoforms.

A problem that comes up is that when we do immunolocalizations, we are dealing with a special set of reactions, with physical chemical experiments, but we are also dealing with the problem of detection of antibody antigen binding, which may be very different from measuring the percentage of active chemical reaction. You may be able to detect antibody antigen binding under conditions permitting a very low percentage of reaction.

With the nematode, one has the advantage of very tight mutants that are really in the structural gene for one kind of myosin isoform. By micro-dissection experiments the gene product or myosin is restricted to the body wall muscle versus the pharnyx, a muscle that is essentially invisible in immunoflorescence experiments with monoclonal antibodies to the body-wall myosins.

However, with the monoclonal antibody specific to myosin B as I defined specificity, careful inspection reveals faint fluorescence in the pharnx. The possibility that we were detecting a very weak secondary reaction arose in this work (577).

A specific immune reaction with the same monoclonal antibody at 100 micrograms per ml. and isolated thick filaments can be observed by electron microscopy. Secondary anti-mouse antibody is also used to detect the reaction. We call this a specific immune reaction since non-immune mouse IgG yields no detectable reaction.

The same experiment was performed with the E190 mutant. The primary antigen, myosin B, is absolutely absent due to genetic deletion. When unreacted mutant filaments and mutant filaments reacting with antibody at 100 micrograms per ml. are compared, the antibody produces a very dense specific immune reaction.

If we lowered the concentration of the monoclonal antibodies to 10 micrograms per ml., we still obtained a very dense reaction with the wild-type filaments. We could not detect reaction with the mutant filaments. An absolute change in concentration prevented detection of the secondary reaction, but permitted us to detect the primary reaction (578).

It turns out the myosin that makes up that mutant filament is also present in wild-type filaments. This type of analysis suggests that the minor isoform is restricted to a portion of the native thick filament. Nevertheless, if you react the mutant filament with the monoclonal to the minor isoform, you can see a 14.3 nm repeat along the entire filament length similar to what Don showed.

It was very difficult for us to chemically detect these secondary reactions. In immunoblot experiments, we utilized over 6 log units of concentration of either of two monoclonal antibodies. With the monoclonal antibody to myosin B, we could detect no reaction with any myosin but the major isoform over the whole range. With the monoclonal antibody which reacts to the minor isoform, under these conditions we could not detect any secondary reaction. Remembering that antibody antigen reactions are biomolecular, we increased the amount of myosin on those blots by a factor of 3 and then repeated the experiment throughout this full range of antibody concentrations.

With either antibody, pushing the reaction with high concentrations of both reactants, 500-1000 micrograms per ml of antibody and 25-50 micrograms of myosin heavy chain in the electrophoretic band, we detected additional reactions by immunoblots. The secondary reaction of the monoclonal for the major body wall isoform was with the minor body wall isoform, also vice versa, just barely seeing the secondary reaction of the monoclonal antibody to the minor myosin of body wall muscles with the major isoform. These secondary reactions are at least 1000 fold weaker than the primary reactions.

I wish to emphasize that in many instances one may detect antibody antigen reactions with the electron microscope or with the fluorescent microscope that are due to the primary specificity, but in addition, be incapable of distinguishing from the primary reaction other reactions that are very weak chemically.

Therefore, one must be concerned not only about accessibility leading to apparent differences in microscopic detection of antibody-antigen reactions, but one must seriously consider that at any given concentration of an antibody, whether reactions may be occurring not only with the primary epitope that chemistry tells you is the primary reactant but also with secondary epitopes which may be very difficult to detect, very easy to ignore as insignificant or be missed entirely in chemical experiments.

CHAPTER 26: GENETIC ANALYSIS OF DUCHENNE DYSTROPHY

Louis Kunkel, Gail Burns, Jeff Aldrige and Samuel Latt

Genetics Division
Children's Hospital
Boston, MA

We have heard many interesting presentations on the physiology and genetic structure of muscle related proteins. The examples have ranged from dystrophic muscle cells in culture to very specific analysis of both actin and myosin genes. I would like to present some of the genetic analyses of the human X chromosome being pursued in the Genetics Division at Children's Hospital in Boston. My presentation will concentrate mainly on our efforts to develop diagnostically useful restriction fragment length polymorphisms (RFLPs) (579) for the human X-linked muscular dystrophies. I will close my presentation with some initial attempts at "walking" (580) in specific X chromosomal regions.

Both the Becker and Duchenne (DMD) dystrophy loci are presumed to be localized to the central dark band (Xp21) of the human X chromosome (581-583). The human X chromosome has been partially purified from the human autosomes by fluorescence activated chromosome sorting and X chromosome enriched recombinant libraries constructed (584,585). Such libraries serve as highly enriched sources of X chromosome-specific DNA sequences. A cloned insert of DNA can be identified as unique and the location in the genome determined by southern hybridization analysis (585) (Figure 95). A summary of all X chromosome DNA fragments prepared within the Genetics Division by our laboratory and the laboratory of Dr. Gail Bruns is presented in Figure 95. Thirty-six fragments of X chromosome DNA span the entire X. Although most are of no known function, some are known to be expressed as cellular RNA and presumably translated into proteins (586). Many more fragments are currently being prepared and localized to increase this composite picture.

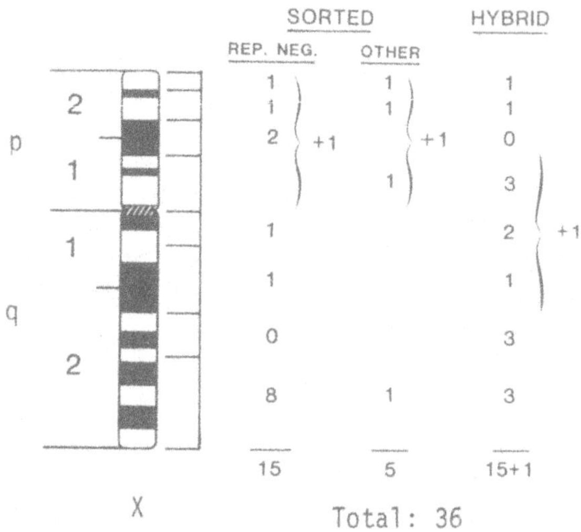

FIGURE 95: Summary of X chromosome localization results. All cloned fragments of DNA were determined to be free of repeated sequence elements (585) and were mapped by hybridization to nitrocellulose filter imprints of human and human-rodent hybrid DNA samples cleaved with restriction endonucleases (585). The human-rodent hybrid mapping panels were either developed within the genetics division or were the generous gift of Dr. T. Mohandas. A schematic X chromosome is presented with various regions highlighted as the range into which a fragment has been localized. Twenty unique fragments were isolated from a flow sorting enriched X chromosome library (585) as either directly repeat sequence negative or indirectly adjacent to repeated sequences or transcribed regions. Sixteen fragments were isolated from a rodent-human hybrid phage library and human X sequences were identified on the basis of being adjacent to human repeated sequence elements. The numbers are a numerical representation of the clones which localized to various regions.

A specific example of physical mapping was undertaken in collaboration with Drs. DeMartinville and Francke of Yale University. Eleven known Xp DNA fragments (prepared within the Genetics Division) were tested against various rodent-human hybrid DNA samples with structurally abnormal or rearranged X chromosomes. From this collaborative study, two cloned fragments were presumptively localized to the region Xp21 (based on the estimated deletion position in the cells used); both of the probes should be physically close to the DMD and Becker dystrophy loci. Newly prepared fragments will be localized in a similar manner with a goal of positioning approximately 40 fragments within or nearby the Xp21 region.

Once positioned to a specific region, a cloned fragment is most useful if it allows genetic distinction of the two X chromosomes in a woman heterozygous for an X-linked disorder. RFLP's (579) represent one means of distinguishing homologus chromosomes in a genetic analysis of families. We have chosen a strategy of RFLP identification which maximizes the likelihood of finding a high frequency RFLP allele system with a minimum of effort (587). Such analysis has been used to test 17 X-specific fragments for recognition of RFLP alleles. An example of the RFLP search strategy is presented in Figure 96. This autoradiograph of the hybridization pattern of the probe D2 to eight different enzyme digests demonstrates the restriction fragment length variation for the enzyme PvuII. The central female DNA sample in the PvuII digests exhibits two hybridizing fragments of 6.6 and 6.0kb, whereas the other two samples only exhibit the smaller 6.0kb fragment. This probe (D2) recognizes a putative RFLP for the enzyme PvuII. From similar analysis, nine new two allele RFLPs have been identified for nine regions of the human X chromosome. Five of these regions are in Xp.

To determine the allele frequencies of the various RFLP detecting probes, DNA samples were obtained from various unrelated heterozygote females segregating human X-linked diseases. The hybridization pattern of another Xp fragment to these female DNA samples is presented in Figure 97. The probe 99-6 hybridizes to a 11kb Pst I fragment from most X chromosomes, but on 29% of X chromosomes, a Pst I site has been lost yielding a larger 22kb hybridizing fragment. Similar analysis has been performed for all X chromosome RFLP detecting probes. The allele status of each woman has been determined, and her offspring contacted and DNA prepared from collected blood samples. Those probes useful for linkage analysis in a specific family were hybridized to restriction enzyme digested DNA samples. An example of this analysis is presented in Figure 98. A woman heterozygous for DMD had two sons affected with DMD. She was also heterzygous for the 22 and 11kb Pst I fragments recognized by 99-6 and the 6.0 and 6.6kb PvuII fragments recognized by the probe D2. Both affected boys received the DMD X and the 6.0kb PvuII fragment hybridizing with the probe D2, a result consistent with no recombination between these two regions on the X. The third region of the X hybridizing with the probe 99-6 does exhibit recombination with DMD (in contrast with the behavior of this probe and DMD in another larger pedigree). Although both boys inherited the DMD X, they each received a different 99-6 allele (one, the 11kb Pst I fragment, the other the 22kb Pst I fragment). This result is consistent with a recombination event between the DMD locus and the 99-6 region. The results presented in Figure 98 are also consistent with the localization of D2 closer to DMD than 99-6.

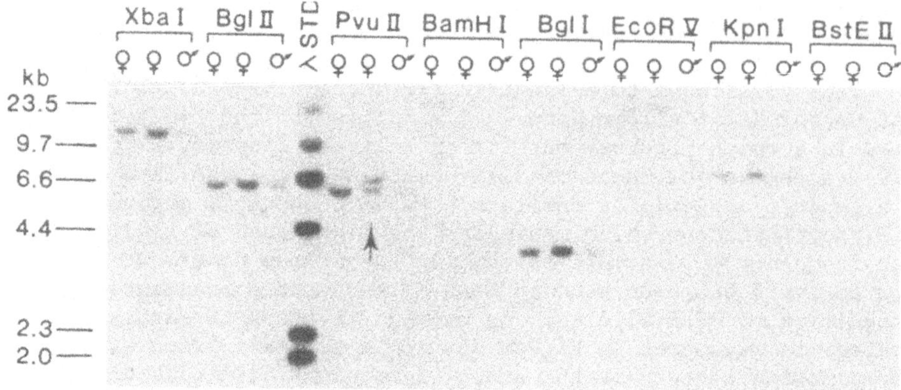

FIGURE 96: Autoradiograph of the screen for RFLP alleles detected by the probe D2. Eight restriction enzymes were used to cleave the same three human DNA samples; two female, one male. Approximately one microgram of digested DNA was loaded into each lane and the fragments separated on the basis of molecular weight by agarose gel electrophoresis. The samples were transferred to nitrocellulose and the filter hybridized with ^{32}P-labeled probe D2. Above each lane is the enzyme used to digest the DNA samples indicated by female, female and male symbols. The arrow indicates the one female DNA sample cleaved with the enzyme PvuII which exhibits a putative RFLP for the probe D2.

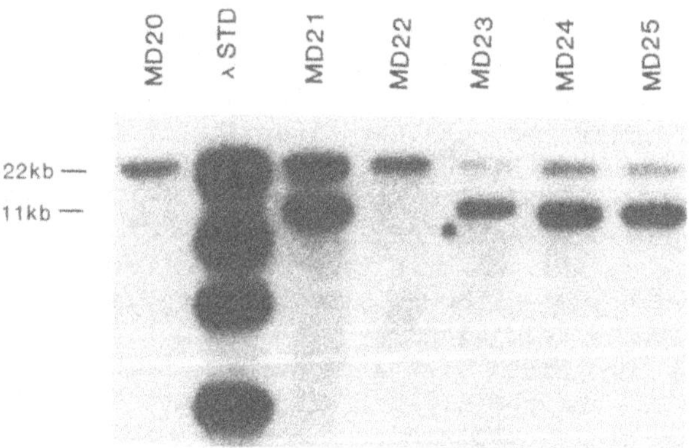

FIGURE 97: Hybridization of the probe 99-6 to various carrier female DNA samples cleaved with Pst I. Six unrelated carrier females for DMD were ascertained and DNA samples prepared. Each DNA was cleaved with the Pst I and the digested DNA (2 ug) hybridized with the probe 99-6. Four females are heterozygous for the 11 and 22 kb fragments, while the other two are homozygous for the 22 kb fragment.

Forty-seven human DNA samples were cleaved with the appropriate enzymes and probes with each of 4 Xp localized RFLP detecting cloned fragments. A summary of hybridization results is presented in the preliminary physical and genetic map of Xp in Figure 99. The two RFLP detecting probes 99-6 and D2 physically map to Xp21->Xp22; B24 to Xp21 and 58 to Xcen->Xp21. These loci are presented relative to DMD and the recombination fractions are given. The placing of 99-6 distal to D2 is based on two crossover events observed for 99-6 with DMD but no crossovers in these same individuals when D2 was tested. The results are preliminary, but the general physical relationship should be maintained when additional individuals are tested. The previously published clones L128 and RC8 (582) would localize near 58 and 99-6 respectively. Although a total of 47

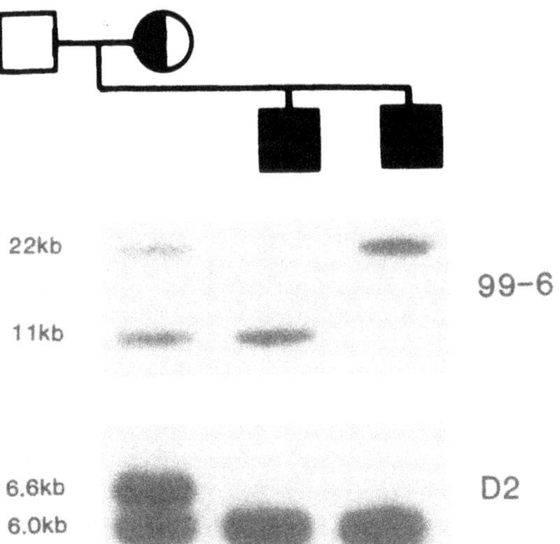

FIGURE 98: Inheritance of 99-6 and D2 alleles in the same DMD family. DNA samples isolated from a carrier female and her two affected sons were cleaved separately with both Pst I and PvuII restriction endonucleases. The mother is heterozygous for both the 99-6 Pst I RFLP and the D2 PvuII RFLP as indicated in the lane under her symbol. Both boys received the same D2 (6.0kb) allele whereas, they received different 99-6 alleles (one 22kb, one 11kb). The two hybridization experiments were done separately and the results combined here as panels marked 99-6 or D2.

individuals were typed for their allele status for the various Xp probes, no probe was informative for more than 18 meiotic events. Additional families are currently being tested to increase the significance of these results.

The ideal situation would be to have all RFLP detecting probes informative in every family. Towards this goal we have initiated "walking" experiments within the DNA region surrounding each of these cloned DNA fragments, to generate a polymorphic haplotype.

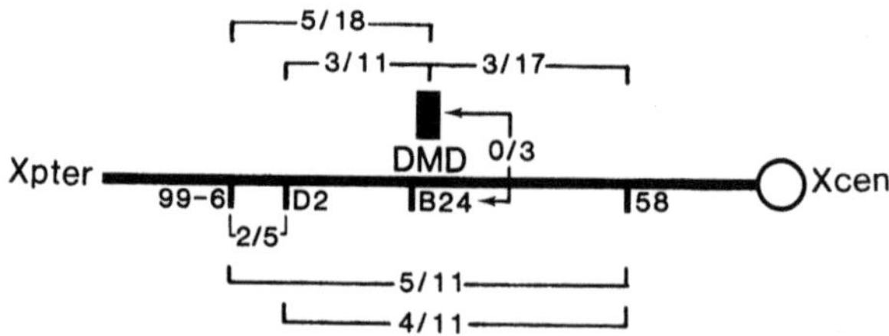

FIGURE 99: Summary of the fraction recombinates observed for 4 RFLP detecting Xp probes in DMD families. The linear arrangement of the cloned fragments is presented relative to the presumed Xp21 DMD locus. Fragments were first positioned by physical localization with mapping panels as either towards the centromere or towards Xpter from DMD. The key hybrid DNA sample was one containing a translocation involving Xp21 with X chromosome representation from Xp21->Xqter. The fraction recombination is presented as the number of recombinates observed in a total number of possible meiotic events tested. The brackets refer to the regions being compared. The positioning of D2 and 99-6 is based on the fact that in two families, the D2 alleles cosegregated with DMD, whereas 99-6 exhibited two recombinates in these same DNA samples. The probe B24 has a low rare allele frequency and was only informative in one small DMD family.

The source of overlapping genome clones was a newly constructed partial MboI digest human X chromosome library (manuscript in preparation). Eight small cloned DNA fragments (2-4kb) from Xp have been each expanded to at least 15kb, and small unique segments are being subcloned in pBR322. These new probes should themselves detect RFLP alleles and hence increase the heterozygosity detectable in each region. Family studies with these new probes will be initiated when appropriate.

Cloned fragments of X chromosome DNA represent genetic and physical tools to approach the problem of Duchenne muscular dystrophy. The closest probes may lead to the accurate detection of the altered DMD locus in families and affected individuals. Proximity to the locus may ultimately lead to the isolation of the region of DNA altered in DMD and a correlation with the abnormal properties of DMD muscle tissue presented at this meeting.

DR. WOOD: Dr. Kunkel, have you looked at any Becker dystrophy?

DR. KUNKEL: We have not looked at any Becker dystrophy families yet, but it appeared initially that our probe was closely linked to Duchenne dystrophy. That last two families we have tested, though, have exhibited recombinates. We have begun a collaboration with Jim Gusella, who has a series of Duchenne families. We will do Southern blots on those informative family member suing this particular probe to strengthen linkage information. It is possible that there may be more than one locus involved in DMD, hence the discrepancy in our results.

DR. WOOD: What is the criterion for diagnosis in these families? Are they all in wheelchairs, are they all 12 years old?

DR. KUNKEL: Actually some of the cell lines are from boys who are no longer alive, but to my knowledge, they all were in wheelchairs by age 12.

DR. BLAU: I still don't understand how Dr. Kunkel will know as he walks along the X chromosome, when he reaches the Duchenne gene.

DR. KUNKEL: One way is to pinpoint the break in the translocations involving Xp21. There are now more than 10 translocations which break in the Xp21 region, all of which appear cytogenetically indistinguishable from each other. Segregation of a few of these translocation chromosomes in hybrid cells would allow positioning of random fragments to either side of the breakpoint. As "walking" proceeds along the DNA, constant testing of a unique probe against these hybrid cell DNA samples should flag when you have crossed the breakpoint. For example, a probe from one end of a phage clone would hybridize with one translocation but not the other, but a second probe from the same phage would hybridize oppositely.

A second way relies strongly on the putative high mutation frequency for the Duchenne locus. This fact is supported by the number of rearrangements observed in the region. A natural extension of this logic is that a lot of Duchenne males have small deletions of Xp21. Any fragments that localized to these deleted regions would be candidates for close markers or "walking" points to the Duchenne locus. Given sufficient probes from the region and sufficient number of unrelated DMD male DNA samples, a series of overlapping deletions may be found. The smallest area of deletion overlap would pinpoint the DMD DNA region.

Looking at 20 different Duchenne males with the two existing probes from the Xp21 region, we just might get lucky with restriction enzymes that cleave human DNA into very large fragments. Each probe should allow a search of approximately 50kb of DNA from the region surrounding the probe. This is approximately 5% of the Xp21 region and a deletion in one of these males might fall in a region covered by one of these two probes.

CHAPTER 27: THE CHROMOSOMAL ASSIGNMENT OF MUSCLE-SPECIFIC GENES

David Yaffe*, Uri Nudel, Henryk Czosnek, Danielle Melloul, and Batya Aloni

Department of Cell Biology
The Weizmann Institute of Science
Rehobot, Israel

Investigations during recent years indicate that the program of gene expression during the differentiation of the striated muscles is much more complex than had been suggested from earlier studies. It is now evident that muscle differentiation is accompanied by successive transitions from embryonic to fetal to adult isoforms of closely related contractile proteins, as well as transitions from fast to slow muscle-specific isoforms, which are under the control of physiological and hormonal factors (381,588,592). Moreover, some contractile proteins seem to be the main adult isoform in one muscle and a juvenile isoform in another muscle. Recently it was found that the mRNA coding for the isoform of actin which is the adult type in the cardiac muscle (cardiac actin) is transiently present in the newborn skeletal muscle (60). We have found a converse situation in the heart. In the newborn heart, the skeletal muscle actin mRNA is present in significant amounts, decreasing rapidly with maturation (593,594). The biological significance of these changes and how they are controlled is unknown. The understanding of the basic mechanisms

* We wish to thank Ms. Zehava Levy, Sara Neuman and Ora Saxel for their excellent technical assistance; Dr. J. Calvo and X. Young for constructing the plasmid pcv, Drs. C.M. Gorman and B.H. Howard for pSVo CAT; Dr. Silverstein for plasmid pIPB and the Scherring Corporation for a gift of G418.

Supported by the Muscular Dystrophy Association, Inc., USA, by the National Institutes of Health, the U.S. Israel Bi-national Science Foundation, Jerusalem and by the Leo and Julia Forchheimer Center for Molecular Genetics of the Weizmann Institute of Science.

controlling these changes in gene expression during muscle development is important for understanding the physiology of muscle function and muscle malformations.

Several coordinatively expressed genes in bacteria and eukaryotes have been found to be clustered (e.g. histone genes in sea urchin and Drosophila, heat shock gene in Drosophila and the chorion gene in silkworm and Drosophila) (595-598). Information on the organization of genes which are coordinatively expressed may provide clues to the mode of control of their expression as well as to their evolution and their involvement in genetically determined disorders. To determine whether genes which are expressed during terminal differentiation of muscle cells are clustered in a specific chromosomal site, we (in collaboration with F. Ruddle, P. Barker and D. Pravtcheva) first assigned the genes coding for several of the major contractile proteins to mouse chromosomes. This included the genes coding for the skeletal muscle myosin heavy chain, myosin light chain 2, and the skeletal muscle, cardiac and cytoplasmic actins. DNA preparations obtained from mouse-Chinese hamster somatic cell hybrids containing incomplete subsets of mouse chromosomes were analyzed by the Southern blotting technique using gene-specific DNA probes (599,600). The results shown in Table 18 can be summarized as follows:

1. The 3 actin genes are located on 3 different chromosomes. The skeletal muscle actin gene and several yet unidentified actin genes (or pseudogenes) are located on chromosome 3. The cardiac actin gene and several yet unidentified actin genes (or pseudogenes) are located on chromosome 17. The cytoplasmic beta-actin gene is located on chromosome 5.

2. The fast skeletal muscle myosin light chain 2 gene is located on chromosome 7.

3. All detectable myosin heavy chain genes, which cross hybridize with probes containing DNA sequences of the skeletal muscle myosin heavy chain, are located on chromosome 11. The question whether the myosin heavy chain genes are linked in a specific region of this chromosome has not been determined as yet.

Since the genes coding for 3 of the major muscle-specific proteins are not clustered, the mechanism of the control of their expression during terminal differentiation is not based on the activation of a common chromatin domain.

The finding that the skeletal muscle and cardiac actin genes are located on 2 different chromosomes excludes the possibility that the transient co-expression of the cardiac and skeletal muscle actin genes in the newborn heart and skeletal muscle

TABLE 18

Assignment of genes coding for contractile proteins to mouse chromosomes

Chromosome No.	Muscle-specific	Non-muscle	Unidentified
2			4-6 actin DNA sequences
3	Skeletal muscle actin		1 actin DNA sequence
5		Cytoplasmic β-actin	
7	Fast muscle myosin light chain 2		
11	All (?) sarcomeric myosin heavy chains		
17	Cardiac muscle actin		2 actin DNA sequences
X			20-50 copies of actin-related DNA sequence

Based on data from Czosnek et al. (1982, 1983, and unpublished).

(mentioned above) is a result of their close proximity in the DNA. Rather, it suggests independent activation or co-activation by transacting control factors.

The identification of the additional actin DNA sequences located together with the skeletal muscle and cardiac actins on chromosomes 3 and 5, respectively, might contribute valuable information to our knowledge on the actin gene family and its evolution. It is also of obvious interest to determine whether the myosin heavy chain genes, which are located on a single chromosome, are clustered and are arranged in some relation to the order of their expression.

Several hereditary degenerative diseases affecting the skeletal muscles have been assigned to mouse chromosomes (601). These include a disease very similar to human Duchenne muscular dystrophy (602). However, to our knowledge, none of these diseases has been assigned to chromosomes 3, 7, 11 or 17. Thus, the structural genes coding for myosin heavy chain, myosin light chain 2, and the skeletal muscle, cardiac do not seem to be causally involved in those muscle diseases.

Recent progress in recombinant DNA techniques and the discovery that cloned genes can be introduced into eukaryotic cells and be expressed now allow some of the questions relating to the control of gene expression to be investigated at the DNA level.

Expression of Cloned Genes Introduced into Myogenic Cells

Active genes are organized in chromatin in a conformation which render them preferentially sensitive to nucleolytic enzymes (603,604). We have previously shown that genes coding for muscle proteins were relatively insensitive to DNAase I in the nuclei of mononucleated proliferating myogenic cells but became preferentially DNAase I sensitive during the transition to the stage of cell fusion (605). We have also found a close temporal correlation between the formation of multinucleated fibers and the accumulation of the skeletal muscle actin mRNA in L8 myogenic cells (606). These observations indicate that the activation of transcription of these genes occurred during terminal differentiation. Thus, the myogenic cell line system seems to be suitable for the investigation of the activation during cell differentiation of cloned tissue- and stage-specific genes, stably integrated into the mononucleated proliferating precursor cells. A number of rat genes coding for contractile proteins have been isolated and sequenced (594,607-609). These genes can now be used for the transfection experiments. In the experiments reported here we investigated the question whether information regarding the developmentally regulated expression of genes expressed during terminal differentiation of skeletal muscle is an intrinsic property of these genes, encoded in the DNA sequence of the gene or its flanking regions. The results show that DNA sequences located in the 5' region of the skeletal muscle actin gene contain information for the regulated expression of this gene during terminal differentiation of myogenic cells.

Expression of an actin/globin chimeric gene in myogenic cells

To be able to distinguish between the transcripts of the endogenous skeletal muscle actin gene and the gene introduced into the cells via gene transfer, we constructed a chimeric rat skeletal muscle actin/human ε-globin gene. The chimeric gene was composed of about two-thirds of the 5' region of the structural gene coding for rat skeletal muscle actin plus 730 bp upstream from the transcription initiation site and about one-third of the 3' region of human ε-globin gene as described in Figure 100. To select for cells containing the chimeric gene, we co-transfected proliferating L8 mononucleated cells with this plasmid and a plasmid containing a dominant neomycin resistance gene ($pIPB_1$), using the calcium phosphate precipitation technique (610,611). Selection was then made in the presence of the neomycin derivative G418. We isolated 20 neomycin-resistant clones, each originating from a single transfected cell. Ten of these were tested by Southern blot hybridization and all were

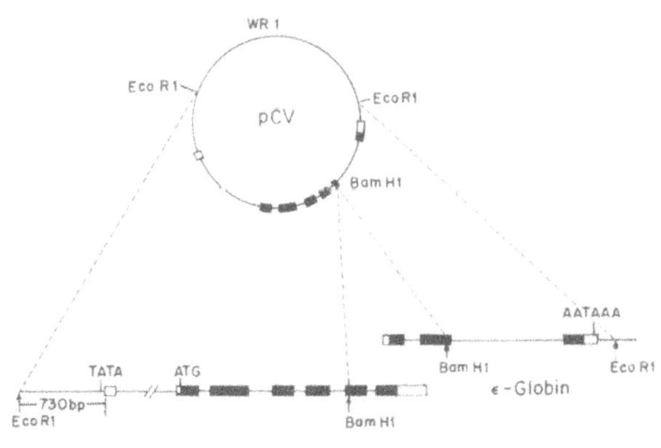

FIGURE 100: Structure of the plasmid pCV containing the chimeric rat skeletal muscle actin human ε-globin gene. The regions of the skeletal muscle actin gene and the ε-globin gene used for the construction of the fused genes are indicated by dashed lines. Empty bars present 5' and 3' untranslated regions. Solid bars represent coding regions. WR1 = plasmid pWR_1 (612).

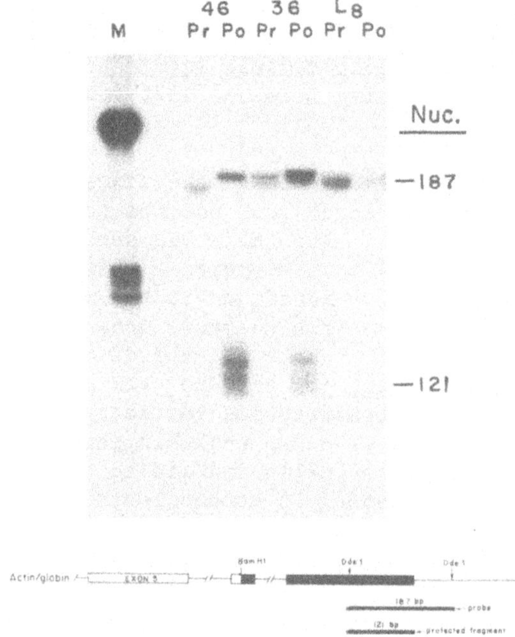

Figure 101: Regulated expression of the actin/globin chimeric gene in myogenic cells. A. Samples containing 40 ug of total RNA isolated from undifferentiated (Pr) and differentiated (Po) cultures of the myogenic clones L8-46 and L8-36, transfected with the actin/globin chimeric gene and control L8 cells, were hybridized with ^{32}P end-labeled DNA fragment extending from a Dde 1 site 121 nucleotides upstream to the putative polyadenylation site of the ε-globin gene to a Dd1 site 66 nucleotides 3' to the polyadenylated site. After hybridization for 16 h at 52°C, each sample was treated with 500 units of endonuclease S1 (30 min at 37°C). The hybrid molecules were then precipitated, electrophoresed on polyacrylamide/urea gel, and fluorographed. RNA from differentiated cultures of clones L8-46 and L8-36 protected a ca. 121 nucleotide long fragment of the probe. Very little protection was obtained in reaction mixtures containing RNA from cultures of mononucleated cells of these lines. No protection was obtained by RNA from control undifferentiated as well as differentiated L8 cultures. The 187 nucleotide fragment is a result of reannealing of the probe during hybridization (162). B. Schematic description of the probe used for the S1 analysis and the fragment protected by the chimeric RNA. Thick empty bars represent exons with skeletal muscle actin DNA sequence. Thick black bars represent exons with ε-globin DNA sequence.

found to contain the actin/globin chimeric gene. The estimated copy number of the transferred gene varied between 1 and 50 (one clone had more than 500 copies).

The expression of the chimeric gene was assayed by the S1 mapping technique, using probes derived either from the skeletal muscle actin cDNA clone p749 or from the ε-globin gene. In a significant number of the clones, the expression of the chimeric gene was found to be developmentally regulated, i.e. the expression of the gene greatly increased (up to more than 50-fold) during the differentiation of the cultures (formation of multinucleated fibers; Figure 101). Furthermore, the temporal relation between differentiation of the cultures and accumulation of the transcription products of the transfected genes was very similar to that of the native skeletal muscle actin gene (Figure 102). This suggests that the two genes are responding to common regulatory factors. S1 endonuclease analysis of the transcripts indicated a correct initiation and termination of the chimeric actin/globin mRNA (612).

Studies of a variety of genes have indicated that the DNA sequences necessary for the transcription of genes are located in the 5' flanking region. To test whether the increased expression of the transferred chimeric gene, which occurred during differentiation was a specific response to cell differentiation, and to determine whether the DNA sequences responsible for the regulated expression of the gene are located in the 5' region of the muscle actin gene, we constructed a plasmid (pα-CAT) containing 730 bp of the 5' flanking region of the rat skeletal muscle actin gene (plus the exon of the 5' untranslated region and 25 bp of the first intron), fused to the bacterial structure gene coding for CAT (Figure 103). The plasmids were introduced into L8 cells, as described above, and clones of myogenic cells containing transferred genes were isolated. CAT activity was measured in extracts from undifferen-

Expression of the Bacterial Chloramphenicol Acetyl Transase (CAT) Gene Spliced to the Muscle Actin Gene Promoter

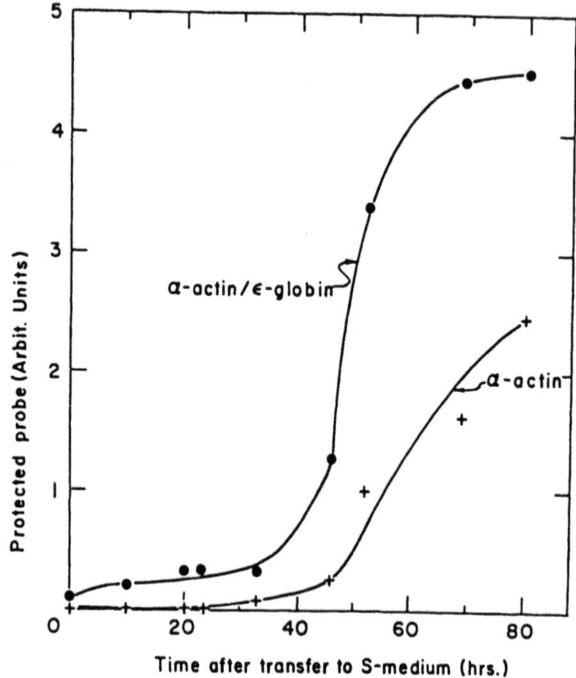

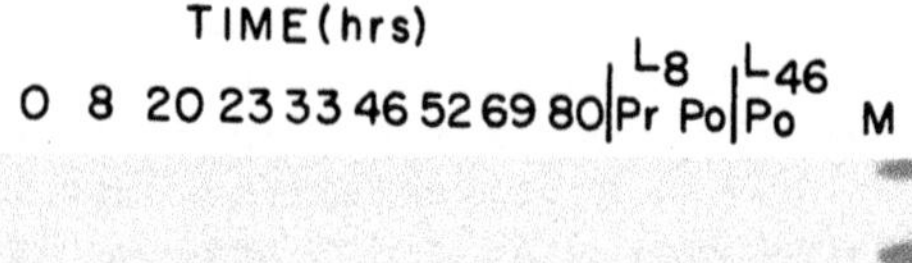

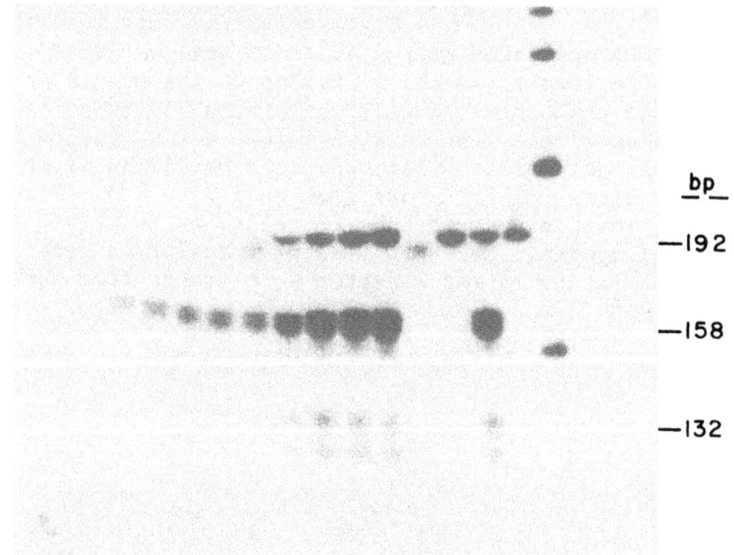

FIGURE 102: Correlation between accumulation of actin/globin gene transcripts and the native skeletal muscle actin mRNA during differentiation of a clone (continued on p. 303).

tiated and differentiated cultures. In the majority of the isolated clones of cells containing the plasmid pα-CAT, CAT activity increased many-fold during differentiation. Only very small changes in CAT activity were observed in clones containing the plasmid pβ-CAT (Figure 104). The results show that the increase in CAT activity during differentiation in clones containing the plasmid pα-CAT was regulated by DNA sequences contained in the fragment derived from the skeletal muscle gene (612).

These experiments demonstrated the existence of DNA sequences in the 5' region of the skeletal muscle actin gene which conferred the developmentally regulated expression of the actin gene. The ability to assay the control of expression of muscle genes by transfection of myogenic cells now makes it possible to define these sequences and perhaps to identify the factors produced during differentiation which regulate the expression of these genes.

Comparison of the sequences of the rat and chick skeletal muscle actin genes (which were separated at least 250 million years ago) reveals very little homology between 5' untranslated regions and between the introns of the two genes. However, the flanking regions between the CAAT box and ca 150 nucleotides upstream from this sequence are considerably conserved. Of particular interest is an almost identical sequence (95% homology) of 20 nucleotides, which includes the CAAT box. These sequences may be involved in the regulation of the tissue-specific expression of the skeletal muscle actin gene (593,613). In order to identify the sequences determining the tissue specificity, we plan to alter

Figure 102 (continued)

of myogenic cells containing the actin/globin chimeric gene (L8-46). A. Cultures of L8-46 mononucleated cells, approaching confluency, were stimulated to differentiate by changing the medium to the fusion promoting 2HI medium (0 time). At the indicated times, cultures were harvested and RNA was extracted and analyzed by the S1 endonuclease method using a cDNA probe which hybridizes with the native actin mRNA (yielding a 192 nucleotide long protected fragment) and with the chimeric mRNA (the major protected fragment - 158 nucleotides). Cell fusion began about 36 h after the change of medium. B. The autoradiograms from the S1 nuclease analysis were scanned by a Beckman DU8 spectrophotometer (using exposures which were in the linear range of the film). The relative intensities of the signals formed by the probes protected by the skeletal muscle actin mRNA and by the cimeric mRNA are shown in the figure (612).

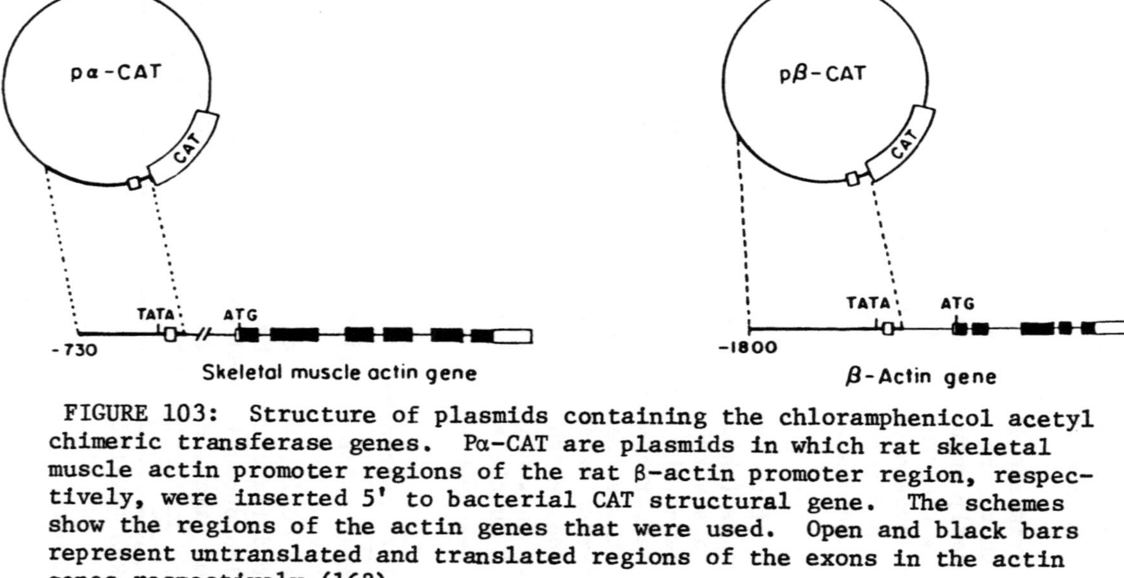

FIGURE 103: Structure of plasmids containing the chloramphenicol acetyl chimeric transferase genes. Pα-CAT are plasmids in which rat skeletal muscle actin promoter regions of the rat β-actin promoter region, respectively, were inserted 5' to bacterial CAT structural gene. The schemes show the regions of the actin genes that were used. Open and black bars represent untranslated and translated regions of the exons in the actin genes respectively (162).

```
                                      CAAT BOX

         5'              CAAT
RAT      TCTAGTGCCCAACACCCAAATATGGCTTGGGAAGGGCAACAACATTCCT   TCGGGCGGTGTGG

CHICK    CGCCGGGCCCGACACCCAAATATGGCGCGGCCGGGGTCG    CATTCCTGTCGCGGGCCGGGCGG

                       TATA                            cap
RAT      AGAGCTCAGGACTATATAAAAACCTGAGGCTAGGGACAGGCGGTCACACGGACGTGAAGCCTCAC

CHICK      TGCTCCCGTCGATA  AAAGGCTCCGGGGCCGG     CGGGCGACCCGAGCTACCCGGAGGAG

                  3'
RAT      TTCCTACCCT

CHICK    CGGGAGGCGT
```

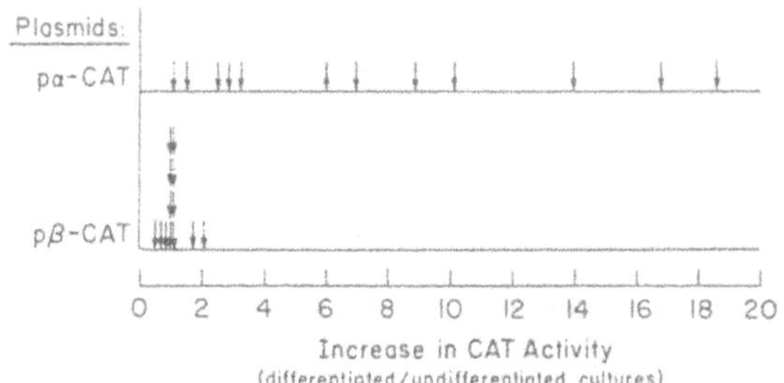

FIGURE 104: The increase in CAT activity following differentiation of myogenic clones containing pα-CAT or pβ-CAT genes. Quantitation of CAT activity was done by measuring the conversion of ^{32}P-labeled chloramphenicol to its acetylated forms. For each transfected clone the same amount of extract from undifferentiated and differentiated cultures was used. The numbers on the abscissa indicate the ratio between CAT activity in extracts from differentiated versus undifferentiated cultures of the same clone. Each arrow represents the ratio of activities from a single clone. Broken arrows represent clones in which no cell fusion occurred after growth for 72 h in the differentiation-stimulating 2HI medium.

selected sequences flanking the skeletal muscle actin gene and test the effects of these modifications on the regulation of expression of the genes following their reintroduction into myoblasts.

The experiments described above demonstrate the existence in the region of the structural gene of DNA sequences which are involved in the control of tissue-specific expression of the skeletal muscle actin. This, however, does not exclude the existence of additional control mechanisms operating on different levels. It should be noted that in most myogenic clones which expressed the transfected gene, small amounts of transcripts were detected even in RNA extracted from cultures of proliferating mononucleated cells. At that stage no native muscle actin mRNA was detected. This may indicate that the control of the transfected gene is more relaxed than that of the native gene. There are several other observations suggested that cloned genes introduced into host cells behave in some respects differently from the corresponding native genes. For example, α2 globulin is normally expressed in the liver and is induced by glucocorticoids. When a clones α2u globulin gene was introduced into Ltk-cells, its expression should be induced by glucocorticoids. However, the native L cell α2u globulin gene remained inactive (612,614). By introducing the gene into somatic cells (i.e., myoblasts) we may circumvent important processes taking place during early embryogenesis, e.g., DNA methylation (615,616). There are several reports in the introduction of tissue specific genes into fertilized mammalian eggs. In most of these experiments, proper regulation of the expression of the gene was not observed. Instead, some of the observations suggest that the site of integration of the donor gene can play an important role in determining the tissue specificity of expression (617,618). To examine the expression of cloned muscle genes following their introduction into the germ line, we have now begun experiments, in collaboration with Dr. M. Shani, in which we injected muscle-specific genes into fertilized mouse eggs which were subsequently implanted into pseudopregnant female mice. The pattern of expression of these genes, in the tissues of the mice which developed from injected eggs in their offspring is being investigated. This is compared with the expression of the same genes introduced into myoblasts.

CHAPTER 28: EXPRESSION OF ISOFORMS FROM CLONED SKELETAL AND CARDIAC ACTIN GENES

Laurence H. Kedes

Department of Medicine
Stanford University School of Medicine
Palo Alto, California

Some of the molecular events in human muscle parallel in many respects the data already presented regarding the expression or co-expression of certain isoforms of contractile protein genes. Contractile protein isoforms can be studied in a model system based on the genetic engineering of cells in which we introduce contractile protein genes into foreign environments and, once they are expressed, ask what they do to the phenotype of the cell. One can also use a muscle cDNA library to study muscle specific genes and their human chromosomal linkages.

We have recently cloned from a human library the full length of cDNAs from the cardiac and skeletal alpha actin genes as well as the cDNAs for the beta and gamma actins. We then cloned their corresponding genomic clones. We found co-expression of skeletal and cardiac actin in human heart and in human skeletal muscle.

We developed both isotype and species specific probes from the 3' untranslated regions of the cDNAs and in so doing had to get around the fact that there is a great deal of evolutionary conservation of the 3' untranslated regions. On the other hand, the isotype sequences for the actins are very distinct from each other. Thus, working within a single species one has no trouble distinguishing skeletal from cardiac actin gene expression but when using a probe across species, one does have cross-hybridization. If one introduces a foreign gene into a new species, one is going to pick up the endogenous gene expression as well. Thus, it is crucial to have isotype specific probes for such experiments because cross-hybridization and contamination of probes sometimes leads to erroneous results.

It has recently become clear that the 3' untranslated regions have strong sequence conservation along evolutionary lines all the way from chicken through human but that these conserved sequences are segmentally arranged in the mRNA. That is, there are sub-regions that are both species specific as well as isotype specific. Accordingly, we prepared such species and isotype specific probes and now can use our probes either to look at expression in many species or to look at the expression of specific genes in heterologus systems.

Figure 105 shows a Southern blot of DNA from the skeletal and cardiac actin cDNA clones and from the genomic clones. The skeletal actin probe hybridizes only to the appropriate fragments of skeletal actin DNA and the cardiac probe hybridizes only to the appropriate fragments of cardiac actin DNA and they don't cross-hybridize. Thus probes are quite specific.

We were plagued for a few years by the problem of a large number of actin coding sequences in the human genome as well as in other mammalian genomes: there are at least 30 or 40 regions of the genome that seem to contain DNA sequences coding for actin. We have determined that there is but a single copy for the human alpha skeletal actin gene and for the cardiac actin gene but there are multiple copies for each of the beta and gamma actin genes. Many of those copies are pseudo-genes, that is genes whose transcription products, if they even exist, would not be capable of making a functional mRNA or protein.

Figure 106 is a Southern blot of human DNA cut with a series of restriction endonucleases. Only a single fragment hybridizes in most of the digests using the actin, isotype-specific, human probe. The reason there are 2 bands in lane 3 is because the probe itself is cut with the restriction enzyme SAC I and in the human genomic DNA you get the two expected bands. Thus actin is a single copy in the haploid human genome. This kind of experiment helps us in interpreting gene expression experiments when questions might arise, such as is there a hidden copy of the isotype that is not being examined or, is there a cross-hybridizing isotype? Since the skeletal actin gene is single copy we don't have that to worry about. A Southern blot demonstrates that the same is true for the human cardiac gene (Figure 107). A series of restriction enzyme digests of human DNA was tested with the isotype specific cardiac actin probe. Again we see single bands in all 5 lanes so we don't have to worry about a hidden isotype being expressed in some of these experiments.

The Relative Distribution of Skeletal & Cardiac Muscle Actins

Given such probes it is possible to look at the expression of cardiac and alpha actin mRNA in various human tissues. Since the RNAs are essentially identical in size, one must develop specific probes.

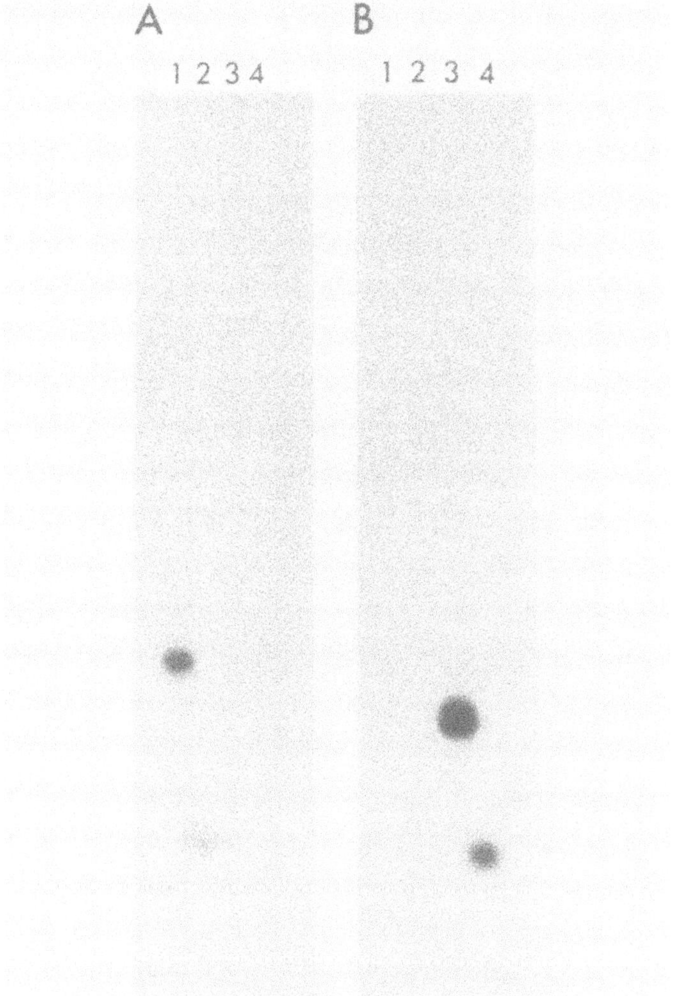

FIGURE 105: Lane 1: Skeletal actin cDNA; Lane 2: skeletal actin 3' untranslated region; Lane 3: cardiac actin cDNA; Lane 4: cardiac actin 3' untranslated region. Hybridization specificity of human muscle skeletal and cardiac actin 3' untranslated region probes. The skeletal and cardiac actin cDNA clones plus the 3' untranslated region sub-clones were digested with appropriate restriction enzymes to generate cDNA fragments free of vector. After electrophoresis on a 1% agarose gel, the fragments were transferred to nitrocellulose and hybridized with a nick-translated skeletal actin 3' probe (A) or cardiac actin 3' probe (B). The DNA digests for the two blots were identical.

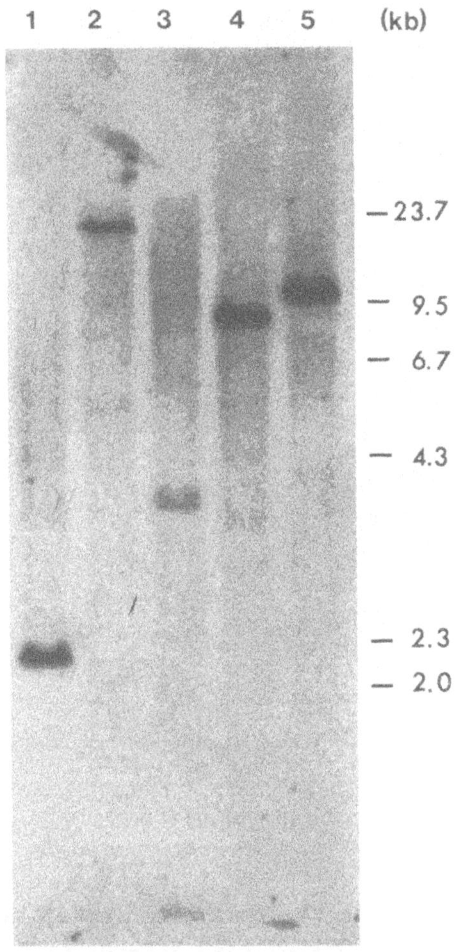

FIGURE 106: Detection of the α-actin gene in the human genome. DNA (8 μg) was digested with Bgl II (1), EcoRI (2), SacI (3), PvuII (4), or Hind III (5) and blot transferred to a nitrocellulose filter. The filter was hybridized with α-actin-specific probe. Size markers are indicated to the right of the figure.

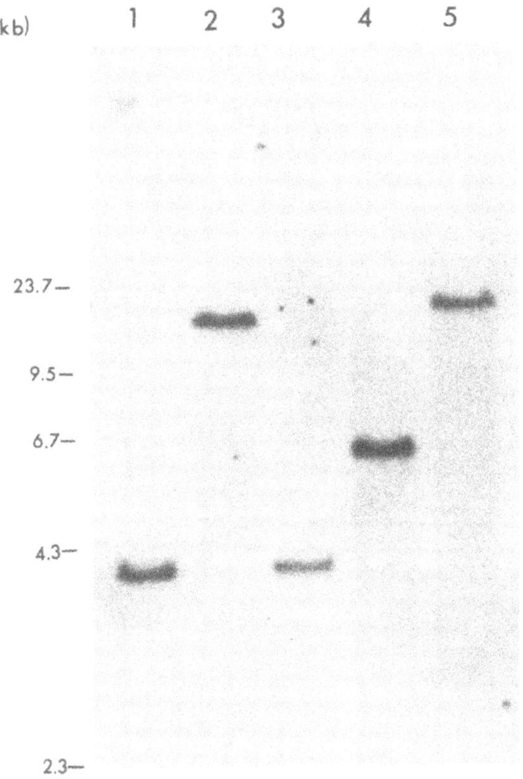

FIGURE 107: Analysis of the cardiac actin gene. Human genomic DNA was digested exactly as described in Figure 106. Blots were hybridized with the human cardiac actin specific probe.

Figure 108 shows a Northern blot of RNA isolated from human skeletal muscle and probed with either skeletal actin specific probe or human cardiac specific probe. The amounts of RNA in each of these lanes is subtly different. Since the probes are essentially of the same specific activity, we can make a relatively good assessment that the ratio of cardiac actin in human leg skeletal muscle is about 5% that of skeletal actin; the ratio is thus about 20:1. Thus 5% of the mRNA in human skeletal muscle seems to be cardiac actin.

Lanes 4 and 8 are the hybridization of those probes with RNA isolated from HeLa cells showing that the specificity for those muscle actins is really complete because it doesn't cross-hybridize with the beta or gamma messengers present in that cell line.

The expression of cardiac actin mRNAs in human skeletal

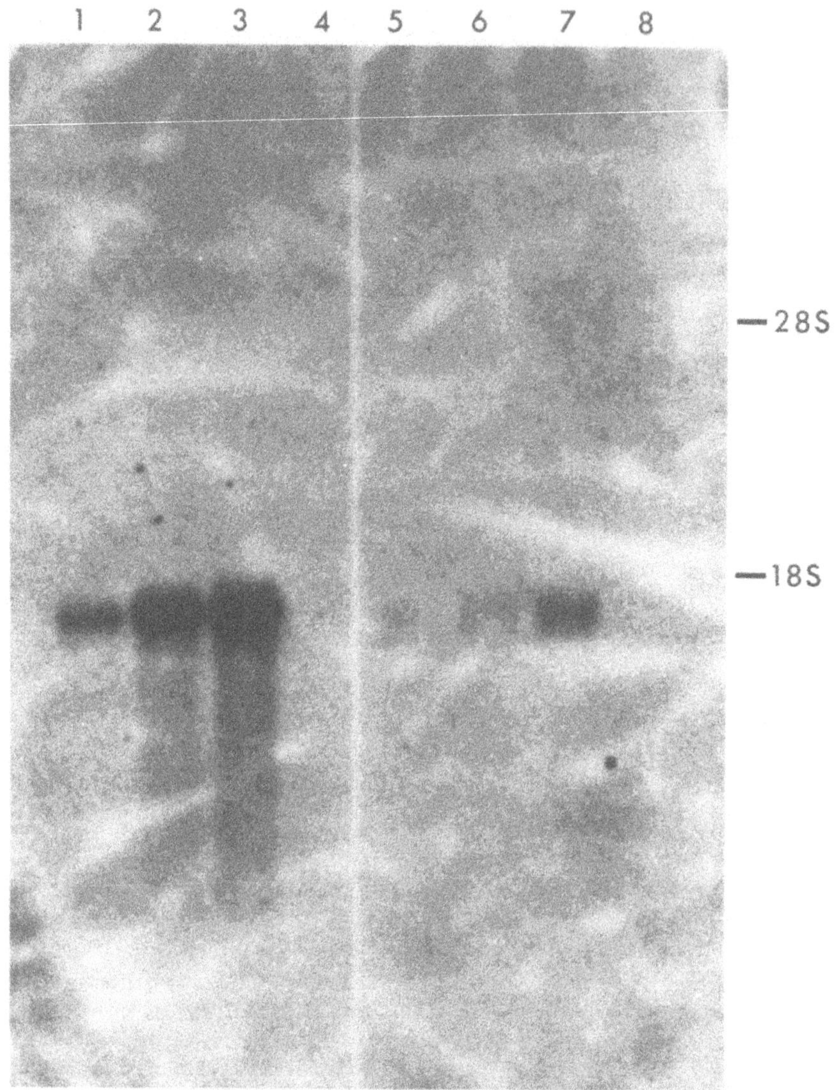

FIGURE 108: RNA blot analysis of skeletal actin and cardiac actin mRNA expression in adult human muscle. Samples of adult human skeletal muscle and HeLa cell total RNA were denatured with glyoxal and size fractionated on a 1% agarose gel. After transfer to diazobenzyloxymethyl-paper, the filters were allowed to hybridize to either the skeletal actin (lanes 1 through 4) or the cardiac actin (lanes 5 through 8) 3' probe. The two probes nick translated to virtually identical specific activities. Lanes 1,2,3,5,6, and 7 contained 1,5,10,5,10, and 20 μg of HeLa cell RNA.

muscle became apparent even before we did this blot because the probe we isolated, the human cardiac actin cDNA, was derived from the leg skeletal muscle library giving direct proof there must in fact be expression of that gene in human skeletal muscle. The number of such clones we isolated in their proportion is really quite close to 20:μl. It was 2 cardiac clones out of about 28 skeletal actin cDNAs.

Similarly when we look at the RNA isolated from human heart, we can measure the relative degree of concentration by the ratio of mRNA expression in these various RNA preparations. Figure 109 is a set of blots of small samples of RNA with different amounts of RNA in micrograms across the top. Each of these represents an autoradiograph of a piece of paper impregnated with RNA hybridized to the various probes that I have been talking about.

Let us concentrate only on panel A for the moment. That represents the result of hybridization of the skeletal alpha actin probe with RNA from HeLa cells, from skeletal muscle and from heart. It is quite clear that there is skeletal alpha actin present in both skeletal muscle and heart but there is about 5 times more skeletal muscle actin in the skeletal muscle than in the heart. In panel B, a hybridization of cardiac actin probe against skeletal muscle we again see there is cardiac actin expressed in both of those tissues. In this instance, the ratio is approximately reversed, about 1 to 5, that is about 5 times more cardiac than skeletal muscle actin is expressed in heart.

Since the probes were of equal specific activity, we can also compare the intensities of these spots between the blots and come up with ratios of expression of skeletal actin in heart and skeletal muscle, skeletal actin vs, cardiac actin, etc. The ratios seen in Table 19 are normalized to the amount of cardiac actin mRNA in human skeletal muscle. The ratio of cardiac to skeletal actin mRNA in skeletal muscle is about 1 to 20, the ratio of skeletal actin expressions in human skeletal and heart muscle is about 5 to 1, and the ratio of cardiac actin expression in human heart and skeletal muscle is also 5 to 1. The surprising result was that the ratio of the skeletal alpha actin mRNA to cardiac actin mRNA in human heart is close to 1 to 1. Almost 50% of the mRNA was skeletal alpha actin.

In addition the real ratio of expression of a total actin mRNA between skeletal muscle and heart is about 2 to 1. Thus there is about twice as much skeletal alpha actin per unit of RNA in skeletal muscle as there is in heart.

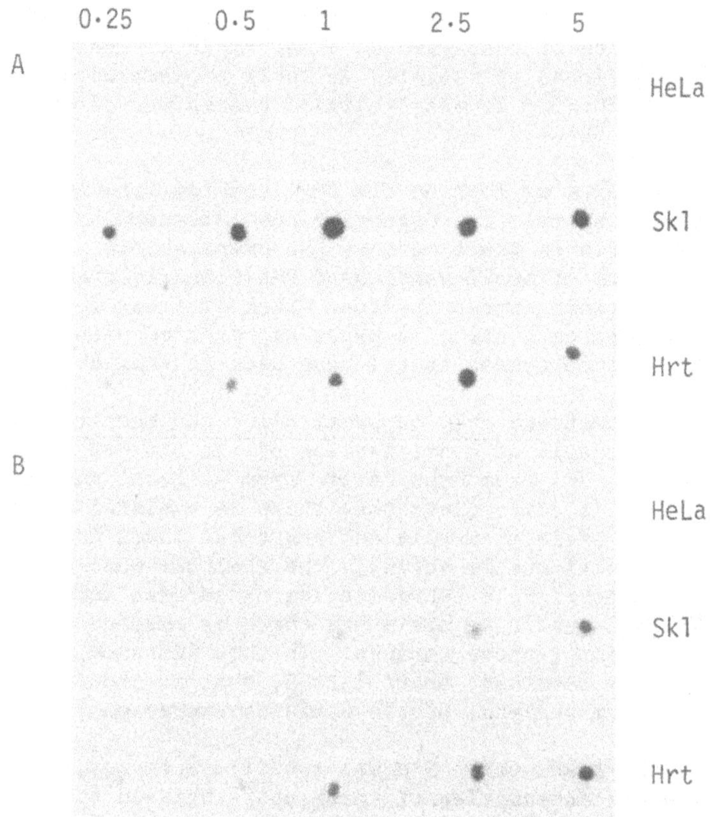

FIGURE 109: RNA dot hybridization measurement of expression of skeletal actin and cardiac actin mRNAs in adult human skeletal muscle and heart. Serial dilutions of RNA isolated from adult human skeletal muscle (Skl) and heart (Hrt) and from HeLa cells were spotted onto nitrocellulose paper in quantities ranging from 5 to 0.25 μg as indicated. DNA fragments corresponding to the skeletal actin 3' probe (A), the cardiac actin 3' probe (B) were nick translated and allowed to hybridize to the indicated panels. The skeletal actin and cardiac actin probes were radiolabeled by nick translation to virtually indistinguishable specific activities, and thus quantitative comparisons between the intensity of autoradiographic exposures between (A) and (B) are a direct measure of relative concentrations of the specific mRNA moieties.

TABLE 19

Relative Expression of Skeletal and Cardiac Actin in Adult Human Skeletal Muscle and Heart[a]

Gene	Relative Expression		
	Heart		Skeletal Muscle
Skeletal Actin	4	← →	20
			↕
Cardiac Actin	5	← →	1
Total Actin[b]	9		21

[a]Data derived from Figures 108 and 109. The level of expression of cardiac actin in skeletal muscle was arbitrarily set at a value of 1 U/μg of total RNA. The arrows indicate the comparisons utilized to calculate the values of relative steady-state mRNA levels.
[b]Predicted relative total actin expression between the two tissues.

Possible Differences in Actin from Normal vs. Severely Damaged Hearts

At Stanford our major source of heart muscle is the cardiac transplant service where they give us their rejects. The hearts we have actually examined have all been ailing hearts, usually large baggy hearts with some sort of myocarditis and fibrosis. Thus we are looking at sick muscle in those hearts. We raise the question whether this 1:1 ratio of skeletal to cardiac actin mRNA may be physiologically regulated. It will be important to establish whether or not cardiac hypertrophy, heart failure, etc., affects the switching of actin as well as, possibly, other isotypes.

Despite our concern about the damaged heart reflecting the normal circumstance in tissue culture systems, we found that the actin expressed is predominantly cardiac. In the upper panel of Figure 110 we probed the skeletal alpha actin probe against three control RNAs and RNA isolated from mouse C2 myoblasts at confluence and over the first three days of fusion. The controls are mouse heart RNA which we know gives no signal against mouse L cells, also an RNA which gives nothing, and by hybridization of the skeletal actin probe against mouse muscle when we expect to see lots of skeletal actin mRNAs. Confluent cells don't express alpha actin and surprisingly the signal here in fusing cells is quite weak compared to what is present in skeletal muscle.

On the other hand when we use the cardiac actin probe against mouse L cells (lower panel of Figure 110) transfected with a human cardiac actin gene or against mouse heart, we see a strong cardiac actin signal. Surprisingly confluent cells have cardiac mRNAs but the cardiac actin comes up very rapidly in the first 24 hours and represents the predominant actin mRNA expressed in fusing C2 cells in culture.

Actin Gene Expression in Muscle Cell Cultures

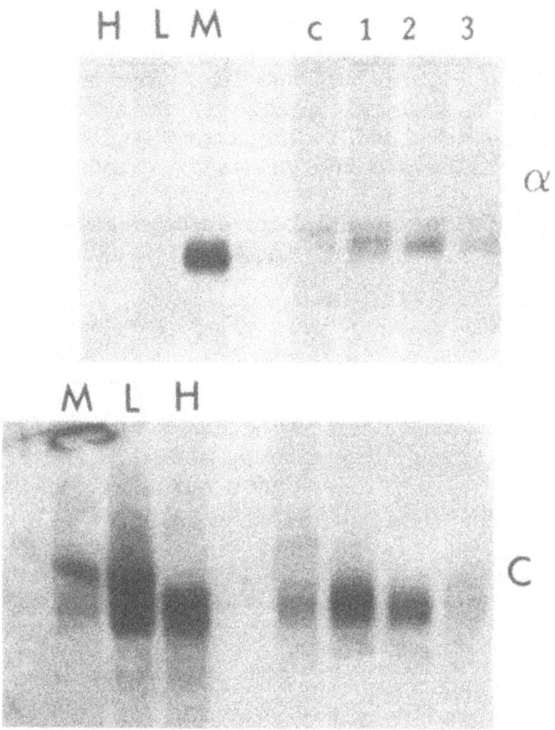

FIGURE 110: Northern blot analysis of alpha-skeletal and alpha-cardiac actin gene expression in mouse C2 muscle cells Panel A. Autoradiograph of RNA blot hybridized with alpha-skeletal actin specific probe. Lanes 1α, L and M are RNAs from mouse heart, L cells and mouse muscle, respectively. Lanes C,1,2,3 were loaded with RNA from C2 cells at confluence and 1,2 or 3 days after fusion. Panel B. Identical experiment as in Panel A except that probe is cardiac-actin specific. Autoradiographs were exposed for 10 days (Panel A) and overnight (Panel B).

Figure 111 shows an essentially parallel result with the human myoblast system. This is a Northern blot of RNA isolated from human myoblasts, confluent cells and cultures at days 2, 4, and 8. Again there is almost no expression of that actin gene and the actin messenger being expressed in those cells, and presumably the actin protein is the cardiac actin.

DR. HOLTZER: Are these all cross-striated myotubes?

DR. KEDES: The degree of fusion was about 60-70% and many of them had cross-striation.

Concerning the function of these isotypes in satellite cells and the issue whether these *in vitro* events in tissue culture really reflect what is going on *in vivo*, I would like to hypothesize that they do, in fact, reflect what is going on *in vivo*.

As satellite cells divide and fuse into myotubes, they may begin to synthesize what some people have been referring to as the embryonic or neonatal isotype. This may be the normal activity of these satellite cells even in adult muscle.

One could test the prediction since rapid growth and regeneration should lead to an increase of the synthesis of cardiac actin mRNA. Therefore the response to growth hormone, injury, and perhaps even stimulation or exercise should show changes in the isoforms as observed with these very sensitive probes. In this regard, it would be interesting to attempt the fusion of human or other myoblasts into normal muscle fibers. One might predict that with very sensitive *in situ* probes one might detect the expression initially of cardiac actin mRNA as opposed to skeletal actin mRNA. Other neonatal or fetal isoforms might be expressed in the same way.

Effects on the Cell Phenotype of Introducing Intact Contractile Protein Genes

We put the human cardiac actin gene into mouse L cells to determine whether that gene is expressed, whether the right messenger is made and finally whether human cardiac actin protein appears, a protein never destined to be expressed in these non-muscle cells. The transfection experiments were performed in collaboration with R. Hickey and A. Skoultchi at Albert Einstein.

Figure 112 shows a blot of the RNA showing that we have

FIGURE 111: Northern blot analysis of skeletal and cardiac actin gene expression in human myoblasts. RNA from human myoblasts (Mb) and from confluent (C) and fusing cells at days 2,4 and 8 was hybridized with either alpha-skeletal or cardiac-actin specific probes.

introduced the gene into mouse TK^- cells because there is mRNA of the right size being expressed in a number of these clones. The probe also picked up some high molecular weight RNAs which we subsequently learned relate to legitimate precursors of cardiac actin.

Dr. Buckingham will point out that before one can insist that there is accurate expression of the cardiac actin gene in terms of the start and stop, it is necessary to prove that the ends of the mRNA really are accurate and homologous to the endogenous or normal cardiac actin production. In this case we know that there is an accurate transcript regarding both initiation and termination of the cardiac actin gene in these mouse L cells.

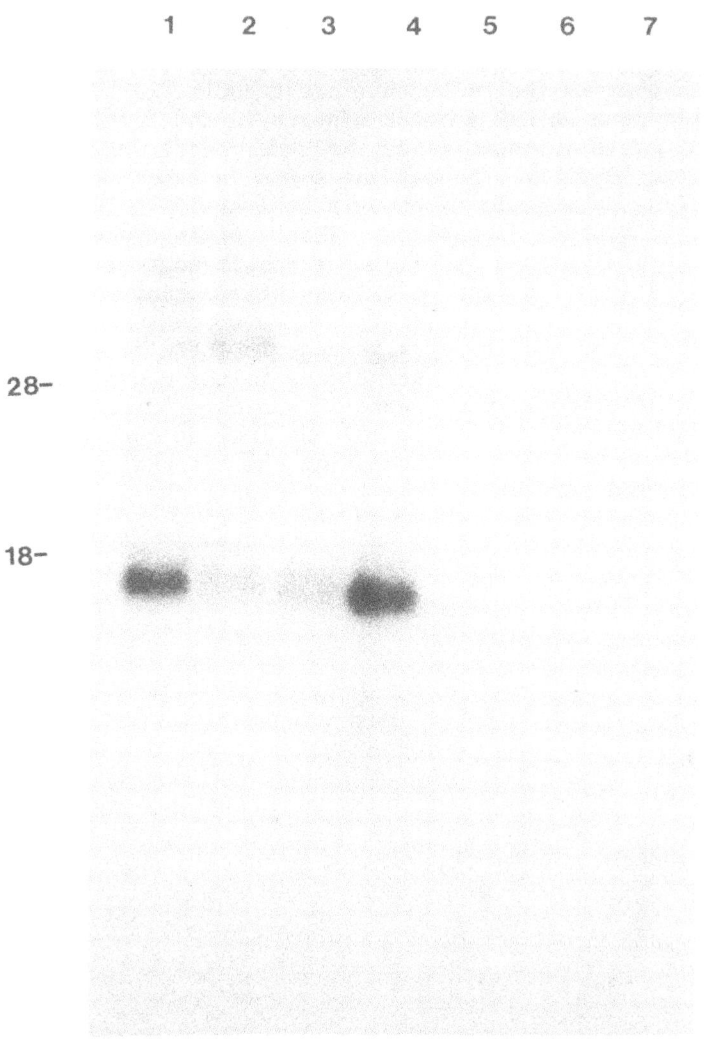

FIGURE 112: Northern blot of total cellular RNA isolated from four independent clones of mouse Ltk(-) cells (Lanes 1-4) co-transfected with HSV tk gene and the human cardiac actin gene. The blot was probed with the cardiac actin isotype specific probe lanes 5-7 and RNAs from Ltk^- cells, Ltk^+ transfectants and HeLa cells respectively.

With such a degree of expression of mRNA, seemingly quantitatively similar to beta and gamma mRNA production, the question naturally arose, are we getting expression of cardiac actin protein in these mouse L cells? The answer is yes as seen in Figure 113. This is the region of an autoradiograph of a two-dimensional gel of S35 methionine labeled L cells that either are or are not transfected with the human cardiac actin gene. I think you will see that in the cells that are transfected with the human cardiac actin gene, a new protein appears in the region where one would expect actin in the L cells, as other people have shown many times is about 20 to 1. The cardiac actin is expressed in terms of S35 labeling at a ratio of about 5 to 1 or 10 to 1 relative to the beta actin protein expression. This protein appears to be relatively stable because labeling for a half hour or 4 hours gave us the same ratio of endogenous cytoskeletal actins.

What about the ability of a sarcomeric actin to integrate into structures in the mouse L cell where it was never really intended to go? We look at that by actually isolating the cytoskeletons of those L cells and separating them from soluble phase.

The Location of Transplanted Sarcomeric Actin

FIGURE 113: Human cardiac actin is expressed in transfected mouse L cells. S^{35} methionine labeled proteins were isolated from mouse L cells transfected with a thymidine kinase gene (left panel) or with both a thymidine kinase gene and the human cardiac gene. The proteins were examined by 2-dimensional gel electrophoresis. α,β indicate the location of the α and β cytoskeletal actin proteins. C indicates the location of the cardiac actin protein.

In Figure 114 the two left panels are autoradiographs of proteins isolated from S35 labeled cells. These are the controls from cells not transfected with the cardiac actin gene demonstrating that beta actin protein is distributed about 1 to 2 between supernatent and the Triton-X-100 insoluble cytoskeleton. We know the cytoskeletons are reasonably pure because vimentin is a protein that normally partitions exclusively in the cytoskeleton. In the transfected cells (right panels) we see that the cardiac actin protein deposits in the cytoskeleton at about the appropriate ratio compared to the beta actin.

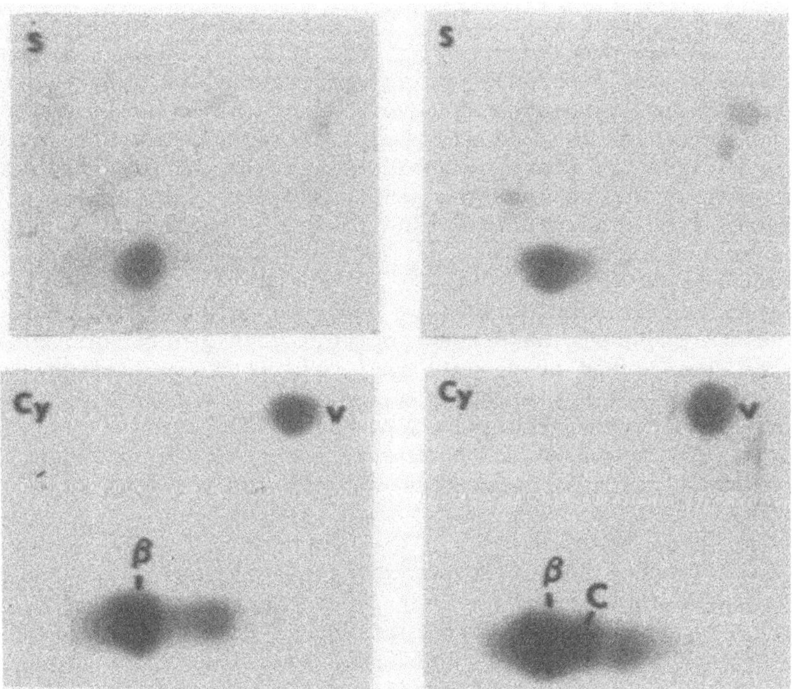

FIGURE 114: Human cardiac actin associates with L-cell cytoskeleton. Autoradiographs of S^{35} methionine labeled proteins isolated from transfected cells as described in Figure 113. Cells were lysed in presence of Triton-X-100 and protiens in the soluble (S) and in soluble cytoskeletal (Cy) phases were examined separately by 2-dimensional gel electrophoresis. V is the position of the cytoskeletal protein, vimentin.

Thus we have demonstrated that the human cardiac actin isoform is capable of a physiological behavior, not necessarily a functional behavior, but at least it deposits and somehow is associated with the cytoskeleton.

Regulation of the Cardiac Actin Gene

we are trying to devise experiments that will tell us whether cardiac actin protein can intermingle directly and physically with the beta and gamma actins or whether they form homopolymers? Since the mouse L cell is a transformed cell line with a cytoskeleton that does not form large actin cables, it is not the most appropriate model for this kind of approach. Therefore, we are trying to introduce the actin and other contractile protein genes into diploid human fibroblasts.

Figure 115 demonstrates that the human cardiac actin gene, just like the rat counterparts, is capable of being regulated in the L6 line of rat myoblasts during differentiation. The RNA isolated from normal myoblasts and myotubes of the L6 cells don't carry any sequences that cross-hybridize with the isotype species specific human actin probe. Myoblasts transfected with the human cardiac gene do not express the gene. However, the cardiac actin gene expression is turned on during fusion as reflected in RNA blots from several clones.

Our result is similar to that reported here by David Yaffe of the Nudel group who have transfected rodent genes. All of the clones we have looked at to date fall only into two classes. Either they are not expressed at all or they are regulated. We found no constitutive expressions to date. The cardiac actin gene is highly regulated and I am sure that there will be interesting parallels, if not identities between the promoter and regulatory regions of the rat and human genes.

Actin-Myosin Interaction

What does this kind of experimental approach tell us about isoforms? Are isoforms of various genes functional in different situations or do they each have different functions? Can a human cardiac actin gene and its protein really function to form the cytoskeleton? Can a beta actin function in a sarcomere? If so, how can we account for what the biophysicists and protein chemists tell us about the importance of those amino acid differences, especially at the amino terminus, between skeletal and cardiac actin vs. beta and gamma actin and their interactions with myosin? The ability to make point mutations and to modify these proteins by making hybrids should expedite the study of myofibrillogenesis and the assembly of cytoskeletal microfilaments.

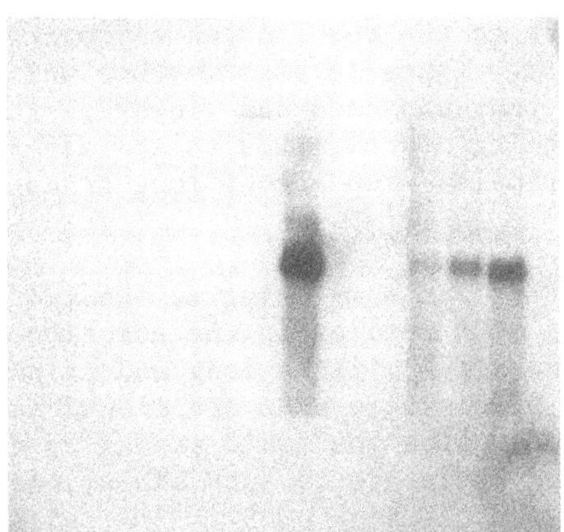

FIGURE 115: Human cardiac actin gene regulation in rat myoblast differentiation. Northern blots were performed with RNAs isolated from rat L6 myoblasts before and after fusion and probed with human cardiac actin specific probe. Six blank lanes on the left contain RNA from myoblasts and differentiating myotubes at 4,5,6,8 and 10 days after onset of fusion. The 3 right lanes contain RNA from L6 myoblasts transfected with the human cardiac actin gene. RNA was isolated from myoblasts and myotubes at 6 and 8 days after fusion. The heavily hybridizing RNA in the middle of the figure is from mouse L cells expressing the human cardiac actin gene.

With Okayama and Berg we made several libraries of cDNA with a vector that has unique structural properties that make it useful. First it is a plasmid that can be linearized by opening a restriction site and creating a poly dt tail. The plasmid can then hybridize with the poly A tail of mRNA from adult striated muscle. After the RNA/DNA hybrid forms on the vector one uses reverse transcriptase to make a copy of the RNA and put on a poly dc tail on those 3' ends. Secondly, this vector has a Hind III restriction end nuclease site that allows you to cut off the poly dc end not attached to the cDNA. Thus one ends up with just a 3/4 length plasmid with a Hind III site exposed and the cDNA tailed with poly dc.

Another small piece of DNA was modified by putting a poly dg tail on one end and a Hind III site on the other. This piece is hybridized to make a circularized molecule that can be used to transfect cells after second strand synthesis.

Two critical technical features of this kind of cDNA cloning vehicle made it useful to us; first, every mRNA is in the same orientation relative to the restriction endonuclease sites known to be in the plasmid. There is also another series of restriction endonuclease sites that can open and linearize the whole molecule. This particular cloning method gives relatively full length cDNAs. The reverse transcription step allows long transcripts, but little short random ones.

They all start at the same point at the end of the poly A tail so that for a given mRNA species in the solution, the vast majority of the reverse transcripts will be long and of uniform length. If one had a solution of a single mRNA and cloned in this vector, then after opening the molecules you would expect to see a single band. Since we always have a mixture of such mRNAs, one would expect to

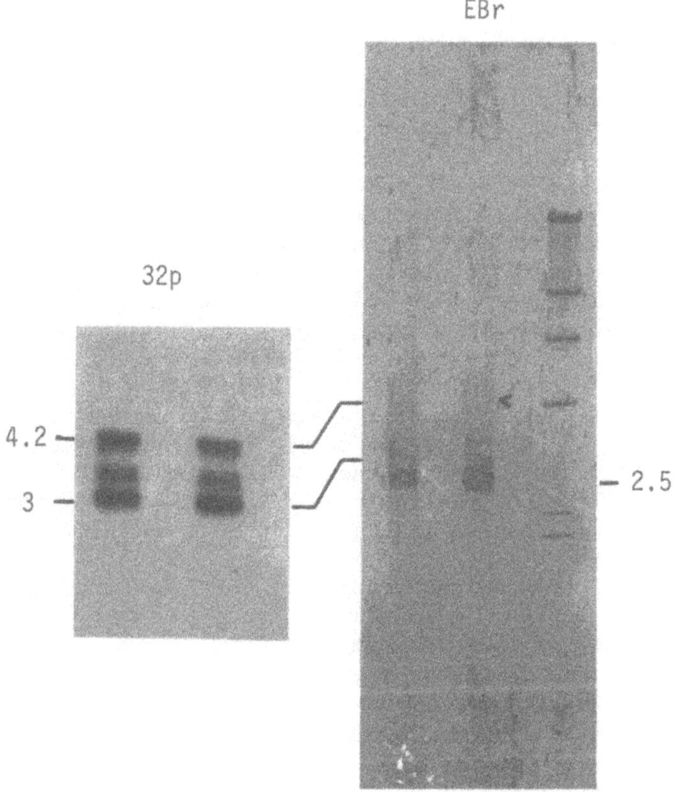

FIGURE 116: Visualization of actin cDNA length heterogeneity in the human muscle library. Two 1-μg samples of the muscle cDNA library were digested with either EcoR1 or Hind III. Ethidium bromide staining of the gel is seen in the right panel, and the corresponding autoradiograms of actin hybridization are seen in the left panel.

get all of the actin messengers of one size, all the myosins of another size, etc. Running those out on a gel we see bands, each representing a specific abundant cloned mRNA.

Figure 116 shows ethidium bromide staining of a linearized cDNA library from human skeletal muscle. Under ultraviolet light there appears a series of bands on the gel and the darkest band is really the linearized plasmid. About 20% of the molecules in the mixture don't contain any inserts, all you get is the plasmid itself recircularized and then a series of larger bands laddered up the gel.

We blotted this RNA and probed it with skeletal actin probe to prove that the bands represent homogeneous messenger classes. We subsequently learned that the 3 bands we detect are each actin cDNAs representing strong reverse transcription stop signals. The reverse transcriptase will get part of the way and then quit. There is some attribute of the structure of that messenger, maybe some secondary folding, that causes the polymerase to fall off and that happens quite frequently at the exact same site so that these 3 bands seen in the left panel each represent skeletal alpha actin mRNAs. We have isolated and cloned all of those, sequenced them and found where the stops were. We have not yet determined why the reverse transcript stopped at these particular points.

We can measure the size of bands and know the size of the mRNA they contain. From Northern blotting experiments we then predict the size of the skeletal alpha actin insert. We cut out the band, recirularize the plasmid and transfect with it. In this way we obtained a full length skeletal alpha actin cDNA.

In similar blots we have detected myosin heavy chain cDNAs and other cDNAs from muscle abundant mRNA classes. These blots and gels yield moderately abundant RNAs, sometimes as many as 50-60 abundant mRNAs. In between the bands are full length copies of less prominent mRNAs. We devised a procedure to take advantage of that. Not only did we cut out visible bands of moderately expressed mRNA, but we sliced up the gel into tiny fractions, eluted the DNA from each and made separate E. coli transfectants after recircularizing the DNA. We then took transfected clones from each plate at random, ran restriction digests of them and compared them. Within any cluster of 12 we always found a predominant cDNA. Sometimes it was 2 out of 12, sometimes 6 out of 12.

In the case of each of those clones we asked whether it expressed in muscle more than in fibroblasts. Figure 117 shows a simple dot blot assay. As a control we can look at what happens when you take a dilution series of RNA from fibroblasts, heart and skeletal muscle and hybridize it with an actin probe. As expected actin is expressed both in muscle and heart in the appropriate ratio. In the next 3 panels we see the result when the probes are pulled out of this library by the method just described. In each case there is no expression detected in fibroblast RNA, but there is expression of one clone in both heart and skeletal muscle and in two others just in skeletal muscle but not heart.

Another clone (Figure 118 panel 4) expressed less well relative to actin but expressed even more in heart than skeletal muscle. Another clone (panel 5) is highly expressed in fibroblast, heart and muscle and one clone (panel 6) weakly expressed in all three.

We have gone through the first 30 of the 100 different places of DNA and the results look essentially the same as those in Figures 117 and 118. Thus we seem to have a relatively efficient way of isolating mRNAs expressed in muscle and identifying those that are specifically expressed in muscle relative to other cell types. In addition, by using DNA from one X vs 4X cell lines,

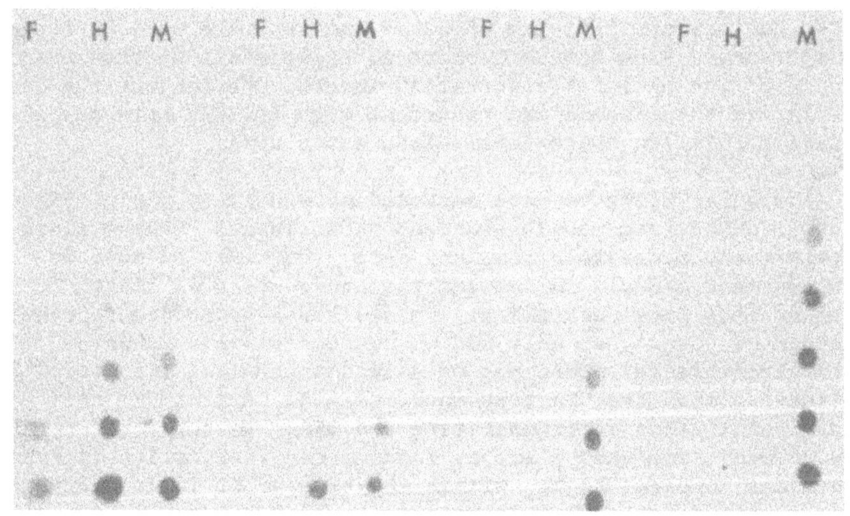

FIGURE 117: Dot blot hybridization of muscle cDNA clones to RNA from fibroblasts (F), heart (H) and muscle (M). Equal quantities of cellular RNA from these three sources were diluted and spotted on nitrocellulose membranes. Duplicate blots were then hybridized independently with radiolabeled cDNA probes. The interpretations of each blot are described in the text.

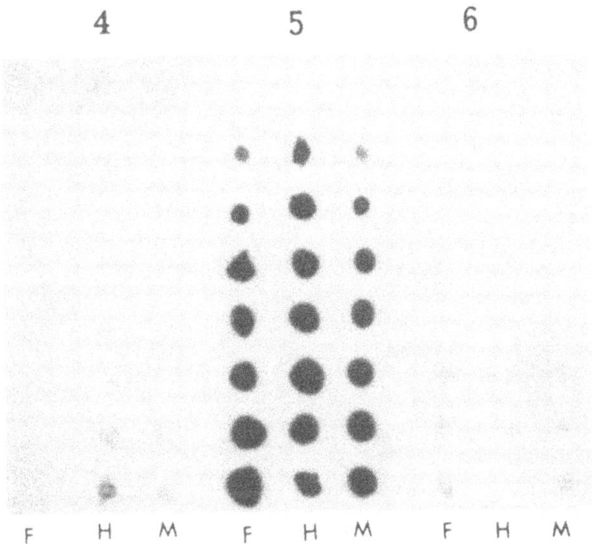

FIGURE 118: See Figure 117:

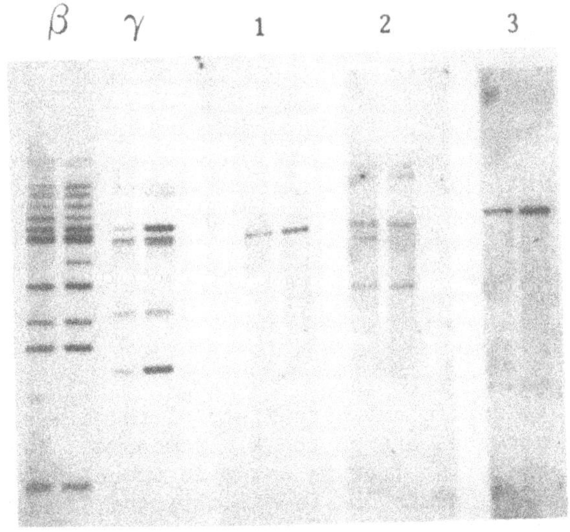

FIGURE 119: Assay of genomic representation and X-linkage of cDNA clones. Equal quantities of DNA from normal human DNA and from XXXX DNA were digested with EcoR1, co-electrophoresed and blotted. Duplicate blots were hybridized with radiolabeled beta-actin or alpha-actin probes or with muscle cDNAs. The interpretation of each of the paired panels is described in the text.

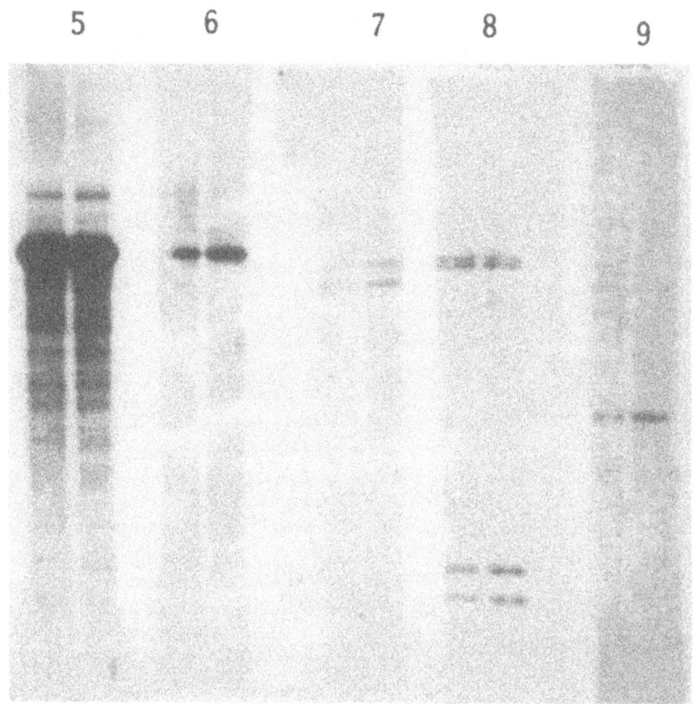

FIGURE 120: See Figure 119.

we have begun to determine whether any of these messengers are coming from genes that are on the X chromosome. To do this we used the beta and gamma isotype specific probes as a control against the human genomic DNA from the 1X and 4X series as a control. Figure 119 shows the normal pattern that we see using the beta or gamma isotype specific probes: a number of bands, one of which is the real gene and the rest of which we believe are pseudo-genes. The intensity of hybridization is between 1X and 4X bands is equal for most bands. There seems to be a gamma coding sequence on the X chromosome. There are two bands in the gamma actin probe blot that appear to be present in a 4 to 1 or 3 to 1 ratio in 4X vs 1X DNA. Those lanes are the controls. What about these cDNAs we pulled out of the library? They gave us a range of answers. Two appear to be good candidates for X-linked genes (panels 1 and 3).

In Figure 120 lane 5 is hybridized with a cDNA that is highly expressed by the dot blot assay. This cDNA is carrying a sequence that is obviously repeated at many sites in the genome that are very similar.

DR. EPSTEIN: Do you expect your cDNA library will include satellite or proliferative myoblast cDNAs?

DR. KEDES: Making a library from proliferative satellite cells might be of interest if they express messengers that differ from those of the myoblasts. We are not contemplating that at present.

DR. HAUSCHKA: The gel in which you showed the expression of the human actin muscle in cardiac messenger looked to me to be producing more message on day 2 than on subsequent days.

DR. KEDES: The explanation is that those cultures were not doing very well at day three.

DR. HAUSCHKA: So that at later times the ratios might change.

DR. KEDES: Yes.

DR. FISCHMAN: I just wanted to mention to Dr. Kedes a recent report in the Journal of Cell Biology by Lacey who injected skeletal muscle G actin into cardiac myocytes. Although it would normally be incorporated into the sarcomeres, as far as one could tell, it was incorporated into the developing cardiac muscle cell.

DR. HOLTZER: If you look at Lacey's micrograph closely, there are two bands. That doesn't make much sense.

DR. FISCHMAN: It was a beginning, however, a very direct approach and simpler than some of the more elaborate approaches that we have heard about.

DR. KEDES: If one wants to begin work at the level of protein interactions to determine what parts of the protein are important, mutating the gene becomes the simplest way.

DR. EPSTEIN: You really should have a background of mutant actin line. Can the absence of beta or gamma actin really function? Having a temperature sense of mutant for actin and replacing it with a sarcomeric actin, you can't mutate.

DR. BLAU: If, however, you see a certain interaction between the protein made by the gene and myosin inside the cell, then you can mutate that gene and look at the interactions, as long as you get a protein-protein interaction.

CHAPTER 29: THE ACTIN AND MYOSIN MULTIGENE FAMILIES

M. Buckingham, S. Alonso, G. Bugaisky, P. Barton,
A. Cohen, P. Daubas, A. Minty, B. Robert and A. Weydert

Department of Molecular Biology
Pasteur Institute
25 rue du Dr. Roux, 75015 Paris, France

The Actin and Myosin Multigene Families: a) a study of the accumulation of their RNA transcripts demonstrates different developmental strategies during skeletal muscle formation, b) a genetic analysis of their chromosomal organization indicates gene dispersion and permits some precise localizations on the genetic map of the mouse.

It is clear that significant advances are being made at present in the application of DNA technology to the detection of monofactorial genetic diseases in humans. The isolation of nucleic acid probes sufficiently close to the locus of a disease to result in the detection of restriction fragment length polymorphisms which will co-segregate with mutations in this locus will permit carrier detection and prenatal diagnosis (619). However, it is also clear that for diseases such as Duchenne muscular dystrophy which has a high incidence (40%) of cases without any previous family history, genetic screening of families at risk is not enough. Identification, and the development of treatment of the basic defect are equally important. A characteristic of dystrophic muscle is the presence of a diminished and disorganized sarcomere (620) with its inevitable effect on the generation of muscle force and on movement. As Dr. Rowland said in his introductory talk, there is no demonstration, at present, that the contractile protein genes are the site of primary lesion in the

* This work was supported by the Centre National de la Recherche Scientifique, the Ministère de l' Industrie et de la Recherche, the Institut National da la Santé de la Recherche Médicale, NATO, the Foundation pour la Recherche Médicale and the Muscular Dystrophy Association of America.

dystrophies. However, whatever the primary lesion may be it has a feedback effect in the end on sarcomere assembly and contractile protein gene expression.

The research in which we are engaged is directed towards understanding at the level of gene regulation, how a skeletal muscle phenotype is initially established, and how it is subsequently modified during development. We have concentrated on the major structural components of the sarcomere, the actins and myosins, and have chosen the mouse as the best model for this fundamental research, because of the relatively advanced state of mouse genetics and embryology. I shall present two types of result: one on the differing patterns of mRNA accumulation during development for the actins and myosins, and the other on an analysis of actin and myosin gene organization, using mouse genetics.

mRNA Accumulation in Tissue Culture

Last year we reported that cardiac actin transcripts accumulate during the formation of skeletal muscle (60) and Figure 121 is to remind you of what happens in tissue culture. As muscle fibers form, cardiac and skeletal actin transcripts co-accumulate. In older myotubes there is a decrease in the relative proportion of cardiac actin mRNA so that by 16 days after the onset of fusion this has fallen to 25% of its original level relative to the skeletal actin transcripts (621). Similarly in this mouse cell line (T-984, Cl 10) (622) the mRNAs for two types of myosin light chain, $LC1_{emb}$, the fetal isoform and $LC1_F$ the adult fast skeletal isoform, co-accumulate. The $LC1_{emb}$ protein co-migrates on two-dimensional gels with the major light chain of adult heart atria ($LC1_A$) (623), and isolation of the mRNA and gene for these isoforms confirm their identity (624). This is therefore in some ways analogous to the actin story. Figure 122 shows two-dimensional gels of the peptides synthesized in an in vitro translation experiment with RNA from fused muscle cell cultures. Both $LC1_F$ and $LC1_{emb}$ mRNAs are detected (625). A similar gel analysis of the proteins synthesized during myotube formation demonstrates the presence of both proteins in a constant ratio: $\left(\frac{LC1_F}{LC1_{emb}} = \text{approx.} \frac{1}{2}\right)$ from the onset of myotube formation to 11 day old myotubes (621). In this respect, therefore, this gene pair differs from the actins.

mRNA Accumulation in vivo

We have also looked at the in vivo situation in skeletal muscle derived from limb buds and later from limbs in fetal and newborn mice. The results of this study for the actins are represented

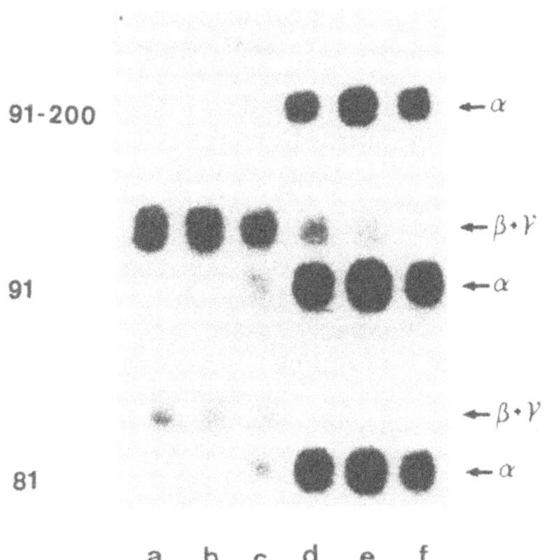

FIGURE 121: Northern blots with RNA samples from cultured muscle cells hybridized with cardiac and skeletal actin probes. a-f: RNA samples prepared from cultures of a mouse muscle cell line (622) before (a,b) at (c) and after myotube formation (d-f). 91-200: A 3' non-coding sequence probe specific for skeletal muscle actin (632). 91: A skeletal muscle actin coding sequence probe (632) cross hybridizing with muscle (α) and non-muscle (β,γ) actin sequences. 81: A cardiac actin coding sequence (60) hybridizing to the cardiac actin mRNA under these experimental conditions (glyoxal gels, blot washed in 0.1 SSC, 45°C, (60).

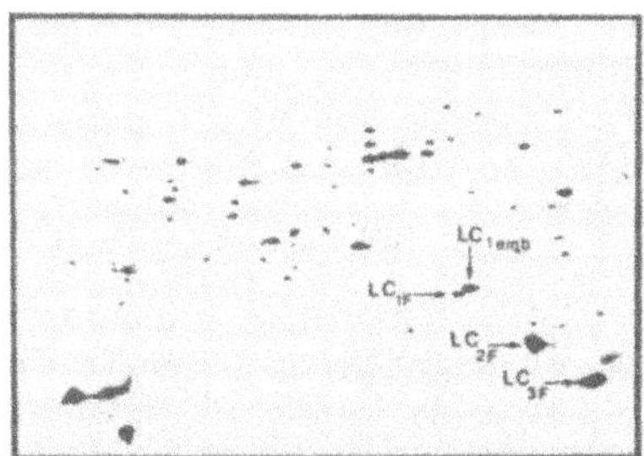

FIGURE 122: *In Vitro* translation of the mRNAs encoding myosin light chains in myotubes of a mouse muscle cell line. The ^{35}S-labeled products of an *in vitro* protein synthesis directed by mRNA from cultured mouse myotubes, analyzed by two-dimensional electrophoresis. The position of the myosin light chains (LC) is indicated.

schematically in Table 20. Two probes were used. One corresponds to the 3' non-coding sequence of skeletal muscle actin mRNA and is specific for these transcripts. The other is a cardiac coding sequence probe which under high stringency conditions hybridizes preferentially to cardiac actin (60). The relative proportion of cardiac actin transcripts is maximal in 18 day fetal muscle, and is significantly lower in 11-12 fetal muscle. This early time point corresponds to the onset of fetal life when fine muscle fibers are beginning to appear in the limb bud tissue. Such early fibers do not appear to contain more cardiac actin mRNA. Between 16-18 days the muscle undergoes the principal increase in mass, both the density and size of fibers increase (626). It would appear that cardiac actin transcripts mainly accumulate in this time, perhaps in response to a requirement for large quantities of actin. In this context it is significant that in the toad, Xenopus where distinct cardiac and skeletal like actin isoforms are first identified during amphibian evolution the two proteins are both present in significant amounts in adult heart and skeletal muscle tissues (627). The question of the functional significance of the 4 out of 375 amino acid differences between the two isoforms is open. However, one can propose that in mammals one or the other isoform predominates in the adult tissue because of a functional advantage, but that such fine-tuning is not crucial and at developmental stages where large quantities of striated muscle actin are required rapidly, both genes are expressed.

The situation for the myosin light chains is different. Similar experiments were performed with 3' coding sequence probes for $LC1_F/LC3_F$ (628) and for the fetal/atrial light chain $LC1_A$(=$LC1_{emb}$) (624). Cross hybridization between these sequences is minimal under the conditions used, although the background hybridization with $LC1_A$ is significantly higher than with other probes. As for the actins, the results are presented schematically in Table 20. Fetal light chain transcripts are relatively more abundant in early fetal muscle and their proportion decreases during later fetal life, so that in new born muscle RNA they are no longer detectable (625) by _in vitro_ translation or Northern blot analysis. This is clearly different from the accumulation pattern for cardiac actin transcripts which are maximal in late fetal life and persist at significant levels for the first week or two after birth. Little is known at present about the $LC1_{emb}$ isoform, although it has diverged considerably from the adult $LC1_F$, in its -COOH terminal coding region (624). One might argue in this case, that its structural/functional role in the sarcomere is significantly different. The alternative, of course, is that its presence reflects a regulatory phenomenon at the gene level in these early myotubes such that the cardiac $LC1_{emb}$ gene is activated rather than or as well as the $LC1_F$ gene without this conferring any functional advantage at the protein level.

TABLE 20
Accumulation of mRNAs Encoding Fetal and Adult Actin and Myosin Isoforms During Skeletal Muscle Development

Skeletal muscle	Foetal			New Born			Adult	Fused muscle cell cultures : Myotubes	
Age (days)	11/12	15/16	18	1/2	5/6	11/12	90	1	11
Myosin Heavy Chains									
foetal MHC	ND	ND	+++	++				ND	ND
adult MHC				+	+++	+++	+++		
Alkali Myosin Light Chains									
foetal $LC1_A$ ($LC1_{emb}$)	++	++	+					+++	+++
adult $LC1_F/LC3_F$		(+)	+++	+++	+++	+++	+++	++	++
Actins									
foetal/cardiac α_c		(+)	++	++	++	(+)	(+)	+++	+
adult skeletal α_{sk}	++	++	+++	+++	+++	+++	+++	+++	+++

The data represented schematically here are derived from the experiments of S_1 protection, dot blots, RNA translation and protein labeling discussed in the text. ND: not done.

The third component which we have investigated in vivo is the myosin heavy chain. Developmental isoforms of this protein, specific to skeletal muscle have been shown to accumulate prior to

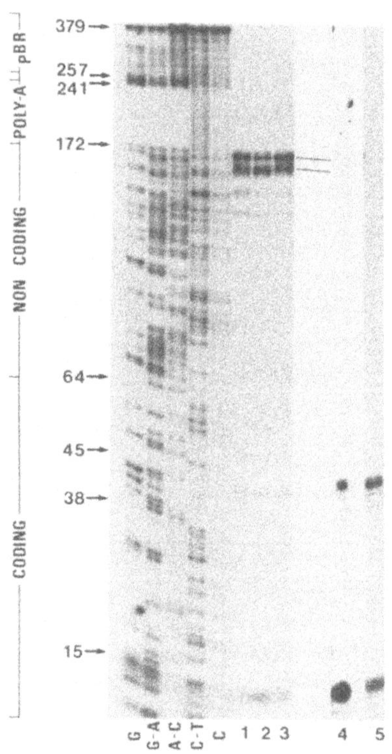

FIGURE 123: S_1 protection experiments showing the sequential accumulation of mRNAs encoding myosin heavy chains in late fetal and newborn skeletal muscle. S_1 protection experiments were performed by Wedert et al (629), using a myosin heavy chain probe corresponding to the -COOH terminal coding and 3' non-coding sequences of an adult fast skeletal muscle mRNA. On the left hand side DNA sequencing on this sequence is shown, on the right, total or partial protection of the labeled probe with different RNA preparations from: 1. adult mouse skeletal muscle; 2-3. newborn (5-6 days) mouse skeletal muscle; 4. newborn (1-3 days) mouse skeletal muscle; 5. fetal (18 days) mouse skeletal muscle. The band at 15 nucleotides is a background level of protection seen also in the absence of RNA.

the adult isoforms (381). S_1 protection experiments using an adult skeletal myosin heavy chain sequence as probe and RNA from fetal and newborn muscle are shown in Figure 123. In 18 day fetal muscle a major fetal heavy chain transcript is detected as a partially protected band (at position 43-45). Immediately after birth adult mRNA appears (at position 159-169), the two bands probably correspond to different polyadenylation sites, and accumulates rapidly so that at 5 days it is already the major species (629). Thus for the myosin heavy chain family there is a sequential accumulation of fetal and adult gene transcripts.

The modalities of RNA accumulation of the three multigene familes - actins, alkali myosin light chains and myosin heavy chains - during muscle development are summarized in Table 20. The main point is that each is different. The actin and LC1 families both accumulate adult cardiac as well as skeletal type transcripts, but with different time courses. The myosin heavy chain family follows a quite different strategy with specific developmental genes, expressed sequentially. This means that a fetal/newborn muscle and possibly its individual fibers will contain mixtures of fetal and adult isoforms for the actins and myosins. It also means that each multigene family is responding differently to the same regulatory signals or to different regulatory signals which effect changes in gene expression during development.

I should now like to turn to the organization of the genes encoding different isoforms of the actins and myosins. We have made use of mouse genetics in order to look at the question of linkage between genes of a given multigene family and between genes expressed in the same phenotype.

Chromosomal Organization of Muscle Genes

The approach depends on the detection of a restriction fragment length polymorphism for the gene in question between two mouse lines or mouse species. The segregation of this polymorphism in recombinant inbred lines or in backcrosses derived from the two parental types, and comparison with that for another gene or for known genetic markers permits linkage relationships to be established (630). Two technical points are worth mentioning. With certain cDNA probes and genes it is not easy to find differences in restriction sites in the region of the probe between inbred mouse lines. Between different mouse species (631) such as _mus spretus_ (_mus 3_) and _mus musculus_ (_mus 1_), polymorphisms are more frequent. The second point concerns the advantages of using backcrosses rather than recombinant inbred lines, in initial localization studies. In the latter a distance of 1 cM (1 cM = approx. 1000 Kb) between two genes permits detection of linkage, whereas the backcrosses 20-30 cM of the chromosome are covered. For these reasons we have used the less orthodox approach of back-crosses between different mouse species to obtain a first chromosomal localization, followed by a second type of cross, usually with recombinant inbred lines. For all markers examined the two have given identical results, indicating that the chromosomal organization of mus 1 and mus 3 is very similar. Figure 124 shows an example of the segregation of a restriction fragment polymorphism for the gene of the atrial light chain $LC1_A$, which is also expressed in fetal skeletal muscle. In Table 21 results obtained for the myosin light chain family are shown. The adult fast skeletal light chains $LC1_F$ and $LC3_F$ are encoded by a single gene, with a common 3' coding sequence and distinct 5' exons (628). This gene, the cardiac ventricular gene $LC1_V$, and the atrial/fetal gene $LC1_A/LC1_{emb}$ (624) are not linked and in fact are localized on different chromosomes.

In Table 22 the results of a genetic analysis for other myosin and actin genes are shown. As for the myosin light chains, no linkage is observed for the cardiac and skeletal muscle actin genes (632). Interestingly, the backcrosses analysis demonstrates that adult skeletal and cardiac myosin heavy chain genes are also not linked and co-segregate with markers on different chromosomes, contrary to what has been suggested from cell hybrid analyses which showed all myosin heavy chain sequences on mouse chromosome 11. Thus our genetic analysis does not demonstrate any linkage between members of an actin or myosin multigene family. Nor does it demonstrate as indicated in Table 22 any linkage between actin and myosin genes expressed together in the same phenotype.

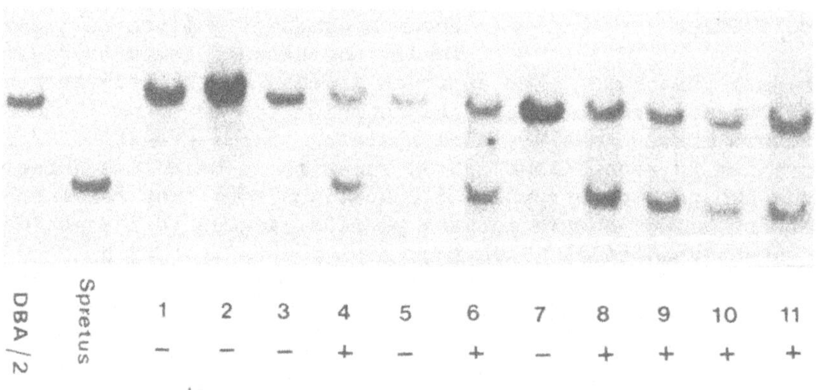

FIGURE 124: Southern blots of genomic DNA from mus 1/ mus 3 backcrosses restricted with Bam Hi, hybridized with an $LC1_A/LC1_{emb}$ light chain probe and washed under stringency conditions (0.1 x SSC, 65°C) which show only the homologous gene.

TABLE 21

Segregation of Alkali MLC Genes in DBA/2: Mus spretus backcrosses

	1	2	3	4	5	6	7	8	9	10	Total Co-segregation	%	Chr.
Idh - 1	-	+	+	+	+	-	-	-	-	+	19/19	100	1
LC_{1F}/LC_{3F}	-	+	+	+	+	-	-	-	-	+	9/20	45	
LC_{1F}/LC_{3F} (pseudogene)	+	-	+	-	+	+	+	+	+	+			
Es 3	+	+	-	-	-	+	-	-	+	-	34/37	96	11
LC_{1A}	-	+	-	-	-	+	-	-	+	-			
Es 14	-	-	+	-	+	+	+	+	-	+	37/37	100	9
LC_{1V}	-	-	+	-	+	+	+	+	-	+			

The results of segregation analyses of restriction length polymorphisms for myosin light chain genes, and of known chromosomal markers, are shown for backcrosses between mus 1 (DBA/2) x (mus 1 (DBA/2) x mus 3 (spretus). Heterozygotes carrying the spretus type polymorphism are scored as (+).

TABLE 22
Non Co-Segregation of Actin and Myosin Striated Muscle Genes in DBA/2: Mus Spretus Backcrosses

	1	2	3	4	5	6	7	8	9	10	11	12	13	14	15	16	17	18	19	20	Chr.
LC_{1F}/LC_{3F}	-	+	+	+	+	-	-	-	-	+	+	-	-	+	+	+	+	-	-	-	**1**
Skeletal actin	+	+	-	+	-	-	+	-	+	-	+	+	-	-	-	+	+	-	+	-	? 8
Adult skeletal MHC	-	+	+	-	+	-	+	-	+	+	+	+	+	-	-	+	-	+	+	-	? 11
LC_{1A}	-	+	-	-	-	+	-	-	+	-	+	+	+	+	-	+	-	+	+	-	**11**
Cardiac actin	+	-	-	-	+	-	+	-	+	-	+	+	-	+	+	+	-	-	+	-	
Cardiac MHC	-	-	-	-	+	+	-	-	+	+	+	-	-	+	+	-	+	+	+	-	**14**
LC_{IV}	-	-	+	-	+	+	+	+	-	+	+	-	-	-	-	-	+	+	-	+	**9**

Heterozygoes (+) are scored for restriction length polymorphisms of the spretus type as in Table 21. Chromosomal assignments in heavy type indicate clear co-segregation with at least one marker. Other assignments are suggested by significant co-segregation, but await confirmation.

Three points can be made from the results presented here. First, we have shown no linkage between genes within the same multigene family. In this respect the atrial/fetal light chain gene is particularly interesting. It has probably been derived from the $LC1_F/LC3_F$ adult gene relatively recently (270×10^6 years), since it is not found in birds, and since its 3' non-coding sequence has retained homology with the adult skeletal gene. Its probable formation from a gene duplication type event has thus been followed by gene dispersion. One can argue that the development of new genes within a multigene family is favored by rapid dispersion since gene conversion events, which will tend to re-homogenize similar sequences and therefore prevent the generation of diversity, will be more frequent between neighboring sequences on the same chromosome. In yeast intrachromosomal recombination events are $\times 10^3$ more frequent than those between chromosomes (633).

The second point concerns developmental patterns of regulation. As discussed in the first part of this talk only the myosin heavy chain family has been shown to have specific developmental isoforms whose transcripts accumulate sequentially during skeletal muscle development. It remains to be seen whether in this case the genes are linked. There is an indication from structural analysis of genomic clones that two cardiac genes, possibly V_1 and V_3 which also show developmental regulation, may be adjacent to each other (634). Such a situation would be reminiscent of the globin family (635) and one can speculate that the non-dispersion in such cases may be significant in the regulation of their sequential expression. The third point concerns the genes of the adult skeletal and cardiac actin and myosins some of which, as discussed, (cardiac actin and $LC1_A/LC1_{emb}$) also play a role as developmental isoforms. The fact that a gene encoding an adult isoform of one tissue is also expressed during the development of another, together with the fact that mRNAs for different actin and myosin isoforms do not accumulate in parallel during skeletal muscle maturation, already suggests that blocks of genes for a given phenotype are not activated together. There is clearly no linkage between genes expressed in the same muscle phenotype. This therefore excludes cis-acting regulatory mechanisms and implies regulation of diffusible transacting factors.

The manipulation of genes _in vitro_ opens the way to the study of activating factors, and in the longer term to the factors which interfere with the normal program of actin and myosin gene expression in dystrophic muscle.

DR. KEDES: I have two comments to make related to actin genes in human chromosomes. The human skeletal muscle actin gene is on chromosome 1 and is single copy, the cardiac actin gene is on chromosome 15 and is single copy. Essentially all the other 20-30 actin coding sequences are beta or gamma sequences including the two smooth muscle sequences. There are beta and gamma pseudogene sequences on the X chromosome. My other comment relates to the concept of the evolution of cardiac and alpha actin genes at the time of the emergence of amphibia. The fact that these two genes may be expressed 50/50 in xenopus laevis, whereas the salamander expresses only a single copy of actin gene in both skeletal and cardiac muscle may be related to the time of the duplication. Those two genes may turn out to be linked in xenopus and equally co-expressed. What may have happened in rodents and man is that these two duplicated linked genes dispersed and are now differentially regulated.

CHAPTER 30: MULTIGENE FAMILIES, DIFFERENTIAL TRANSCRIPTION AND DIFFERENTIAL SPLICING: DIFFERENT ORIGIN OF CONTRACTILE ISO-PROTEINS IN MUSCLE

Emmanuel E. Strehler

Department of Cardiology
Children's Hospital
Boston, MA

I would like to summarize some of the results obtained in Bernardo Nadal-Ginard's lab in the last two years concerning the number, structure and regulation of the genes for the isoforms of rat muscle protein. I will concentrate on the gene(s) for three of these proteins: myosin heavy chain (MHC), myosin light chain 1/3 (LC1/3) and Troponin T (TNT). The work to be presented has been carried out in collaboration with the following investigators in our lab: MHC: Vijak Mahdavi, Danuta Bois, Muthu Periasamy, Robert Wydro and Russell Medford; LC1/3: Muthu Periasamy and Leonard Garfinkel; TNT: Hanh Nguyen, Russell Medford and Antonia Destree.

Myosin Heavy Chain

About two to three years ago a cDNA clone was isolated from a cDNA library made with RNA from fused myotubes derived from L6E9 cells. The rat skeletal muscle cell line is known to express only the embryonic type of MHC. The cDNA clone isolated was subsequently shown to represent embryonic MHC by sequencing, Northern analysis, etc. (636-638). This clone has been used to screen other cDNA libraries made with RNA from different rat tissues in order to get more cDNAs specific for different types of MHC. Figure 125 shows the nucleotide sequence of the carboxy-terminal codons and the 3' untranslated region of six different MHC cDNA clones isolated by this procedure. The tissue- and developmental stage-specificity of the mRNAs represented by these cDNA clones was established mainly by Northern blot analysis and S1 nuclease mapping. They were shown to represent two cardiac, two adult skeletal muscle, one neonatal skeletal muscle and one embryonic skeletal muscle MHC (634,636,638-640) (Figure 125). Two of the cDNAs (Figure 125 c&d) specify an identical carboxyterminal aminoacid sequence and they show 60% match in their 3' untranslated sequence, which is significantly more than what we find when we compare the other cDNAs to each other (Figure 125). We therefore studied these two cDNAs in more detail (640). Northern analysis showed that they both represent MHC mRNAs expressed mostly in adult skeletal muscle, and S1 nuclease mapping confirmed that they are specific for the MHCs of fast red (type IIA) and fast white (type IIB) skeletal muscles (640). In a next step we wanted to find out, by S1 nuclease mapping, how many different MHCs are expressed in muscle during development and in different muscle tissue. For that we deliberately chose a probe from a cDNA region which we knew from sequence analysis to be highly conserved between all our MHC cDNAs. As shown in Figure 126 the probe which was derived from the type IIA specific MHC cDNA clone is fully protected only by RNA from adult muscle tissues (band at the 360 nucleotide level). This MHC type is also expressed in soleus muscle, most likely due to the presence of type IIA fibers in this tissue, but not in cardiac muscle. The other, only partially protected bands correspond to MHC isotypes specific for adult cardiac and slow muscle (band at 75 nucleotides), embryonic skeletal muscle (160 nucleotides), type IIB skeletal muscle (165 nucleotides), and neonatal skeletal muscle (215-280 nucleotides). This probe thus identifies a minimum number of five different MHC isoforms. Additional bands seen in Figure 126 represent either yet undefined MHC genes, or artefacts of the S1 nuclease mapping technique, or both (640).

The sequence divergence of the 3' untranslated regions of our cDNA clones indicates their gene specificity. However, because large parts of the coding regions of the different MHC cDNAs are highly conserved screening of genomic DNA libraries results in the isolation of several different MHC genes (or fragments thereof). So far we have obtained genomic clones specifying at least six different MHC genes. As shown in Figure 127A three of them have been analyzed in some detail by restriction mapping, Northern analysis, Southern blotting using our cDNAs as probes, and by partial sequencing (634,636,638,639,641). These genes are all very large, about 25 kilobases in size. Given the size of the mature MHC mRNA (approx. 7000 nucleotides) this brings the ratio of noncoding to coding sequence in these genes to 3 or 4 to 1. As can be seen in Figure 127B the coding sequences are split into many relatively small exons. Interestingly, the position of the introns at the 5' end are conserved if we compare the embryonic skeletal muscle to the adult cardiac MHC gene. In other words, the coding sequences seem to be interrupted at preferential sites in these genes.

Taken together, our data indicate that most, if not all of the different sarcomeric MHC isoenzymes are encoded by structurally, but different genes. We estimate the total number to be not much more than 7 or 8, including the genes for an embryonic, a neonatal, the two adult fast skeletal and two cardiac muscle MHC. One of

a) GCC AAG AGC CGT GAC ATT GGC GCC AAG GGC CTG AAT GAA GAG TAG ATCTTGCTCTACCCAACCCTAAGGATGCCTGTGAAGCCCTGAGACCTGGAGCCTTTGAAACAGCACCTTCAGGCAGAAACACAATAAAGCAATTTTCCTTCAAGCC$(A)_{37}$
Ala Lys Ser Arg Asp Ile Gly Ala Lys Gly Leu Asn Glu Glu END

b) GCC AAG AGC CGT GAC ATT GGC GCC AAG CAG AAA ATG CAC GAT GAG GAA TAA CCTGTCCAGCAGAAAGAGCCTCGCCGTTGCCATCCCACAATAAATACGAATGTTCGATTTGCCTGC$(A)_{93}$
Ala Lys Ser Arg Asp Ile Gly Ala Lys Gln Lys Met His Asp Glu Glu END

c) GTG AAG AGC CGA GAG GTT CAC ACC AAA GTC ATA AGC GAA GAA TAG CTCAATTCCTTCTGTTGAAAGGTGACAGAAGAAATCACACAATGTGACGTTCTTTGTCACTGTCCTGTATATCAAGGAAATAAAAGCTGCAGATAATTTTGC$(A)_{90}$
Val Lys Ser Arg Glu Val His Thr Lys Val Ile Ser Glu Glu END

d) GTA AAG AGC CGC GAG GTT CAC ACT AAA GTC ATA AGT GAA GAG TAA GGCAGCTCTGATGCTGTAGAATGACCGAAGAAAGGCACAAAATGTGAAGCCTTTGGTCATGCCCCCATGTGATTCTATTTAATCCTATTGTAAGGAAATAAAGAGCCCAAGTTCTTGCAAGC$(A)_{70}$
Val Lys Ser Arg Glu Val His Thr Lys Val Ile Ser Glu Glu END

e) GTG AAG AGC CGC GAG GTT CAC ACC AAA ATC AGT GCA GAG TAA ACGCATCTTGAGGAGGCCGCCAAGTGGCTGAAGGAAAGGCACAGAATGTGCTGCCTTGGGTCGCTTGCTGGGTCGCTTGCCTCTCGTGTTTACTTTTCTCCCACTGCTGACTGAATAAAACCACAACTCATTGTAATT(A)
Val Lys Ser Arg Glu Val His Thr Lys Ile Ser Ala Glu END

f) GCT AAA ACC CGG GAC TTC ACC TCT AGC CGG ATG GTG GTC CAT GAA AGT GAA GAA TGA GCATGTCCTCTTGGTGAGGGGCAGAAGATATGCAGAATGTATGTTTTCCGTGGCCTCCTGACCACCTGCTTAATTTCCACGTAACCCCTTTCCACATGCAATAAATTTGCCTTGTTCAAG
Ala Lys Thr Arg Asp Phe Thr Ser Ser Arg Met Val Val His Glu Ser Glu Glu END

FIGURE 125: Protein carboxyterminal codons and 3' untranslated regions of rat MHC cDNA clones. a) Fetal/adult cardiac (ventricular); b) adult cardiac (ventricular); c) adult skeletal (fast); d) adult skeletal (fast); e) fetal skeletal; f) embryonic skeletal. Underlined sequences indicates polyadenylation signal.

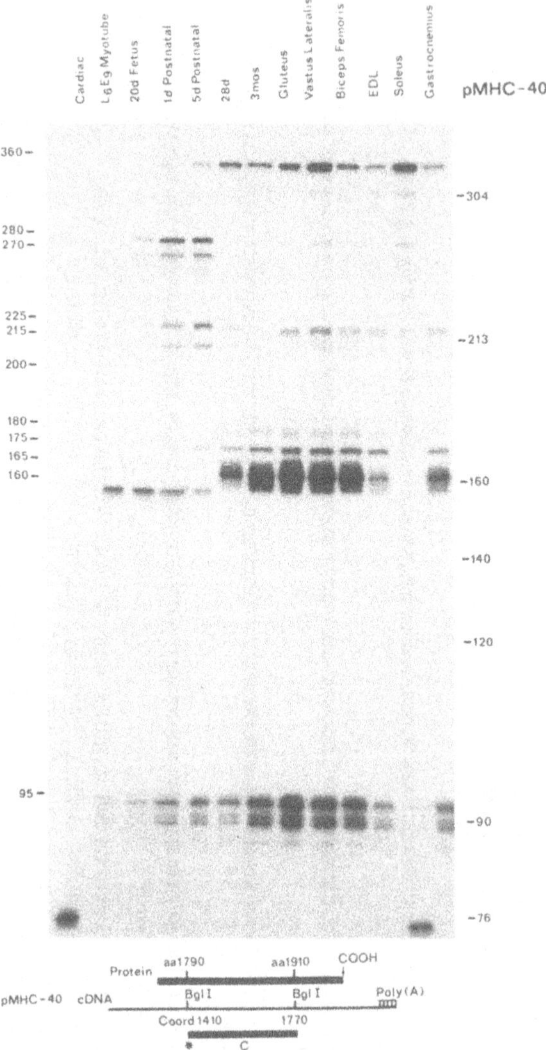

FIGURE 126: Detection of different MHC mRNA species from various muscle tissues and developmental stages by S1 nuclease protection. The probe (c, bottom of figure) was derived (360 base pair BgII restriction fragment specifying amino acids 1790 to 1910) from the fast muscle (type IIA) specific MHC cDNA clone pMHC40 (bottom of figure). After 3' end labeling the non-coding strand (position of label indicated by asterisk) was hybridized to RNA from various sources (indicated on top of each lane), S1 nuclease digested and the protected fragments run on a polyacrylamide gel under denaturing conditions. Fragment sizes are indicated in numbers of nucleotides.

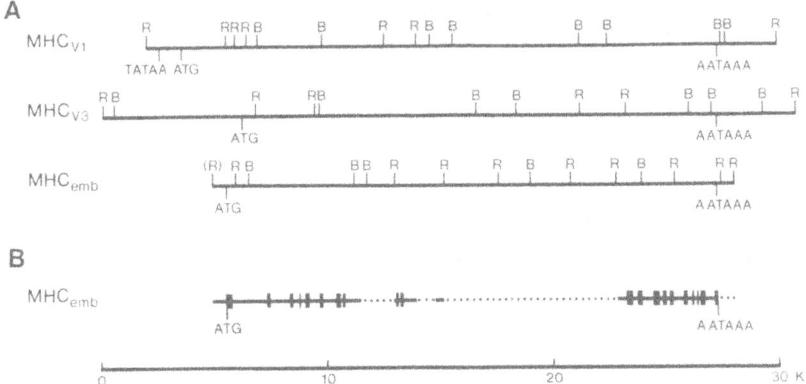

FIGURE 127: Restriction maps and some structural features of rat MHC genes A. EcoRI(R) and BamHI(B) restriction maps are shown in the adult ventricular (V1), fetal/adult ventricular(V3) and embryonic(emb) MHC genes. The genes are aligned with respect to their polyadenylation signals (AATAAA). TATAA and ATG indicate TATA box and initiation codon, respectively. (R): Artificially (linker addition) created EcoRI site. B. Partial structure of the embryonic MHC gene as determined by sequencing. Black boxes indicate exons, solid lines intervening sequences. Dotted lines: sequence not determined.

the cardiac MHC genes (the β-type) is also expressed in the slow soleus muscle (642). There are most probably not going to be many more striated muscle MHC genes. These sarcomeric MHC genes form a so-called multigene family. This family has been mapped to chromosome 17 in the human and to chromosome 11 in the mouse (643). We know that at least two of its members (the two cardiac genes) are closely linked in the genome and are separated from each other by only a few kilobases of chromosomal DNA (644).

Myosin Light Chain 1/3

Adult skeletal muscle LC1 and LC3 are striking in the fact that their 141 carboxyterminal aminoacids are identical and that they differ from each other only at their aminoterminal ends (Figure 128). How does this look at the nucleotide level? We isolated cDNA clones for both LC1 and LC3. The same striking sequence identity in the parts encoding the 141 carboxyterminal aminoacids and, most important, also in the entire 3' untranslated regions, was found on the nucleotide level (644). This sequence identity, particularly of the 3' untranslated regions, suggested that the mRNAs for LC1 and LC3 are transcribed from a single gene. We have isolated overlapping genomic DNA clones covering the complete LC1 and 3 gene locus in order to

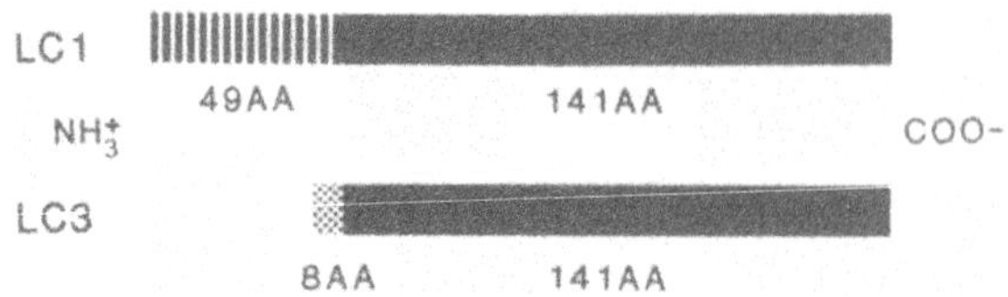

FIGURE 128: Schematic representation of the myosin light chain 1 and 3 proteins. LC1 and 3 share 141 amino acids at the carboxy (COO^-) terminus. LC1 has 49 amino terminal (NH_3+) specific amino acids which are different from the 8 amino terminal amino acids of LC3.

prove this hypothesis (644). As shown in Figure 129 this single LC1/3 gene displays some very unusual features. Most strikingly, the exons encoding the specific 5' ends of LC1 and LC3 are separated by huge introns from the common exons. Note also the presence and location of two "miniexons" encoding aminoacids 1-8 of LC3 and 41-49 LC1 (Figure 129): the LC1 specific miniexon lies downstream of the LC3 specific miniexon and 5' untranslated region. The most interesting question concerns the regulation of this single gene both at the level of transcription and RNA splicing. Figure 130 shows two models explaining how the two different mRNAs for LC1 and LC3 could be produced. If there is only one promoter region upstream of the LC1 specific 5' end-exon a very large primary transcript is made which has to be differentially spliced in order to bring together the exons specifying either the LC1 or the LC3 mRNA (Figure 130A). Alternatively, there could be two promoters, one specific for LC1 and one specific for LC3, in which case differential transcription leads to two different primary transcripts (Figure 130B). However, even in this case differential splicing is involved in the production of the mature mRNAs since the decision still has to be made as to which miniexon will be maintained in the mature mRNA. So far our data on the LC1/3 gene do not allow us to discriminate between the two possibilities for transcription. It is clear, however, that the fast skeletal muscle myosin light chains 1 and 3 are encoded by a single gene and that alternative splicing is involved in the production of the two mature mRNAs.

A cDNA clone specific for TNT has been isolated and characterized in our lab some years ago (645). Using this cDNA as a probe we were able to fish a genomic DNA clone containing sequences coding for TNT. This clone was subsequently analyzed by restriction mapping, Northern blotting and sequencing (646) and was found to contain the coding information for TNT from aminoacid 41 to the carboxyterminus, as well as the complete 3' untranslated region of the TNT mRNA. Interestingly, the last exon encoding the carboxyterminal aminoacids (243-259) and the

Troponin T

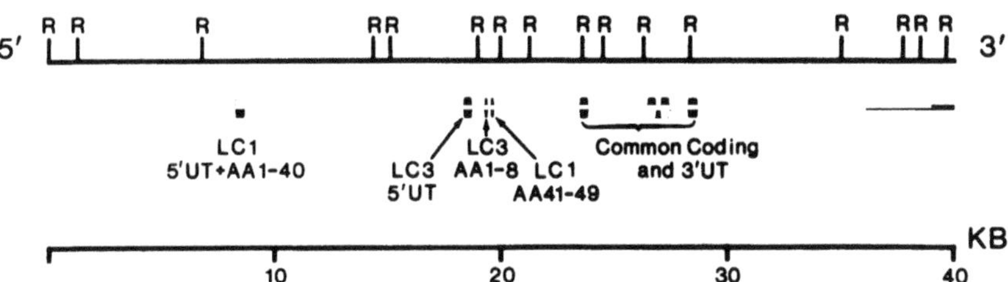

FIGURE 129: Structure of the single gene encoding both LC1 and LC3. The EcoRI(R) restriction map is shown on top of the structural map in which the black boxes represent the exons. UT: untranslated region. AA: amino acids.

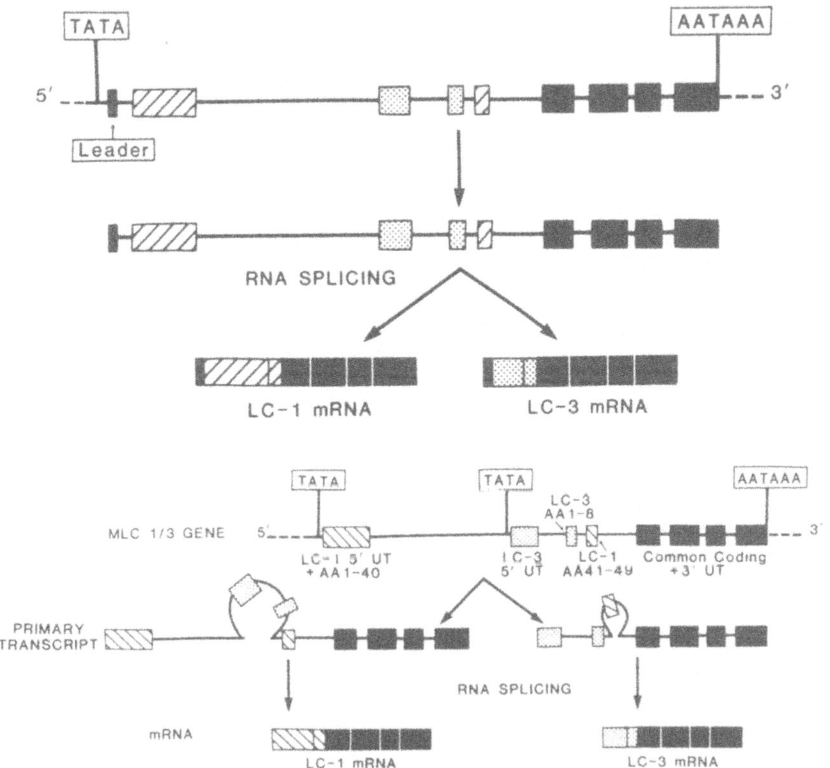

FIGURE 130: Models to explain the expression of LC1 and LC3 mRNAs from their single gene. A. The gene (top) has only one promotor (TATA) 5' of a leader sequence common to both LC1 and LC3 mRNAs. A single large primary transcript is made (middle) which is subsequently processed by differential splicing to yield the two different mature mRNAs (bottom). B. The gene contains two promotors (TATA) specific for LC1 and LC3, respectively. Differential transcription leads to two distinct primary transcripts which still need to be accurately and differentially spliced (as indicated) in order to produce the two mature mRNAs. Striped, dotted and black boxes indicate LC1-specific, LC3-specific and LC1/3-common exons respectively.

3' untranslated region lies almost 3kb downstream of the exons specifying aminoacids 41-228. Since, of course, one did not want to sequence 3kb just to find the miniexon coding for the missing 14 aminoacids 229-242, Northern analysis was performed using two subfragments of that 3kb region as probes in order to pinpoint the location of the miniexon. Surprisingly, however, both subfragments were positive in this analysis. Is the small exon encoding amino acids 229-242 split again in two even smaller miniexons? There was no other way to find out but by sequencing the whole region. As a surprising result it was found that the exon for amino acids 229-242 is represented twice in this stretch of DNA (Figure 131); however, with differing nucleotide sequences. One of the exons shows 100% matching sequence with the corresponding region in our original TNT cDNA clone. By comparing our sequence data with rabbit sequences published recently by Putney et al. (647) it was found (648) that one of the small exons (the one represented in our cDNA) encodes aminoacids 229-242 of the so-called alpha type of TNT and the second one the corresponding aminoacids of the beta type TNT (Figure 131). Again, two distinct mRNAs (differing in the small region encoding the aminoacids 229-242) arise from a single gene. The only way to get expression of either alpha or beta TNT is by accurate differential splicing of the primary transcript. We know that alpha and beta TNT are differentially expressed in different muscle tissues and in different stages of development. This means that the splicing mechanism has to be regulated in a tissue- and developmental stage-specific manner. But what does the 5' end of the TNT gene look like? In order to be able to answer this question we first tried to get full length cDNAs for TNT. This was attempted by primer extension, whereby you take a piece of your "old" cDNA as primer, hybridize it to RNA and try to finish up the cDNA with

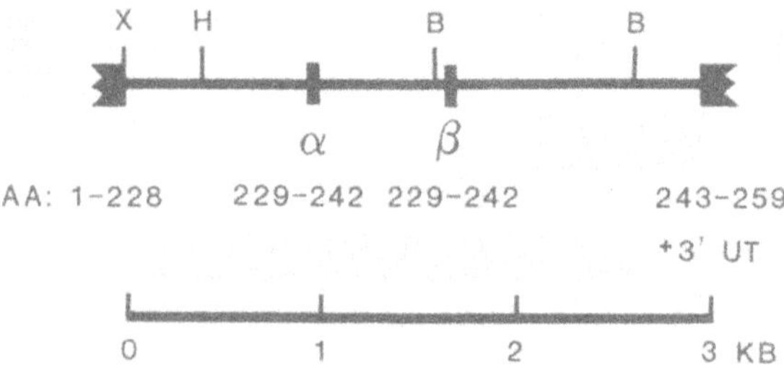

FIGURE 131: Isotype switch region within the troponin T gene. Restriction sites of XbaI (X), HindIII (H) and BamHI (B) are shown. Broken black boxes indicate the location of the exons specifying the amino terminal (AA 1-228) and the carboxyterminal amino acid and the 3' untranslated region (AA 243-259 + 3' UT) on either side of the miniexons encoding the α or β-specific amino acids 229-242 (small black boxes).

reverse transcriptase. Following this procedure we got a couple of extended cDNA clones, which were then sequenced (649).

Unexpectedly, almost every clone showed a different nucleotide sequence at the very 5' end. So far four different TNT cDNAs varying only in their 5' end sequence have been identified. It seems likely that the different 5' end sequences are encoded in separate exons in the same TNT gene, so that the pattern of differential splicing leading to the mature TNT mRNAs becomes even more complex than suspected before.

In conclusion, our recent results on the structure and expression of the muscle protein genes indicate the additional complexity of these genes needed to provide for the different muscle protein isoforms. It is evident that the tissue- and development-specific expression of the mRNAs for muscle isoproteins can be regulated in multiple ways and at different levels in the genome. Considering our data on differential splicing it becomes clear that the intervening sequences are probably not just superfluous pieces of DNA but are perhaps involved in regulating the differential expression of multiple mRNAs from the same gene. One has to keep this in mind if one wants to look for regulatory sequences in these genes.

DR. WOOD: There are two fundamental ways in which enzyme switches might work. One is asynchronized, meaning that the old form sits around in an _in vitro_ or _in vivo_ system for a period of days or weeks while the new form is being synthesized. Then you have the more synchronized kind of introduction of a new isoform where it seems that the block of the old gene occurs coincidentally with the turning on of the new one. I was just wondering if any of the speakers might want to comment on the types of regulation that might be involved in those two forms of asynchronized and synchronized expression of new isoforms.

DR. PETTE: It is not quite clear. We did some incorporation studies, and there is no evidence for the necessity of proliferation in order to get isoenzyme switches. Of course, this does not exclude fusion.

DR. EPSTEIN: Do we really know that splicing occurs at the RNA level and that the genes are remaining intact, or could there be different nuclei in which DNAs may be spliced differentially?

DR. STREHLER: We know, at least for LC1/3 and TNT, that the genes are not rearranged. We don't know however, whether a single cell makes the different isoforms. It is also very difficult to prove that the primary transcript is really as large as it would have to be coming from a gene such as the one for LC1/3.

DR. FISCHMAN: I would like to ask Dr. Strehler if there is any direct evidence from *in vitro* translation studies with the RNA from a muscle in which you suspect there are six forms of troponin T.

DR. STREHLER: There is evidence for more than two forms of troponin T. We do not have any evidence for six different troponin Ts.

DR. FISCHMAN: Our present immunologic evidence indicates that fast myosin light chain 2 is slightly different in the cultured cells. Could it be that the cultured cells are making a fast light chain 2 so that it is affecting the immunological properties of the protein?

DR. STREHLER: Our evidence points to the direction of only one gene for the fast light chain 2. The sequencing doesn't point to the involvement of mechanisms like differential splicing in the processing of the primary transcript. However, we don't have the complete sequence of the gene yet.

DR. EPSTEIN: I was going to comment on Dr. Rowland's statement that the contractile proteins and their isoforms are probably not involved in the pathogenesis of muscular dystrohy. I think we could imagine a constant myopathy and even a progressive myopathy on the basis of myosin isoforms. A structural gene mutation that knocks out the major myosin heavy chain isoform might still lead to the production of thick filaments of normal length but made up with only one myosin isoform. If the gene should be switched off in the middle of muscle maturation with respect to the myosin heavy chain isoforms, the addition of thick filaments to the pre-existing sarcomeres would stop. We are now examining whether any thick filaments are not formed in some of our mutants and what the composition of the existing thick filament is. In the nematode muscle system there is some relationship between the presence of the two myosin heavy chain isoforms and thick filament integration into sarcomeres.

DR. BLAU: Isn't it true you also had a mutant in myosin isoform that results in decreased cell proliferation?

DR. EPSTEIN: Not that I know of. There are mutants that affect the muscle cell lineage, specific kinds, but they are in other genes.

DR. EMERSON: The question now is whether the information for the transcriptional regulation resides in the sequences which are close by the DNA, or whether there are more complicated mechanisms for activating the transcription of genes. One would predict DNA sequence homologies close by these genes which are shared by the set of transcriptional regulated genes.

DR. KEDES: Are there really only 15-17 new proteins that distinguish a myoblast from proteins in the myofiber or are you just talking about contractile proteins.

DR. EMERSON: I was talking about both proteins which are in the abundant class.

DR. KEDES: How do you know you don't get any cross-hybridization? Are some RNAs in common that represent the genes. If they represent both it must be the same gene.

DR. EMERSON: It is not cross hybridization for those 17. Part of the analysis is Northern gels and size of the transcript and comparing that with the 17 and doing a Southern blot and asking whether there are any shared genomic bands in a high stringency analysis for both of those. That is how we bring it down to a set of 17. Within that, the set is much larger, there are overlapping clones. Virtually all of these in the set have been eliminated.

DR. BUCKINGHAM: I would suspect that you are seeing different transcripts which are being switched on at the same time. There might be some type of cross-hybridization going on.

DR. EMERSON: Since in the adult probe we use only 40% homologous with any known myosin heavy chain sequence, there could be no cross hybridization.

DR. STREHLER: There is a consensus sequence in the embryonic globin gene that is not species specific but is found across species in human and rat. That really points to the direction we should look for breaking off the sequence.

DR. EMERSON: In Ordahl's description he showed in a chicken/rat sequence that there was a conservation of a block of sequences of 20 nucleotides between chicken and rat. It falls into that class of consensus sequences.

DR. FISCHMAN: Have you looked for non-homologus sequences in the neonatal stage, post-hatch stage that might support or refute the concept of a neonatal myosin?

DR. EMERSON: All of the clones have been derived either from adult animal or embryonic culture.

PART VI

SUMMARY AND SYNTHESIS

CHAPTER 30: SUMMARY AND SYNTHESIS

R. Rodney Howell

Department of Pediatrics
University of Texas Medical Branch
Houston, TX

In discussing the basic phenotype expression of Duchenne Muscular Dystrophy, Dr. Rowland mentioned the prolonged pursuit of a hypothesized defect in the plasma membrane and of a presumed disturbance in one or more of the contractile proteins. Thus far neither lead has been very productive. Indeed the so far identified gene loci for contractile proteins are located on chromosomes other than the X chromosome. I gather, however, that neither membrane nor contractile protein can be clearly dismissed as a potential culprit at the present time.

We have heard a great deal about shifts in actin, myosin and tropomyosin isotypes including the persistence of neonatal forms in dystrophic muscle. Dr. Hoh with his remarkable suspended rat demonstrated shifts in the muscle protein types during disuse. Are there abnormalities physiologically and how do these relate to the dystrophic conditions?

Questions about the switching on and off of nuclei remain to be settled as well as the recruitment of new nuclei to produce different forms of myosin.

A newer hypothesis has emerged from the observations of Dr. Blau. She is proposing a genetic disorder in the satellite cells that make them unable to proliferate at the required rate to keep up with the normal demands of growth.

The phenotype that she observed in cultures and called the dystroblast displays the characteristics of an aged or senescent myoblast. She is planning to attempt to correct the situation in the dystrophic myoblast by cell fusion of a normal satellite cell with a dystroblast.

There is some indication that the dystroblast could be a marker for the dystrophic gene and thus may be extremely useful in identifying carriers. A disturbance with trophic factors offers another possible avenue in which to pursue the elusive phenotype expression of the dystrophic gene.

Dr. Hauschka presented a series of rules for studying the trophic factors in different cultures _in vitro_. We heard about the effect of insulin and transferrins and also about the role of certain oxypurines in the growth of cells. Hypoxanthine excretion in the muscle _in vivo_ appears to be a useful measure of muscle exercise and of the metabolic condition of the muscle. It would be of great interest to know the exact mechanism by which the oxypurines produce muscle stimulation.

I would be very interested to hear from our colleagues who presented their work on transferrin about exactly how they perceive this might be related to the dystrophic condition.

Transferrin, required for the growth of muscle cells _in vitro_, can be substituted by iron and is accompanied by a rapid switch to oxidative metabolism. Have transferrin receptors been demonstrated? How might abnormalities in transferrin be related to the dystrophic conditions?

I was surprised not to hear more discussion of the potential value of other metals in this situation. X-ray fluorescence might be a valuable tool to apply to these cells because simultaneously you can assess the state not only of iron but of calcium, copper, zinc and some other important metals.

Dr. Lowey has called for more enzymatic data on myosin and other contractile proteins. While it is clear that they have enzymatic functions, it is not clear what those functions are. Dr. Lowey has pointed out that assessing the enzyme function of myosin is a difficult job but very important to do.

Dr. Garrels' 2D gels provide an extremely powerful tool for the identification of proteins as gene products and to characterize differences in disease states by screening relatives. The confounding effects of polymorphisms could be gotten around by the analysis of multiple gels.

Each of the genetic myopathies that Dr. Miranda described depend on the defective expression of an enzyme. The fact that phosphorylase which is deficient in the mature person with McArdle's disease was found to be active in the embryo tissue and in culture demonstrates quite elegantly the importance of differential enzyme regulation.

This work also brings to the fore our present ignorance in the face of the importance of understanding the mechanisms of gene activation.

We heard that thyroid and other hormones increase the amount of mRNA for the heavy myosin gene. To know the exact mechanism of switching on that gene would be of considerable value.

Dr. Pette produced a switch in muscle fiber types with electrical stimulation. We need to know more about the effects on dystrophic cells of repeated electrical stimulation and the possible practical value of electrical stimulation of muscles or exercise training in the treatment of dystrophic children.

Dr. Blau presented a very provocative experiment with human amniotic fibroblasts and mouse myocytes and demonstrated at least two important and interesting things to me; one was that she could activate protein synthesis without DNA replication and that she could demonstrate that human muscle proteins are expressed in the amniocytes.

Dr. Buckingham showed striking evidence in her linkage and breeding studies that she could show co-expression of widely scattered genes as well as individual expression of genes that were closely linked to the chromosomes. She also believes that certain early forms of myosin might be importantly related to the dystrophic condition. I would be very interested in hearing from her about how she thinks that that might be.

Dr. Kedes' library for muscle protein from an amputated leg should be of great value and may help in identifying the gene product in Duchenne dystrophy. I hope Dr. Kedes will explain how he proposes to identify the gene for Duchenne dystrophy and how Dr. Blau's system may help in that effort.

I think Dr. Kunkel has discussed what he plans to do with the deletions in the X chromosome as a step toward cloning the Duchenne gene and discovering its function.

After hearing the vast amount of material that has been presented here I suspect that at a practical level for diagnosing the disease and counseling patients and families we will very likely rely on information from restriction fragment length polymorphisms and modification of *in vitro* systems as Dr. Blau has suggested long before we identify and understand the function of the dystrophic gene.

CODA

Dr. Howell's excellent summary has provided us some important questions to consider. Reflecting his own interest in the genetic basis of muscular dystrophy, they pertain to the degree to which the results presented here bear on the clinical problems.

Genes, Gene Regulation and Muscle Disease

Dr. Howell reminded us that the muscle contractile proteins under discussion here may not be linked directly to the genetic problem. Recognizing that the gene for Duchenne and Becker's dystrophy is located on the X chromosome while all available evidence now places the genes for muscle contractile proteins elsewhere, what is the significance of current research on contractile proteins?

We do not know what the gene for dystrophy is and we clearly do not have the defective gene product. What we do have is the very strong possibility that the dystrophic gene, whatever it may be, is regulated as part of a developmental sequence of gene expression. If we can understand the basis for this regulation we may then at least come to know and understand when and how the dystrophic gene is activated or suppressed.

The contractile proteins myosin, actin, tropomyosin, etc., are coded for by a family of genes that are developmentally regulated. Thus, at embryonic, neonatal and adult stages of development the presence or absence of the appropriate gene product (protein) is expressed or not expressed. In other words the study of these genes can show us whether or not a muscle is displaying an abnormal pattern of gene regulation. If for example the dystrophic gene is a member of the adult set of genes (see below) rather than the embryonic set, then at least we will be able to relate the manifestation of the disease to the developmental history of the individual.

If, on the other hand, the defective gene turns out to be a regulatory one these studies on contractile protein gene regulation will have an even greater bearing on our understanding of the pathogenesis of the disease.

The isoforms of myosin, actin, etc., are distinct proteins or subunits of the same functional protein. In most cases each is coded for by a separate gene. Thus, the isoforms appear and disappear at precise stages of muscle development and maturation. In many animal and in some human dystrophies, there is an inappropriate expression of embryonic and/or neonatal isoforms. While in normal adult muscle one finds only adult isoforms for the various proteins, in dystrophy one may find as well the expression of embryonic/neonatal isoforms. There may also be a shift in the dystrophic organism to slow rather than to fast type gene expression.

Protein Isoforms and Their Significance

If it turns out that there is no "abnormal" protein in DMD, it is possible that the problem may simply be an altered timing of gene expression. In other words there may not be anything abnormal other than the timing...the regulation of gene expression. Our task, then, will be to learn how to restore a normal sequence of gene expression in dystrophic muscles.

Dr. Howell focused attention on the significance of trophic factors. Whether they come from innervating nerves, from blood borne hormones or other agents, or from adjacent fibroblasts, or other cells in the vicinity, they may influence the regulation of muscle gene expression. It is well known for example that the nerve supply can control muscle gene expression. The underlying mechanism, however, continues to be elusive. An insight here may provide the key to reversal of an inappropriate sequence of gene expression in diseased muscle.

Trophic Factors and Muscle Growth

A further possibility is that the muscle degeneration of dystrophy may be a consequence of inadequate growth. A defect in the muscle satellite cell has now been suggested as an etiologic possibility. Satellite cells in muscle represent the potential for regrowth, for regeneration both in normal and diseased muscles. These cells are normally dormant but must be responsive to growth factors. What activates a satellite cell? How is this cell population sustained? What factors contribute to satellite cell death or to early senescence? Recent work on growth factors such as transferrin and their selective localization in muscle offers us a hopeful beginning toward understanding the role of trophic factors in regulation of muscle growth via control of satellite cell proliferation.

While the search for a specific gene sequence responsible for diseased muscle is well underway, cell culture researchers continue to pursue the defect from the protein side. A major challenge is to achieve full expression of the dystrophic phenotype in cell culture. Surprisingly, muscle cells taken from dystrophic sources and placed in culture are mostly normal; the dystrophic characteristics are not expressed. Actually we should not be surprised since the Columbia University group showed years ago, as Dr. Howell reminds us, that cultured muscle expresses embryonic genes for particular enzymes. The embryonic genes seem to be normal but their adult reincarnations appear defective. If the disease strikes as the adult gene is turned on, we must learn how to turn on the adult genes in culture. So far we have not been able to achieve the conditions necessary for a "full disclosure" of the adult gene set.

Knowledge of the different genes is a "payoff" from earlier studies of contractile protein gene expression. Knowing that the proteins exist in different isoforms, ranging from embryonic through adult, enables us to tell what stage of expression the cultured muscle cell is in. Once we have the conditions for a routine expression of muscular dystrophy in cell culture we will have a good chance to search out the putative abnormal gene product. But even if the defect is not a protein but some regulatory sequence we will still be ahead. We may utilize such cultures to screen drugs and other molecules that may reverse some of the disease symptoms. Finally, when the gene for dystrophy is isolated, a muscle culture system in which the gene can be expressed will still be required.

Dr. Howell mentioned the fact that some muscles may be more resistant to the disease than others. This is an extremely important point. While most fibers will eventually become involved with the disease process, relative resistance may provide critical clues. The complexity of the nomenclature currently used to describe muscle fiber types reflects our limited understanding of the differences.* The problem is compounded by the fact that the characteristics of fiber types differ among animal forms and that none precisely reproduces the situation in the human.

Muscle Fiber Heterogeneity and Resistance to Disease

*Gauthier, G.F.: Skeletal Muscle Fiber Types, Chapter 8 in Myology. Engle, A.G. and Banker, B.Q. (eds.) McGraw-Hill, New York, 1985 (In press).

From all of the foregoing presentations and discussions, progress toward an understanding of the pathogenesis of Duchenne Muscular Dystrophy is evident on several fronts. The enormous complexity of muscle and the vast number of things that can go wrong in this hard working tissue have required a wide ranging interdisciplinary, as well as international, effort. The colloquium attempted to focus on mutually enlightening dialogue on the problem from the various, somewhat disparate points of view and methods of approach.

REFERENCES

1. Rowland, L.P., ed. Pathogenesis of human muscular dystrophies. Amsterdam: Excerpta Medica, 1977.

2. Walton, J.N., Mastaglia, F.L., eds.: The muscular dystrophies. Brit Med Bull 36:105-203, 1980.

3. Serratrice, G., Cros, D., Desnvelle, D., Gastaut, J.L., Pellissier, J.F., Pugett, S.A., eds.: Neuromuscular diseases. New York: Raven Press, 1984.

4. Rowland, L.P.: Biochemistry of muscle membranes in Duchenne muscular dystrophy. Muscle & Nerve 3:3-20, 1980.

5. Scotland, D.L., ed.: Disorders of the motor unit. John Wiley, New York, 1982.

6. Rowland, L.P.: The membrane theory of Duchenne dystrophy. Ital J Neurol Sci In press.

7. Kingston, H.M., Harner, P.S., Pearson, P.L., Davies, K.E., Williamson, R. and Page, D.: Localization of gene for Becker muscular dystrophy. Lancet 2:1200, 1983.

8. Mokri, B., Engle, A.G.: Duchenne dystrophy: electron microscopic findings pointing to a basic or early abnormality in the plasma membrane of the muscle fiber. Neurology 25:1111-1120, 1975.

9. Bonilla, E., Schotland, D.L. and Wakagama, V.: Freeze fracture studies in human muscular dystrophy. In: Schotland, D.L. ed. Diseases of the Motor Unit, John Wiley, New York, 475-488, 1982.

10. Wolf, S. and Murray, A.K. eds.: Composition and Function of Cell Membranes. Plenum Press, New York, 1981.

11. Viginos, P.J., Jr., and Lefkowitz, M.: A biochemical study of certain skeletal muscle constituents in human progressive muscular dystrophy. J Clin Invest 38:873-881, 1959.

12. Samaha, F.J.: Actomyosin alterations in Duchenne muscular dystrophy. Arch Neurol 28:405-407, 1973.

13. Samaha, F. and Gergely, J.: Biochemical abnormalities of the sarcoplasmic reticulum in muscular dystrophy. N Engl J Med 280:184-188, 1969.

14. Furukawa, T. and Peter, J.B.: Superprecipitation and ATPase activity of myosin B in Duchenne muscular dystrophy. Neurol 21:920-924, 1971.

15. Furukawa, T., Peter, J.B.: Muscular dystrophy and other myopathies. Troponin activity of natural actomyosin from skeletal muscle. Arch Neurol 26:385-390, 1972.

16. Samaha, F.J., Davis, B. and Nagy, B.: Duchenne muscular dystrophy: ATP and creatine phosphate content in muscle. Neurol 26:385-390, 1981.

17. Penn, A.S., Cloak, R. and Rowland, L.P. Myosin from normal and dystrophic human muscle immunochemical and electrophoretic study. Arch Neurol 27:159-173, 1972.

18. Samaha, F.S.: Tropomyosin and troponin in normal and dystrophic human muscle. Arch Neurol 26:547-550, 1972.

19. Sugita, H. and Toyokura, Y.: Alteration of troponin subunits in progressive muscular dystrophy. Proc Japan Acad 52:256-263, 1976.

20. Fitzsimons, R.P., Hoh, J.F.Y.: Embryonic and fetal myosins in human skeletal muscle. Presence of fetal myosins in Duchenne dystrophy and infantile spinal muscular atrophy. J Neurol Sci 52:367-384, 1981.

21. Takagi, A., Ishihura, S., Nonaka, I. and Sugita, H.: Myosin light chain components in single muscle fibers of Duchenne muscular dystrophy. Muscle & Nerve 5:399-404, 1982.

22. Takamuri, M., Mori, K., Ide, Y. and Tsujihata, M.: Contractile and chemosensitive properties of muscle treated with calcium ionophore, A23187. J Neurol Sci 51:207-215, 1981.

23. Sugita, H., Okimoto, K., Ebashi, S., Okinaka, S.: Biochemical alteration in muscular dystrophy: special reference to sarcoplasmic reticulum. In: Milhorat, A.T., ed.: Exploratory concepts in muscular dystrophy. Amsterdam, Excerpta Medica, 321-326, 1967.

24. Peter, J.B. and Worsfold, M.: Muscular dystrophy and other myopathies. Sarcotubular vesicles in early disease. Biochem Med 2:364-371, 1969.

25. Takagi, A., Schotland, D.L. and Rowland, L.P.: Sarcoplasmic reticulum in Duchenne muscular dystrophy. Arch Neurol 28:380-384, 1973.

26. Seiler, D., Kuhn, E., Fiehn, W.: Abnormalities of the sarcoplasmic reticulum in myopathies. In: Hausmanowa-Petrusewicz, I., ed. Structure and function of normal and diseased muscle and peripheral nerve. Warsaw: Poland Medical Publishers, 211-215, 1974.

27. Samaha, F.J., Congedo, C.Z.: Two biochemical types of Duchenne dystrophy: sarcoplasmic reticulum membrane proteins. Ann Neurol 1:125-130, 1977.

28. Dux, L., Martonosi, A.: Membrane crystals of Ca^{2+} ATPase in sarcoplasmic reticulum of normal and dystrophic muscle. Muscle & Nerve 6:566-573, 1983.

29. Sorenson, S., Eastwood, A.B., Charash, W.E. and Reuben, J.P.: Duchenne dystrophy: abnormal generation of tension and Ca^{++} regulation in skinned and single fibers. Neurol 28:447-457, 1978.

30. Takagi, A.: Sarcoplasmic reticulum of Duchenne muscular dystrophy: a study of skinned muscle fibers. In: Serratrice, G., et al, eds. Neuromuscular Diseases. Raven Press, New York, 123-125, 1984.

31. Banerji, A.P., Karandikar, P.V., Varadkar, A.M., Desai, A.D., Potnis, A.V.: Muscle transkelotase in normal fetuses and Duchenne dystrophy. Clin Chim Acta 86:307-311, 1978.

32. Miike, T.: Maturation defect of regeneration fibers in cases with Duchenne and congenital muscular dystrophy. Muscle & Nerve 6:545-552, 1983.

33. Rowland, L.P.: Pathogenesis of muscular dystrophies. Arch Neurol 23:315-321, 1976.

34. Sewry, C.A., Dubowitz, V.: Calcium and necrosis. In: Serratrice, G. et al, eds. Neuromuscular Diseases. Raven Press, New York, 131-137, 1984.

35. Engel, A.C., Biesecker, G.: Complement activation of muscle fiber necrons. Ann Neurol 12:289-296, 1982.

36. Walsh, E.S., Hurko, O., Quinn, C.A. and Brown, S.M.: X-chromosome coded antigens in Duchenne muscular dystrophy. In: Serratrice, G. et al, eds.: Neuromuscular Diseases. Raven Press, New York, 119-122, 1984.

37. Pato, C.N., Davis, M.H., Dovatty, M.J., Bryant, S.H. and Gruenstein, E.: Increased membrane permeability to chloride in Duchenne muscular dystrophy fibroblasts and its relation to muscle fibers. Proc Nat Acad Sci USA 80:4732-4736, 1983.

38. Kent, C.: Increased rate of cell substratum detachment of fibroblasts from patients with Duchenne muscular dystrophy. Proc Nat Acad Sci USA, 80:3086-3090, 1983.

39. Jones, G.E., Witkowski, J.A.: A cell surface abnormality in Duchenne muscular dystrophy: intercellular adhesiveness of skin fibroblasts from patients and carriers. Human Genet 63:232-237, 1983.

40. Devlin, R. and Emerson, C.: Coordinate regulation of contractile protein synthesis during myoblast differentiation. Cell 13:599-611, 1978.

41. Paterson, B. and Strohman, R.C.: Myosin synthesis in cultures of differentiating chicken embryo skeletal muscle. Dev Biol 29:113-138, 1972.

42. Paterson, B. and Bishop J.: Changes in mRNA population of chick myoblasts during myogenesis in vitro. Cell 12:751-765, 1977.

43. Strohman, R.C., Moss, P., Micou-Eastwood, J., Spector, D., Przybyla, A. and Paterson, B.: Messenger RNA for myosin polypeptides: Isolation from single myogenic cell cultures. Cell 10:265-273, 1977.

44. Devlin, R. and Emerson, C.: Coordinate accumulation of contractile protein mRNAs during myoblast differentiation. Dev Biol 69:202-216, 1979.

45. Shani, M., Zevin-Sonkin, D., Saxel, O., Carmon, Y., Katcoff, D., Nudel, U. and Yaffe, D.: The correlation between the synthesis of skeletal muscle actin, myosin heavy chain and myosin light chain and the accumulation of corresponding mRNA sequences during myogenesis. Dev Biol 86:483-492, 1981.

46. Dollenmeier, P., Turner, D.C. and Eppenberger, H.M.: Proliferation and differentiation of chick skeletal muscle cells cultured in a chemically defined medium. Exp Cell Res 135:47-51, 1981.

47. Holtzer, H., Croop, J., Toyama, Y., Bennet, G., Fellini, S. and West, C.: Differences in differentiation programs between presumptive myoblasts and their daughters, the definitive myoblasts and myotubes. In: Plasticity of Muscle. D. Pette, editor. Walter de Gruyter & Co., Berlin, New York, 1980.

48. Nadal-Ginard, B.: Commitment, fusion and biochemical differentiation of a myogenic cell line in the absence of DNA synthesis. Cell 15:855-864, 1978.

49. Nguyen, H.T., Medford, R.M. and Nadal-Ginard, B.: Reversibility of muscle differentiation in the absence of commitment: Analysis of a myogenic cell line temperature-sensitive for commitment. Cell 34:281-293, 1983.

50. Gauthier, G.F., Lowey, S. and Hobbs : Fast and slow myosin in developing muscle fibers. Nature (Lond.) 274:25-29, 1978.

51. Matsuda, R., Bandman, E. and Strohman, R.C.: Regional differences in the expression of myosin light chains and tropomyosin subunits during development of chicken breast muscle. Dev Biol 95:484-491, 1983.

52. Crow, M.T., Olson, P.S. and Stockdale, F.: Myosin light chain expression during avian muscle development. J Cell Biol 96:763-774, 1983.

53. Obinata, T., Reinach, F.G., Bader, D.M., Masaki, T., Kitani, S. and Fischman, D.: Immunological analysis of C-protein isoform transitions during the development of chicken skeletal muscle. Dev Biol 101:116-124, 1984.

54. Rushbrook, J. and Stracher, A.: Comparison of adult, embryonic and dystrophic myosin heavy chains from chicken muscle by sodium dodecyl sulfate/polyacrylamide gel electrophoresis and peptide mapping. Proc Natl Acad Sci USA, 76:4331-4334, 1979.

55. Whalen, R.G., Schwartz, K., Bouveret, P. Sell, S.M. and Gros, F.: Contractile protein isozymes in muscle development: Identification of an embryonic form of myosin heavy chain. Proc Natl Acad Sci USA, 76:5197-5201, 1979.

56. Bandman, E., Matsuda, R. and Strohman, R.C.: Developmental appearance of myosin heavy and light chain isoforms in vivo and in vitro in chicken skeletal muscle. Dev Biol 93:508-518, 1982.

57. Bader, D., Masaki, T. and Fischman, D.: Immunochemical analysis of myosin heavy chain during avian myogenesis in vivo and in vitro. J Cell Biol 95:763-770, 1982.

58. Benfield, P.A., Lowey, S., LeBlanc, D.D. and Waller, G.S.: Myosin isozymes in avian skeletal muscles. II. Fractionation of myosin isozymes from adult and embryonic chicken pectoralis muscle by immuno-affinity chromatography. J Musc Res Cell Motility 4:717-723, 1983.

59. Sweeney, L.J., Clark, W.A., Umeda, P.K., Zak, R. and Manasek, F.J.: Immunoflorescence analysis of the primordial myosin detectable in embryonic striated muscle. Proc Natl Acad Sci, USA, 81:797-799, 1984.

60. Minty, A.J., Alonso, S., Carvatti, M. and Buckingham, M.E.: A fetal skeletal muscle actin mRNA and its identity with cardiac actin mRNA. Cell 30:185-192, 1982.

61. Matsuda, R., Spector, D.H. and Strohman, R.C.: Regenerating adult chicken skeletal muscle and satellite cell cultures express embryonic patterns of myosin and tropomyosin isoforms. Dev Biol 100:478-488, 1983a.

62. Butler-Browne, G.S., Bugaisky, L.B., Cuenoud, S., Schwartz, K. and Whalen, R.G.: Denervation of newborn rat muscles does not block the appearance of adult fast myosin heavy chain. Nature (Lond.) 299:830-833, 1982.

63. Toyota, N. and Shimada, Y.: Isoform variants of troponin in skeletal and cardiac muscle cells cultured with and without nerves. Cell 33:297-304, 1983.

64. Matsuda, R., Spector, D. and Strohman, R.C.: Denervated skeletal muscle displays discordinate regulation for the synthesis of several myofibrillar proteins. Proc Natl Acad Sci USA, 81:1122-1125, 1984.

65. Amphlett, G., Perry, S.V., Suska, H., Brown, M. and Vrbova, G.: Cross innervation and the regulatory system of rabbit soleus muscle. Nature (Lond.) 257:602-604, 1975.

66. Hoh, J.F.Y.: Neural regulation of mammalian fast and slow muscle myosins: An electrophoretic analysis. Biochem 14:742-747, 1975.

67. Weeds, A.G. and Burridge, K.: Myosin from cross-reinnervated cat muscles. Evidence for reciprocal transformation of heavy chains. FEBS Lett 57:203-208, 1975.

68. Ecob, E.S., Butler-Browne, G.S. and Whalen, R.W.: The adult fast isozyme of myosin is present in a nerve-muscle tissue culture system. Differentiation 24: 24-87, 1983.

69. Paterson, B. and Eldridge, J.: Science. In press, 1984.

70. Strohman, R.C., Micou-Eastwood, J., Glass, C.A. and Matsuda, R.: Human fetal muscle and cultured myotubes derived from it contain a fetal-specific myosin light chain. Science 221:955-957, 1983.

71. Rothman, S.M. and Bischoff, R.: Electrophysiology of Duchenne dystrophy myotubes in tissue culture. Ann Neurol 13:176-179, 1983.

72. Campion, D.: The muscle satellite cell: A review. Internat Rev Cytol 87:225-251, 1984.

73. DiMauro, S., Bresolin, N. and Papadimitriou, A.: Fuels for exercise: clues from disorders of glycogen and lipid metabolism. In: Neuromuscular Diseases, edited by G. Serratrice et al., pp. 45-50, Raven Press, New York, 1984.

74. Engel, A.G.: Metabolic and endocrine myopathies. In: Disorders of Voluntary Muscle, 4th ed., edited by J.N. Walton, pp. 671-674, Churchill Livingstone, New York, 1981.

75. Kula, R.W., Shafiq, S.A., Sher, J.H. and Qazi, Q.H.: I-cell disease (Mucolipidosis II). Differential expression in satellite cells and mature muscle fibers. J Neurol Sci 63:75-84, 1984.

76. Shanske, S., Miranda, A.F., Penn, A.S. and DiMauro, S.: Mucolipidosis II (I Cell Disease); Studies of muscle biopsy and muscle cultures. Pediat Res 15:1334-1339, 1981.

77. Askansas, V., Engel, W.K., DiMauro, S., Mehler, M. and Brookes, B.R.: Adult-onset acid maltase deficiency; Morphologic and biochemical abnormalities reproduced in cultured muscle. New Engl J Med 294:573-578, 1976.

78. Bresolin, N., Miranda, A.F., Chang, H.W., Shanske, S. and DiMauro, S.: Phosphoglycerate kinase deficiency myopathy: Biochemical and immunological studies of the mutant enzyme. Muscle & Nerve In press.

79. DiMauro, S., Bresolin, N., Miranda, A.F., and Chang, H.W.: Glycogen storage disease: New enzyme defects. In: Neuromuscular Diseases edited by G. Serratrice, et al pp. 67-70, Raven Press, New York, 1984.

80. DiMauro, S., Dalakas, M., and Miranda, A.F.: Phosphoglycerate kinase (PGK) deficiency: another cause of recurrent myoglobinuria. Ann Neurol 13:11-19, 1983.

81. Miranda, A.F., DiMauro, S., Antler, A., Stern, L.Z. and Rowland, L.P.: Glycogen debrancher deficiency is reproduced in muscle cultures. Ann Neurol 9:283-288, 1981.

82. Miranda, A.F., Shanske, S., Hays, A.P. and DiMauro, S.: Immunocytochemical analysis of normal and acid maltase-deficient muscle cultures. Arch Neurol In press.

83. DiMauro, S., Hays, A.P., Bresolin, N.: Disorders of glycogen metabolism of muscle. In: CRC Critical Reviews in Clinical Neurobiology edited by A.D. Roses. CRC Press, Inc., Boca Raton, FL., In press.

84. Engel, A.G.: Metabolic and endocrine myopathies. In: Disorders of Voluntary Muscle, 4th ed., edited by J.N. Walton, pp. 671-674, Churchill Livingstone, New York, 1981.

85. D'Ancona, G.G., Worm, J. and Croce, C.: Genetics of type II glycogenosis: Assignment of the human gene for acid alpha-glucosidase to chromosome 17. Proc Natl Acad Sci USA, 76:4526-4529, 1979.

86. Solomon, E., Swallow, D., Burgess, S. and Evans, L.: Assignment of the human acid alpha-glucosidase gene (alpha-GLU) to chromosome 17 using somatic cell hybrids. Ann Hum Genet 42:273-281, 1979.

87. Weil, D., Cong, W.V., Gross, M.S. and Frezal, J.: Localisation du gene de l'alpha-glucosidase acide (GWa) sur le segment q21 q ter du chromosome 17 par l'hybridation cellulaire interspecifique. Hum Genet 52:249-257, 1979.

88. Beratis, N.G., LaBadie, G.V. and Hirschhorn, K.: Genetic heterogeneity in acid alpha-glucosidase deficiency. Am J Hum Genet 35:21-33, 1983.

89. Hers, H.G.: Alpha-glucosidase deficiency in generalized glycogen storage disease (Pompe's disease). Biochem J 86:11-16, 1963.

90. Pompe, J.C.: Over idiopatische hypertrophie von het hart. Ned T Geneesk 76:304-311, 1932.

91. Reuser, A.J.J. and Kroos, M.: Adult form of glycogenosis type II. A defect in an early stage of acid alpha-glucosidase realization. FEBS Lett 146:361, 1982.

92. Miranda, A.F., Peterson, E.R. and Masurovsky, E.B.: Developmentally-regulated isozymes in innervated human muscle culture. J Neuropath Exp Neurol 42:350, 1983.

93. Reuser, A.J.M., Koster, J.F., Hoogeveen and Galijaard, H.: Biochemical, immunological and cell genetic studies in glycogenosis type II. Am J Hum Genet 30:132-143, 1978.

94. Steckel, F., Gieselman, V., Waheed, A., Hasilik, A., von Figura, K., Elferink, R.O., Kalsbeek, R. and Tager, J.M.: Biosynthesis of acid alpha-glucosidase in late-onset forms of glycogenosis type II (Pompe's disease). FEBS Lett 150:69-76, 1982.

95. Mehler, M. and DiMauro, S.: Residual acid maltase activity in late-onset acid maltase deficiency. Neurol 27: 178-184, 1977.

96. Hays, A.P., Miranda, A.F., Mehler, M. and DiMauro, S.: Immunocytochemical studies of acid maltase in human fibroblast and muscle cultures. In Vitro 15:204, 1979.

97. DiMauro, S., Hartwig, G.B., Hays, A.P., Eastwood, A.B., Franco, R., Olarte, M., Chang, M., Roses, A.D., Fetell, R., Schoenfeldt, R.S. and Stern, L.Z.: Debrancher deficiency: neuromuscular disorder in 5 adults. Ann Neurol 5:422-436, 1979.

98. Illingsworth, B.: Glycogen storage disease. Am J Clin Nutr 9:683-690, 1961.

99. Justice, P., Ryan, C., Hsia, D.Y.Y. and Krmpotik, E.: Amylo-1, 6-glucosidase in human fibroblasts: Studies in type III glycogen storage disease. Biochem Biophys Res Commun 39:301-306, 1970.

100. Chen, S.H., Malcolm, L.A., Yoshida, A., Giblett, E.: Phosphoglycerate kinase: an X-linked polymorphism in man. Am J Human Genet 23:87-91, 1971.

101. Valentine, N.N., Hsieh, H.S., Paglia, D.E., Anderson, H.M., Banghan, M.A., Jaffe, E.R. and Garson, O.M.: Hereditary hemocytic anemia associated with phosphoglycerate kinase deficiency in erythrocytes and leukocytes. New Engl J Med 280:528-534.

102. Kitamura, M., Iijima, N., Hashimato, F. and Hirasuka, A.· Hereditary deficiency of subunit H of lactate dehydrogenase. Clin Chim Acta 34:419-423, 1971.

103. Sato, K., Satoh, K., Sato, T., Imai, F. and Morris, H.P. Isozyme patterns of glycogen phosphorylase in rat tissues and transplantable hepatomas. Cancer Res 36:487-495, 1976.

104. DiMauro, S., Arnold, S., Miranda, A.F. and Rowland, L.P.: McArdle disease: The mystery of reappearing phosphorylase activity in muscle culture: A fetal isozyme. Ann Neurol 3:60-66, 1978.

105. Proux, D. and Dreyfus, J-C.: Phosphorylase isoenzymes in tissues: Prevalence of the liver-type in man. Clin Chem Acta 48:167-172, 1973.

106. Sato, K., Imai, F., Hatayama, I. and Roelofs, R.I.: Characterization of glycogen phosphorylase isozymes present in cultured skeletal muscle from patients with McArdle disease. Biochem Biophys Acta 78:663-668, 1977.

107. Will, H., Krause, E.G., Bohm, M., Guski, H. and Wollenberger, A.: Kinetische Eigenschaften der Isoenzyme der Glycogen-phosphorylase b aus Herz-und Skelettmuskulatur des Menschen. Acta Biol Med Germ 33:149-160, 1974.

108. Davis, C.H., Schilselfeld, L.H., Wolf, D.P., Leavitt, C.A. and Krebs, E.G.: Interrelationships among glycogen phosphorylase isozymes. J Biol Chem 242:4824-4833, 1967.

109. Miranda, A.F., Nette, E.G., Hartlage, P.L. and DiMauro, S.: Phosphorylase isozymes in normal and myophosphorylase-deficient human heart. Neurol 29:1538-1541, 1979.

110. Bresolin, N., Miranda, A.F., Jacobson, M.P., Lee, J.H., Capilupi, T. and DiMauro, S.: Phosphorylase isozymes of human brain. Neurochem Path In press.

111. McArdle, B.: Myopathy due to a defect in muscle glycogen breakdown. Clin Sci 10:13-33, 1951.

112. Mommaerts, W.F.H.M., Illingsworth, B., Pearson, C.M., Guillory, R.J. and Seradarian, K.: A functional disorder of muscle associated with the absence of phosphorylase. Proc Natl Acad Sci USA, 45:791-797, 1959.

113. Schmid, R. and Mahler, R.: Chronic progressive myopathy with myoglobinuria: demonstration of a glycogenolytic defect in muscle. J Clin Invest 38:2044-2058, 1959.

114. Cornelio, F., Bresolin, N., DiMauro, S., Mora, M. and Balestrini, M.R.: Congential myopathy due to phosphorylase deficiency. Neurol 33:1383-1385, 1983.

115. DiMauro, S., and Hartlage, P.L.: Fatal infantile form of muscle phosphorylase deficiency. Neurol 28:1124-1129, 1978.

116. Schlisefeld, L.H.: Comparative studies of phosphorylase isozymes from rabbit. Ann NY Acad Sci USA, 210: 181-191, 1973.

117. Roelofs, R.I., Engel, W.K. and Chauvin, P.B.: Histochemical phosphorylase activity in regenerating muscle fibers from myophosphorylase-deficient patients. Science USA, 177:795-797, 1972.

118. Meienhofer, M.C., Askanas, V., Proux-Daegelen, D., J-C, and Engel, W.K.: Muscle-Type phosphorylase activity present in muscle cells cultured from three patients with myophosphorylase deficience. Arch Neurol 34: 779-781, 1977.

119. Miranda, A.F., Shanske, S., Hays, A.p. and DiMauro, S.: Immunocytochemical analysis of normal and acid maltase-deficient muscle cultures. Arch Neurol In press.

120. Davidson, M., Mongini, T., Foster, S.A., DiMauro, S. and Miranda, A.F.: Initiation of muscle-type phosphorylase (PPL) and phosphoglycerate mutase (PGAM) synthesis is not nerve-dependent. In Vitro 19:272, 1983.

121. Kahn, A., Cottreau, D. and Dreyfus, J-C.: Phosphofructokinase in human fetus. Pediatr Res 14:1162-1167, 1980.

122. Kahn, A., Meienhofer, M., Cottreau, D., Lagrange, J-L, and Dreyfus, J-C.: Phosphofructokinase (PFK) isozymes in man: studies of adult human tissues. Hum Genet 48:93-108, 1979.

123. Vora, S.: Isozymes of phosphofructokinase. In: Isozymes: Current Topics in Biological and Medical Research, Vol. 6, edited by M.C. Ratazzi, J.G. Scandalios and G.S. Whitt, pp. 119-167, Liss, New York, 1982.

124. Vora, S., Seaman, C., Durham, S. and Piomelli, S.: Isozymes of human phosphofructokinase: Identification and subunit structural characterization of a new system. Proc Natl Acad Sci USA, 77:62-66, 1980.

125. Weil, D., Cottreau, D., van Cong, N., Rebourcet, R., Foubert, C., Gross, M-S., Drefus, J-C. and Kahn, A.: Assignment of the gene for F-type phosphofructokinase to human chromosome 10 by somatic cell hybridization and specific immunoprecipitation. Ann Hum Genet 44:11-16, 1980.

126. Vora, S., Durham, S., deMartinville, B., George, D.L., Francke, U.: Assignment of the human gene for muscle phosphofructokinase (PFKM) to chromosome 1 (region cen q32) using somatic cell hybrids and monoclonal anti-M antibody. Somat Cell Genet 8:95-104, 1982.

127. Vora, S. and Francke, U.: Assignment of the human gene for liver-type 6-phosphofructokinase isozyme (PFKL) to chromosome 21 by using cell hybrids and monoclonal anti-L antibody. Proc Natl Acad Sci USA, 78:3738-3742, 1981.

128. Vora, S., Miranda, A.F., Hernandez, E. and Francke, U.: Regional assignment of the human gene of platelet-type phosphofructokinase (PFKP) to chromosome 10p: Novel use of polyspecific rodent antisera to localize human enzyme genes. Hum Genet 63:374-379, 1983.

129. Colling-Saltin, A.S.: Some quantitative biochemical evaluation of developing skeletal muscles in the human fetus. J Neurol Sci 39:187-198, 1971.

130. Davidson, M., Collins, M., Byrne, J. and Vora, S.: Alterations in phosphofructokinase isozymes during early human development. Biochem J 214:703-719, 1983.

131. Layzer, R.B., Rowland, L.P. and Ranney, H.M.: Muscle phosphofructokinase deficiency. Arch Neurol 17:512-523, 1967.

132. Tarui, S., Okuno, G., Ikura, Y., Tanaka, T., Suda, M. and Nishikawa, M.: Phosphofructokinase deficiency in skeletal muscle: A new type of glycogenosis. Biochem Biophys Res Commun 19:517-523, 1965.

133. Vora, S., Davidson, M., Seaman, C., Miranda, A.F., Noble, N.A., Tanaka, K.R., Frenkel, E.P. and DiMauro, S.: Heterogeneity of themolecular lesions in inherited phosphofructokinase deficiency. J Clin Invest 72:1995-2006, 1983.

134. Davidson, M., Miranda, A.F., Bender, A., DiMauro, S. and Vora, S.: Muscle phosphofructokinase deficiency. Biochemical and immunological studies of phosphofructokinase isozymes in muscle culture. J Clin Invest 72:545-550, 1983.

135. Omenn, G.S. and Hermodson, M.A.: Human phosphoglycerate mutase isozyme marker for muscle differentiation and for neoplasia. In: Isozymes III: Developmental Biology, edited by C.M. Markert, pp. 119-167, Academic Press, New York, 1975.

136. DiMauro, S., Miranda, A.F., Khan, S., Gitlin, K. and Friedman, R.: Human muscle phosphoglycerate mutase deficiency: newly discovered metabolic myopathy. Science 212:1277-1279, 1981.

137. DiMauro, S., Miranda, A.F., Olarte, M., Friedman, R. and Hays, A.P.: Muscle phosphoglycerate mutase deficiency. Neurol 32:484-591, 1982.

138. Boone, C.M., Chen, T.R. and Ruddle, F.H.: Assignment of LDH-A locus in man to chromosome C-11 using somatic cell hybrids. Proc Natl Acad Sci USA, 692:510-514, 1972.

139. Mayeda, K., Weiss, L., Lindahl, R. and Dully, M.: Localization of the human lactate dehydrogenase B gene on the short arm of chromosome 12. Am J Hum Genet 26:58-64, 1974.

140. Kanno, T., Suda, K., Takeuchi, I., Kanda, S., Honda, N., Nishimura, Y. and Oyama, K.: Hereditary deficiency of lactate dehydrogenase M-subunit. Clin Chim Acta 108:267-276, 1980.

141. Nishimura, Y., Honda, N., Ohyama, K., Ichiyama, A., Yanagisawa, M., Sudo, K. and Kanno, T.: Lactate dehydrogenase A subunit deficiency. In: Isozymes: Current Topics in Biological and Medical Research. Vol. 11 Medical and other applications, edited by M. Ratazzi, J.G. Scandalios and G.S. Whit, pp. 51-64, Alan R. Liss, Inc., New York, 1983.

142. Haselik, A.A., Waheed, A., von Figura, K.: Enzymatic phosphorylation of lysosomal enzymes in the presence of UDP-N-acetylglucosamine. Absence of the activity in I-cell fibroblasts. Biochem Biophys Res Commun 98:761-767, 1981.

143. Leroy, J.G., Ho, M.W., McBrinn, M.C., Zielke, K., Jacob, J., O'Brien, J.S.: I-Cell diseases: biochemical studies. Pediat Res 6:752-757, 1972.

144. Mauro, A.: Satellite cells of skeletal muscle fibers. J Biophys Biochem Cytol 9:493-495, 1961.

145. Strohman, R.C., Micou-Eastwood, J., Glass, C.A. and Matsuda, R.: Human fetal muscle and cultured myotubes derived from it contain a fetal-specific myosin light chain. Science 221:955-957, 1983.

146. Miranda, A.F., Peterson, E.R., and Masurovsky, E.B.: Developmentally-regulated isozymes in innervated human muscle culture. J Neuropath Exp Neurol 42:350, 1983.

147. Peterson, E.R.: Tissue Culture Association Manuel, Vol. 4, edited by V.J. Evans, V.P. Perry, and M.M. Vincent, pp. 921-923. Tissue Culture Assoc., Inc., Rockville, MD, 1978.

148. Peterson, E.R., and Crain, S.M.: Maturation of human muscle after innervation by fetal mouse spinal cord explants. In: Muscle Regeneration, edited by A. Mauro, pp. 429-441, Raven Press, New York, 1979.

149. Ecob, M.S., Butler-Browne, G.S. and Whalen, R.G.: The adult fast isozyme of myosin is present in a nerve-muscle tissue culture system. Different 25:84-87, 1983.

150. Strohman, R.C., Bandman, E., Walker, C.R., Spector, D.: Regulation of myosin accumulation by muscle activity in cell culture. J Muscle Res Cell Motil 2:269-282, 1981.

151. Sherman, S.J. and Catteral, W.A.: Electrical activity and cytosolic calcium regulate levels of tetrodotoxin-sensitive sodium channels in cultured rat muscle cells. Proc Natl Acad Sci USA, 81:262-266, 1984.

152. Shimada, Y., Fischman, D.A. and Moscona, A.: Formation of neuromuscular junctions in embryonic cell cultures. Proc Natl Acad Sci USA, 715-721, 1969.

153. Fitzsimons, R.B., and Hoh, J.F.Y.: Embryonic and fetal myosins in human skeletal muscle. The presence of fetal myosins in Duchenne muscular dystrophy and infantile spinal muscular atrophy. J Neurol Sci 52:367-384, 1981a.

154. Fitzsimons, R.B. and Hoh, J.F.Y.: Myosin isoenzymes in fast-twitch and slow-twitch muscles of normal and dystrophic mice. J Physiol 343:539-550, 1983.

155. Close, R.: Force:velocity properties of mouse muscles. Nature (Lond.) 206:718-719, 1965.

156. Douglas, W.B., Jr. and Baskin, R.J.: Contractile properties of developing mouse dystrophic muscle. Am J Physiol 220(5):1344-1354, 1971.

157. Luff, A.R.: Dynamic properties of the interior rectus, extensor digitorum longus, diaphragm and soleus muscles of the mouse. J Physiol 313:161-171, 1981.

158. Hoh, J.F.Y., Kwan, B.T.S., Dunlop, C. and Kim, B.H.: Effects of nerve cross-union and cordotomy on myosin isoenzymes in fast-twitch and slow-twitch muscles of the rat. In: Plasticity of Muscle, Pette, D., editor, Walter de Gruyter & Co., Berlin-New York, 339-352, 1980.

159. Close, R.: Properties of motor units of fast and slow skeletal muscles of the rat. J Physiol 193:45-55, 1967.

160. Kugelberg, E.: Histochemical composition, contraction speed and fatiguability of rat soleus motor units. J Neurol Sci 20:177-198, 1973.

161. Lewis, D.M., Parry, D.J. and Rowlerson, A.: Isometric contractions of motor units and immunohistochemistry of mouse soleus muscle. J Physiol 325:393-401, 1982.

162. Endo, M., Kitazawa, T., Yagi, S., Iino, M., Kakuta, Y. and Horiuti, K.: Functional changes in skeletal muscle of the dystrophic mouse and chicken. In: Muscular Dystrophy: Biomedical Aspects. Ebashi, S. and Ozawa, E., editors, Japan Scientific Societies Press, Tokyo and Springer-Verlag, Berlin, 185-192, 1983.

163. Sandow, A. and Brust, M.: Contractility of dystrophic mouse muscle. Am J Physiol 194:557-563, 1958.

164. Brust, M.: Relative resistance to dystrophy of slow skeletal muscle of the mouse. Am J Physiol 210:445-451, 1966.

165. Harris, J.B. and Wilson, P.: Mechanical properties of dystrophic mouse muscle. J Neurol Neurosurg Psychiat 34:512-520, 1971.

166. Parry, D.J. and Parslow, H.G.: Fiber type susceptibility in the dystrophic mouse. Exp Neurol 73:674-685, 1981.

167. Parry, D.J. and Desypris, G.: Slowing of twitch of dystrophic mouse muscle is partially due to altered activity pattern. Muscle & Nerve 6:397-407, 1983.

168. Martonosi, A.: Sarcoplasmic reticulum. IV. Microsomal Ca^{++} transport in genetic muscular dystrophy of mice. Proc Soc Exp Biol Med 127:824-828, 1968.

169. Mrak, R.E. and Fleischer, S.: Normal function in sarcoplasmic reticulum from mice with muscular dystrophy. Muscle & Nerve 5:143-151, 1982.

170. Fitzsimons, R.B. and Hoh, J.F.Y.: Isomyosins in human type 1 and type 2 skeletal muscle fibers. Biochem J 193:229-233, 1981b.

171. Brooke, M.M. and Kaiser, K.K.: Three "Myosin Adenosine Triphosphatase" systems: The nature of their pH lability and sulfhydryl dependence. J Histochem Cytochem 18: 670-672, 1970.

172. McDonald, B.L., Dawkins, R.L. and Robinson, J.: Myosin autoantibodies reacting with selective muscle fiber types. Muscle & Nerve 2:37-43, 1979.

173. Dalla Libera, L., Sartore, S., Pierobon-Bormioli, S. and Schiaffino, S.: Fast-white and fast-red isomyosins in guinea pig muscles. Biochem Biophys Res Commun 96:1662-1670, 1980.

174. Pierbon-Bormioli, S., Sartore, S., Libera, L.D., Vitadello, M. and Schiaffino, S.: "Fast" isomyosins and fiber types in mammalian skeletal muscle. J Histochem Cytochem 29:1179-1188, 1981.

175. Whalen, R.G., Sell, S.M., Butler-Browne, G.S., Schwartz, K., Bouveret, P. and Pinse-Harstrom, I.: Three myosin heavy chain isozymes appear sequentially in rat muscle development. Nature 292:805-809, 1981.

176. Hoh, J.F.Y. and Yeoh, G.P.S.: Rabbit skeletal myosin isoenzymes from fetal, fast-twitch and slow-twitch muscles. Nature 280:321-323, 1979.

177. Nonaka, I., Takagi, A. and Sugita, H.: The significance of type 2C muscle fibers in Duchenne Muscular Dystrophy. Muscle & Nerve 6:397-407, 1983.

178. Brooke, M.H., Williamson, E., Kaiser, K.K.: The behavior of 4 fiber types in developing and reinnervated muscle. Arch Neurol 25:360-366, 1971.

179. Nonaka, I. and Chou, S.M.: Histochemical study on muscle in Werdnig-Hoffman disease. Clin Neurol (Tokyo) 18:491-498, 1978.

180. Jansson, E. and Kaijser, L.: Muscle adaptation to extreme endurance training in man. Acta Physiol Scand 100:315-324, 1977.

181. Jansson, E., Sjodin, B. and Tesch, P.: Changes in muscle fiber type distribution in man after physical training. Acta Physiol Scand 104:235-237, 1978.

182. Billeter, R., Weber, H., Lutz, H., Howland, H., Eppenberger, H.M. and Jenny, E.: Myosin types in human skeletal muscle fibers. Histochem 65:249-259, 1980.

183. Mastaglia, F.L. and Kakulas, B.A.: Regeneration in Duchenne Muscular Dystrophy - a histological and histochemical study. Brain 92:809-818, 1969.

184. Mastaglia, F.L., Papadimitriou, J.M. and Kakulas, B.A.: Regeneration of muscle in Duchenne Muscular Dystrophy - an electron microscope study. J Neurol Sci 11:425-444, 1970.

185. Marechel, G., Schwartz, K., Beckers-Bleukx, G. and Ghins, E.: Isozymes of myosin in growing and regenerating rat muscles. Eur J Biochem 138:421-428, 1984.

186. Sartore, S., Gorza, L. and Schiaffino, S.: Fetal myosin heavy chains in regenerating muscle. Nature 298:294-296, 1982.

187. Carraro, U., Dalla Libera, L. and Catani, C.: Myosin light and heavy chains in muscle regenerating in absence of the nerve: Transient appearance of the embryonic light chain. Exp Neurol 79:106-117, 1983.

188. Roe, R.D., Yamaji, K. and Sandow, A.: Contractile responses of dystrophic muscles of mouse and man. In: "Exploratory Concepts in Muscular Dystrophy and Related Disorders." A.T. Milhorat, editor, Excerpta Medica Amsterdam, pp. 299-304, 1967.

189. McComas, A.J. and Thomas, H.C.: Fast and slow twitch muscles in man. J Neurol Sci 7:301-307, 1968.

190. Buchthal, F., Schmalbruch, H. and Kamieniecka: Contraction times and fiber types in neurogenic paresis. Neurol (Minneap.) 21:58-67, 1971.

191. McComas, A.J., Sica, R.E.P. and Currie, S.: An electrophysiological study of Duchenne Dystrophy. J Neurol Neurosurg Psychiat 24:469-474, 1971.

192. Jolesz, F. and Sreter, F.A.: Development, innervation and activity-pattern induced changes in skeletal muscle. Ann Rev Physiol 43:531-52, 1981.

193. Salmons, S. and Henriksson, J.: The adaptive response of skeletal muscle to increased use. Muscle & Nerve 4:94-105, 1981.

194. Sreter, F.A., Pinter, K., Jolesz, F. and Mabuchi, K.: Fast to slow transformation of fast muscles in response to long-term phasic stimulation. Exp Neurol 75:95-102, 1982.

195. Brown, W.E., Salmons, S. and Whalen, R.G.: The sequential replacement of myosin subunit isoforms during muscle type transformation induced by long term electrical stimulation. J Biol Chem 258:14686-14692, 1983.

196. Mabuchi, K., Szvetko, D., Pinter, K. and Sreter, F.A.: Type IIB to type IIA fiber transformation in intermittently stimulated rabbit muscles. Am J Physiol 242:373-381, 1982.

197. Anderson, P. and Henriksson, J.: Training induced changes in the subgroups of human type II skeletal muscle fibers. Acta Physiol 99:123-125, 1977.

198. Hoh, J.F.Y. and Chow, C.J.: The effect of the loss of weight-bearing function on the isomyosin profile and contractile properties of rat skeletal muscles. In "Molecular Pathology of Muscles and Nerves." Kidman, A.D., Tomkins, J.K., Cooper, N.A. and Morris, C., editors, Humana Press, New Jersey, pp. 371-384, 1983.

199. Kugelberg, E.: Adaptive transformation of rat soleus motor units during growth. Histochemistry and contraction speed. J Neurol Sci 27:269-289, 1976.

200. Martin, W.D. and Ormond, E.H.: Effects of chronic rotation and hyperactivity on muscle fibers of soleus and plantaris muscles of the rat. Exp Neurol 49:758-771, 1975.

201. Iannuzzo, C.D., Gollnick, P.D. and Armstrong, R.B.: Compensatory adaptations of skeletal muscle fiber types to a long-term functional overload. Life Sci 19:1517-1524, 1976.

202. Fardeau, M., Godet-Guillain, J., Tome, F.M.S., Carson, S. and Whalen, R.G.: Congenital neuromuscular disorders: a critical review. In "Current Topics in Nerve and Muscle Research." Aguayo, A.J. and Karpati, G., editors, Excerpta Medica, Amsterdam, pp. 164-177, 1979.

203. Volpe, P., Damiani, E., Margreth, A., Pelligrini, G. and Scarlato, G.: Fast to slow change of myosin in nemaline myopathy: electrophreitc and immunologic evidence. J Neurol Sci 47:463-72, 1980.

204. Essen, B., Fohlin, L., Thoren, C. and Saltin, B.: Skeletal muscle fiber types and sizes in anorexia nervosa patients. Clin Physiol 1:395-403, 1981.

205. Silverman, H. and Atwood, H.L.: Increase in oxidative capacity of muscle fibers in dystrophic mice and correlation with overactivity in these fibers. Exp Neurol 68:97-113, 1980.

206. Parslow, H.G. and Parry, D.J.: Slowing of fast-twitch muscle in the dystrophic mouse. Exp Neurol 73: 674-685, 1981.

207. Fidzianska, A.: Ultrastructural changes in muscle in spinal muscular atrophy - Werdnig-Hoffmann's disease. Acta Neuropath (Berl.) 27:247-256, 1974.

208. Fidzianska, A.: Morphological differences between the atrophied small muscle fibers in amyotrophic lateral sclerosis and Werdnig-Hoffmann disease. Acta Neuropath (Berl.) 34:321-327, 1976.

209. Tsukagoshi, H., Yanagisawa, N. and Oguchi, K.: Morphometric quantification of the cervical limb motor cells in various neuromuscular diseases. J Neurol Sci 47:463-472, 1980.

210. Kumagai, T. and Hashizume, Y.: Morphological and morphometric studies of the spinal cord lesion in Werdnig-Hoffmann disease. Brain & Dev 4:87-96, 1982.

211. Whalen, R.G., Schwartz, K., Bouveret, P., Sell, S.M. and Gros, F.: Contractile protein isozymes in muscle development: Identification of an embryonic form of myosin heavy chain. Proc Natl Acad Sci (USA) 76:5197-5201, 1979.

212. Ecob, M., Brown, A., Bryers, P., Butler-Browne, G., Young, C. and Whalen, R.G.: Regeneration and differentiation of adult mammalian muscle in a nerve-muscle culture system. Expl Biol Med 9:93-101, 1984.

213. Fitzsimons, R.B. and Hoh, J.F.Y.: Fetal myosins in skeletal muscle from a patient with myalgia and fatigue. Lancet, February, 480-483, 1982.

214. Butler-Browne, G.S., Bugaisky, L.B., Cuenoud, S., Schwartz, K. and Whalen, R.G.: Denervation of newborn rat muscles does not block the appearance of adult fast myosin heavy chain. Nature 299:830-833, 1982.

215. Ashmore, C.R. and Doerr, L.: Oxidative metabolism in skeletal muscle of normal and dystrophic chicks. Biochem Med 4:246-259, 1970.

216. Ashmore, C.R. and Doerr, L.: Postnatal development of muscle fiber types in normal and dystrophic skeletal muscle of the chick. Exp Neurol 30:431-446, 1971.

217. Asmundson, V.S. and Julian, L.M.: Inherited muscle abnormality in the domestic fowl. J Hered 47:248-252, 1956.

218. Peterson, D.W., Hamilton, W.H. and Lillyblade, A.L.: Composition of hypertrophic and atrophic muscle in genetic muscular dystrophy of the chicken. Proc Soc Exp Biol Med 127:300-305, 1968.

219. Cosmos, E. and Butler, J.: Differentiation of fiber types in muscle of normal and dystrophic chickens. A quantitative and histochemical study of the ontogeny of muscle enzymes. In: "Exploratory Concepts in Muscular Dystrophy and Related Disorders," Milhorat, A.T. ed. Excerpta Medica, Amsterdam, pp. 197-204, 1967.

220. Wilson, B.W., Randall, W.R., Patterson, G.T. and Entrikin, R.K.: Major physiological and histochemical characteristics of inherited dystrophy of the chicken. Ann NY Acad Sci 317:224-246, 1974.

221. Koenig, J. and Fardeau, M.: Etude histochimique des muscle grands dorsaux l'anterieur et posterieur du poulet et des modifications observees apres denervation et reinnervation homologue ou croisee. Arch Anat Micr Morphoog Exp 62:249-267, 1973.

222. Toutant, T.J., Toutant, M.N., Renaud, D. and LeDouarin, G.H.: Enzymatic differentiation of muscle fiber types in embryonic latissimus dorsi of the chick: Effects of spinal cord stimulation. Cell Diff 8:375-382, 1979.

223. Bandman, E.: Myosin component of the latissimus dorsi and the pectoralis major in the dystrophic chicken. Muscle and Nerve. In press.

224. Moss, F.P. and Leblond, C.P.: Satellite cells as the source of nuclei in muscles of growing rats. Anat Rec 170: 421-436, 1971.

225. Snow, M.H.: Myogenic cell formation in regenerating rat skeletal muscle injured by mincing II - An autoradiographic study. Anat Rec 188:201-218, 1977.

226. Snow, M.H.: An autoradiographic study of satellite cell differentiation into regenerating myotubes following transplantation of muscles in young rats. Cell Tiss Res 186:535-540, 1978.

227. Allbrook, D.B., Han, M.F., Hellmuth, A.E.: Population of muscle satellite cells in relation to age and mitotic activity. Pathol 3:233-243, 1971.

228. Aloisi, M., Mussini, I. and Schiaffino, S.: Activation of muscle nuclei in denervation and hypertrophy. In: Basic Research in Myology. B.A. Kaklulas, ed. Exerpta Medica Amsterdam, pp. 338-342, 1973.

229. Cardasis, C.A., Cooper, G.W.: An analysis of nuclear numbers in individual muscle fibers during differentiation and growth: a satellite cell-muscle fiber growth unit. J Exp Zool 191:347-357.

230. Kelly, A.M.: Satellite cells and myofiber growth in the rat soleus and extensor digitorum longus muscles. Dev Biol 61:1-10, 1978.

231. Schmalbruch, H. and Hellhammer, U.: The number of nuclei in adult rat muscles with special reference to satellite cells. Anat Rec 189:169-176, 1977.

232. Schultz, E.: A quantitative study of the satellite cell population in postnatal mouse lumbrical muscle. Anat Rec 180:589-595, 1974.

233. Snow, M.H.: Satellite cell distribution within the soleus muscles of the adult mouse. Anat Rec 201:463-469, 1981.

234. Wakayama, Y., Schotland, D., Bonilla, E. and Orecchio, E.: Quantitative ultrastructural study of muscle satellite cells in Duchenne dystrophy. Neurol 29:401-407, 1979.

235. Korneliussen, H.: Identification of muscle fiber types in "semi-thin" sections stained with p-phenylene-diamine. Histochemie 32:95-98, 1972.

236. Hansen-Smith, F.M. and Carlson, B.M.: Cellular responses to free grafting of the extensor digitorum longus muscle of the rat. J Neurol Sci 41:149-173, 1979.

237. Summers, P. and Parsons, R.: An electron microscopic study of satellite cells and regeneration in dystrophic mouse muscle. Neuropathol Appl Neurobiol 7:257-268, 1981.

238. Benoit, P.W. and Belt, W.D.: Destruction and regeneration of skeletal muscle after treatment with a local anesthetic, bupvacaine (Marcaine). J Anat 107:547-556, 1970.

239. Epstein, H.F. and Wolf, S. eds: Genetic Analysis of the X Chromosome. Plenum Press, New York, 1982.

240. Appel, S.H. and Roses, A.D.: The muscular dystrophies. In: The Metabolic Basis of Inherited Disease. Stanbury, J.B., Wyngaarden, J.B. and Frederickson, D.S., editors, McGraw-Hill Co., New York, 1260-1281, 1978.

241. Hauschka, S.D.: Clonal analysis of vertebrate myogenesis. II. Environmental influences upon human muscle differentiation. Dev Biol 37:329-344, 1974a.

242. Hauschka, S.D.: Clonal analysis of vertebrate myogenesis. III. Developmental changes in the muscle-colony-forming cells of the human fetal limb. Dev Biol 37:345-368, 1974b.

243. Golbus, M.S., Stephens, J.D., Mahoney, M.J., Hobbins, J.C., Haseltine, F.P., Caskey, C.T. and Banker, B.Q.: Failure of fetal creatine phosphokinase as a diagnostic indicator of Duchenne muscular dystrophy. N Eng J Med 300:860-861, 1979.

244. Blau, H.M. and Webster, C.: Isolation and characterization of human muscle cells. Proc Natl Acad Sci USA 78: 5623-5627, 1981.

245. Paterson, B. and Strohman, R.C.: Myosin synthesis in cultures of differentiating chicken embryo skeletal muscle. Dev Biol 29:113-138, 1972.

246. Yaffe, D.: Rat skeletal muscle cells. In: Tissue Culture Methods and Applications. Kruse, P.F., Jr. and Patterson, M.K., Jr., editors. Academic Press, New York, 106-114, 1973.

247. Yaffe, D. and Saxel, O.: A myogenic cell line with altered serum requirements for differentiation. Differentiation 7:159-166, 1977.

248. Blau, H.M., Webster, C., Chiu, C.-P., Guttman, S., Adornato, B. and Chandler, F.: Isolation and characterization of pure populations of normal and dystrophic human muscle cells. In: Muscle Development: Molecular and Cellular Control, Cold Spring Harbor Laboratory, New York, 543-556, 1982.

249. Blau, H.M., Webster, C., Chiu, C.-P., Guttman, S. and Chandler, F.: Differentiation properties of pure populations of human dystrophic muscle cells. Exp Cell Res 144:495-503, 1983b.

250. Franklin, G.I., Cavanagh, N.P.C., Hughes, B.P., Yasin, R. and Thompson, E.J.: Creatine kinase isoenzymes in cultured human muscle cells. I. Comparison of Duchenne muscular dystrophy with other myopathic and neurogenic diseases. Clinica Chemica Acta 115:179-189, 1981.

251. Cavanagh, N.P.C., Franklin, G.I., Hughes, B.P., Yasin, R., Phillips, E., van Beers, G. and Thompson, E.G.: Creatine kinase isoenzymes in cultured human muscle cell. II. A study of carrier females for Duchenne muscular dystrophy by needle and open biopsy. Clinica Chimica Acta 115:191-198, 1981.

252. O'Farrell, P.H.: High resolution two-dimensional electrophoresis of proteins. J Biol Chem 250:4007-4021, 1975.

253. Ionasescu, V., Ionasescu, R., Feld, R., Witte, D., Cancilla, P., Kaeding, L. and Stern, L.Z.: Alterations in creatine kinase in fresh muscle and cell cultures in Duchenne dystrophy. Annals of Neurol 9:394-399, 1981.

254. Thompson, E.J., Yasin, R., van Beers, G., Nurse, K. and Al-Ani, S.: Myogenic defect in human muscular dystrophy. Nature 268:241-243, 1977.

255. Blau, H.M., Webster, C. and Pavlath, G.K.: Defective myoblasts identified in Duchenne muscular dystrophy. Proc Natl Acad Sci USA 80:4856-4860, 1983a.

256. Thompson, E.J.: Tissue culture of dystrophic muscle cells. Brit Med Bull 36:181-185, 1980.

257. Walsh, F.S. and Ritter, M.A.: Surface antigen differentiation during human myogenesis in culture. Nature 289:60-64, 1981.

258. Brooke, M.H. and Engel, W.K.: The histographic analysis of human muscle biopsies with regard to fiber types. 4. Children's Biopsies. Neurol 19:591-605, 1969.

259. Cardasis, C.A.: Isolated single mammalian muscle fibers aid in the study of satellite cell and myonuclear populations. In: Muscle Regeneration Alex Mauro, editor, Raven press, New York, 155-166, 1979.

260. Kelly, A.M.: Variations in satellite cell distribution in developing and mature muscles of the rat. In: Muscle Regeneration Alex Mauro, editor, Raven Press, New York, 167-176, 1979.

261. Wakayama, Y. and Schotland, D.L.: Muscle satellite cell populations in Duchenne dystrophy. In: Muscle Regeneration Alex Mauro, editor, Raven Press, New York, 121-129, 1979.

262. Stockdale, F.E. and Holtzer, H.: DNA synthesis and myogenesis. Exp Cell Res 24:508-520, 1961.

263. Hauschka, S.D.: Cultivation of muscle tissue. In: Growth, Nutrition, and Metabolism of Cells in Culture G.H. Rothblat and V.J. Cristofalo, editors. Vol. 2, 67-130, Academic Press, New York, 1972.

264. Hauschka, S.D.: Clonal analysis of vertebrate myogenesis. II. Environmental influences upon human muscle differentiation. Develop Biol 37:329-344, 1974.

265. Hauschka, S.D. and Konigsberg, I.R.: The influence of collagen on the development of muscle colonies. Proc Nat Acad Sci USA 55:119-126, 1966.

266. Yaffe, D.: Cellular aspects of muscle differentiation in vitro. In: Current Topics in Developmental Biology 4:37-77, 1969.

267. Ozawa, E. and Hagiwara, Y.: Avian and mammalian transferrins are required for chick and rat myogenic cell growth in vitro, respectively. Proc Japan Acad 57,B:406-409, 1981.

268. Hagawara, Y. and Ozawa, E.: Class specificity of avian and mammalian sera in regards to myogenic cell growth in vitro: Possible role of transferrin in the specificity. Develop Growth & Differen 24:115-123, 1982.

269. Ii, I., Kimura, I. and Ozawa, E.: A myotrophic protein from chick embryo extract: Its purification, identity to transferrin and indispensibility for avian myogenesis. Develop Biol 94:366-377, 1982.

270. Florini, J.R. and Roberts, S.B.: A serum-free medium for the growth of muscle cells in culture. In Vitro 15:983-992, 1979.

271. Ewton, D.Z. and Florini, J.R.: Relative effects of the somatomedins, MSA, and growth hormone on myoblasts and myotubes in culture. Endocrin 106:577-583, 1980.

272. Ewton, D.Z. and Florini, J.R.: Effects of the somatomedins on myoblast differentiation in vitro. Develop Biol 86:31-39, 1981.

273. Linkhart, T.A., Lim, R. and Hauschka, S.D.: Regulation of normal and variant mouse myoblast proliferation and differentiation by specific growth factors. C.S.H. Conference on Cell Proliferation. Vol. 9 "Growth of Cells in Hormonally Defined Media" 867-876, 1982.

274. Hauschka, S.D.: Developmental analysis of vertebrate myogenesis. III. Developmental changes in the muscle-colony-forming cells of the human fetal limb. Develop Biol 37:345-368, 1974.

275. Rutz, R. and Hauschka, S.D.: Clonal analysis of vertebrate myogenesis. VII. Heritability of muscle colony type through sequential subclonal passages in vitro. Develop Biol 91:103-110, 1982.

276. Hauschka, S.D., Rutz, R. and Haney, C.: Regional distribution and cell lineage states of myogenic cells during early stages of vertebrate limb development. In: Muscle Development: Molecular and Cellular Control. CSHL Press, New York, 367-376, 1982.

277. Ozawa, E. and Kohawa, K.: Muscle trophic factor: I. Assay of a muscle trophic factor by measurement of muscle cell nuclei. Muscle & Nerve 1:230-235, 1978.

278. Kohama, K. and Ozawa, E.: Muscle trophic factor: II. Ontogenic development of activity of a muscle trophic factor in chicken serum. Muscle & Nerve 1:236-241, 1978.

279. Markelonis, G.J., Kemerer, V.F. and Oh, T.H.: Sciatin: purification and characterization of a myotrophic protein from chicken sciatic nerves. J Biol Chem 255:8967-8970, 1980.

280. Popiela, H. and Ellis, S.: Neurotrophic factor: Characterization and partial purification. Develop Biol 83:266-277, 1981.

281. Saito, K., Hagiwara, Y., Hasegawa, T. and Ozawa, E.: Indispensability of iron for the growth of cultured chick cells. Develop Growth & Differ 24:571-580, 1982.

282. King, G.L., Kahn, C.R., Rechler, M.M. and Nissley, S.P.: Direct demonstration of separate receptors for growth and metabolic activities of insulin and multiplication-stimulating activity (an insulin-like growth factor) using antibodies to the insulin receptor. J Clin Invest 66:130-140, 1980.

283. McKeehan, W.L., Hamilton, W.G. and Ham, R.G.: Selenium is an essential trace nutrient for the growth of W1-38 diploid human fibroblasts. Proc Natl Acad Sci USA 53:288-293, 1976.

284. Ham, R.G. and McKeehan, W.L.: Development of improved media and culture conditions for clonal growth of normal diploid cells. In Vitro 14:11-22, 1978.

285. Ball, E.H. and Sanwall, B.D.: Synergistic effect of glucocorticoids and insulin on the differentiation of myoblasts. J Cell Physiol 102:27-36, 1980.

286. Emerson, C.P., Jr.: Control of myosin synthesis during myoblast differentiation. In: Pathogenesis of Human Muscular Dystrophy. L.P. Rowland, editor. Excerpto Media Press, Amsterdam, 799-809, 1977.

287. Chiquet, M., Puri, E.C. and Turner, D.C.: Fibronectin mediates attachment of chicken myoblasts to a gelatin-coated substratum. J Biol Chem 254:5475-5482, 1977.

288. Turner, D.C., Lawton, J., Dollenmeier, P., Ehrismann, R. and Chiquet, M.: Guidance of myogenic cell migration by oriented deposits of fibronectin. Develop Biol 95:497-504, 1983.

289. Peterson, E.R. and Crain, S.M.: Maturation of human muscle after innervation by fetal mouse spinal cord explants in long-term cultures. In: Muscle Regeneration. A. Mauro, editor. Raven Press, New York, 429-441, 1979.

290. Ecob, M.S.: The application of organotypic nerve cultures to problems in neurology with special reference to their potential use in research into neuromuscular diseases. J Neurol Sci 58:1-15, 1983.

291. Hayashi, I. and Kobylecki, J.: Growth of myoblasts in hormone-supplemented serum-free medium. In: C.S.H. Conference on Cell Proliferation. Vol. 9, Growth of Cells in Hormonally Defined Media, 857-865, 1982.

292. Dollenmeier, P., Turner, D.C. and Eppenberger, H.M.: Proliferation and differentiation of chick skeletal muscle cells cultured in a chemically defined medium. Exp Cell Res 135:47-61, 1981.

293. Hauschka, S.D., Linkhart, T.A., Clegg, C. and Merrill, G.: Clonal studies of mouse and human muscle. In: Muscle Regeneration. A. Mauro, editor. Raven Press, New York, 311-322, 1978.

294. Linkhart, T.A., Clegg, C.H. and Hauschka, S.D.: Myogenic differentiation in permanent clonal mouse myoblast cell lines: regulation by macromolecular growth factors in the culture medium. Develop Biol 86:19-30, 1981.

295. Linkhart, T.A., Clegg, C.H. and Hauschka, S.D.: Control of mouse myoblast commitment to terminal differentiation by mitogens. J Supramolec Struct 14:483-498, 1980.

296. Chamberlain, J., Jaynes, J. and Hauschka, S.D.: Manuscript in preparation, 1984.

297. Linkhart, T.A., Clegg, C.H., Lim, R., Merrill, G., Chamberlain, H. and Hauschka, S.D.: Control of mouse myoblast commitment to terminal differentiation by mitogens. In: Muscle Development: Molecular and Cellular Control. CSHL Press, New York, 366-374, 1982.

298. Bulinski, J.C., Kumar, S., Titani, K. and Hauschka, S.D.: Peptide antibody specific for the amino terminus of skeletal muscle α-actin. Proc Nat Acad Sci USA 80: 1506-1510, 1983.

299. Lim, R.W. and Hauschka, S.D.: EGF responsiveness and receptor regulation in normal and differentiation-defective mouse myoblasts. Develop Biol In press.

300. Merrill, G.F., Witter, E.F. and Hauschka, S.D.: Differentiation of thymidine kinase deficient mouse myoblasts in the presence of 5'-bromodeoxyuridine. Exp Cell Res 129:191-199, 1980.

301. Lim, R.W. and Hauschka, S.D.: A rapid decrease in epidermal growth-factor binding capacity accompanies the terminal differentiation of mouse myoblasts in vitro. J Cell Biol 98:739-747, 1984.

302. Konigsberg, I.R.: Diffusion-mediated control of myoblast fusion. Develop Biol 26:133-152, 1971.

303. O'Neill, M.C. and Stockdale, F.E.: A kinetic analysis of myogenesis in vitro. J Cell Biol 52:52-56, 1972.

304. Yaffe, D.: Developmental changes preceding cell fusion during muscle differentiation. Exp Cell Res 66: 33-48, 1971.

305. Nadal-Ginard, B.: Commitment, fusion and biochemical differentiation of a myogenic cell line in the absence of DNA synthesis. Cell 15:855-864, 1978.

306. Bayne, E.K. and Simpson, S.B.: Influence of environmental factors on the accumulation and differentiation of prefusion G1 lizard myoblasts in vitro. Exp Cell Res 126:15-30, 1980.

307. Devlin, B.H. and Konigsberg, I.R.: Reentry into the cell cycle of differentiated skeletal myocytes. Develop Biol 95:175-192, 1983.

308. Nguyen, H.T., Medford, R.M. and Nadal-Ginard, B.: Reversibility of muscle differentiation in the absence of commitment: Analysis of myogenic cell line temperature-sensitive for commitment. Cell 34:281-293, 1983.

309. Merrifield, P.A., Compton, R.S. and Konigsberg, I.R.: Cell cycle dependence of differentiation in synchronous skeletal muscle myocytes. In: Molecular Aspects of Myogenesis and Myogivrillogenesis in Cell Culture: Normal and Diseased Muscle. H.M. Eppenberger and J.C. Perriard, editors. S. Karger Press, New York, In press, 1984.

310. Quinn, L.S. and Nemeroff, M.: Analysis of the myogenic lineage in chick embryos. III. Quantitative evidence for discrete compartments of precursor cells. Differentiation 24:111-123, 1983.

311. Carrel, A.: Artificial activation of the growth in vitro of connective tissue. J Exptl Med 17:14-19, 1913.

312. Ozawa, E., Kimura, I., Hasegawa, T., Ii, I., Saito, K., Hagiwara, Y. and Shimo-Oka, T.: Iron-bound transferrin as a myotrophic factor. In: Muscular Dystrophy: Biomedical Aspects (Egashi, S. and Ozawa, E. eds.), pp. 53-60, Japan Sci Soc Press, Tokyo/Springer-Verlag, Berlin, 1983.

313. Ozawa, E. and Kohama, K.: Partial purification of a factor promoting chicken myoblast multiplication in vitro. Proc Japan Acad 49:852-856, 1973.

314. Hagiwara, Y., Kimura, I. and Ozawa, E.: Chick embryo extract, muscle trophic factor and horse sera as environments for chick myogenic cell growth. Devel Growth and Differ 23:249-254, 1981.

315. Kimura, I., Hasegawa, T., Miura, T. and Ozawa, E.: Muscle trophic factor is identical to transferrin. Proc Japan Acad 57B:200-205, 1981.

316. Kimura, I., Hasegawa, T. and Ozawa, E.: Indispensability of iron-bound chick transferrin for chick myogenesis in vitro. Devel Growth and Differ 24:369-380, 1982.

317. Ii, I., Kimura, I. and Ozawa, E.: A myotrophic protein from chick embryo extract: Its purification, identity to transferrin, and indispensability for avian myogenesis. Devel Biol 94:366-377, 1982.

318. Hasegawa, T., Saito, K., Kimura, T. and Ozawa, E.: Fe^{3+} promotes in vitro growth of myoblasts and other cells from chick embryos. Proc Japan Acad 57B:206-210, 1981.

319. Saito, K., Hagiwara, Y., Hasegawa, T. and Ozawa, E.: Indispensability of iron for the growth of cultures chick cells. Devel Growth and Differ 24:571-580, 1982.

320. Ozawa, E. and Hagiwara, Y.: Avian and mammalian transferrin are required for chick and rat myogenic cell growth in vitro, respectively. Proc Japan Acad 57B:406-409, 1981.

321. Shimo-Oka, T., et al.: Manuscript in preparation.

322. Neuman, R.E. and Tytell, A.A.: Iron replacement of lactalysate and embryo extract in growth of cell cultures. Proc Soc Exp Biol & Med 107:867-880, 1961.

323. Barnes, D. and Sato, G.: Serum-free culture: a unifying approach. Cell 22:649-655, 1980.

324. Aisen, P.: The transferrins. In: Iron in biochemistry and medicine, II. (Jacobs, A. and Worwood, M. eds.) pp. 87-129, Academic Press, London and New York, 1980.

325. Ozawa, E.: Trophic effects on chick muscle cells of a factor promoting chick myoblast multiplication. Proc Japan Acad 53b:130-132, 1978.

326. Ozawa, E. and Hagiwara, Y.: Degeneration of large myotubes following removal of transferrin from culture medium. Biomed Res 3:16-23, 1982.

327. Saito, K., Hagiwara, Y.: Unpublished data.

328. Ii, I., Kimura, I., Hasegawa, T. and Ozawa, E.: Transferrin is an essential component of chick embryo extract for avian myogenic cell growth in vitro. Proc Japan Acad 57B:211-216, 1981.

329. Ii, I.: Unpublished data.

330. Ii, I.: Unpublished data.

331. Linkhart, T.A., Clegg, C.H. and Hauschka, S.D.: Myogenic differentiation in permanent clonal mouse myoblast cell line: regulation by macromolecular growth factors in the culture medium. Devel Biol 86:19-30, 1981.

332. Herskovits, J.J., Masters, C.J., Wassarman, P.M. and Kaplan, N.O.: On the tissue specificity and biological significance of aldolase C in the chicken. Biochem Biophys Res Comm 26:24-29, 1967.

333. Lebherz, H.G. and Rutter, W.J.: Distribution of fructose diphosphate aldolase variants in biological systems. Biochemistry 8:109-121, 1969.

334. Lebherz, H.G.: Ontogeny and regulation of fructose diphosphate aldolase isoenzyme in "red" and "white" skeletal muscles of the chick. J Biol Chem 250:5976-5981, 1975.

335. Lebherz, H.G., Petell, J.K., Shackelford, J.E. and Sardo, M.J.: Regulation of concentrations of glycolytic enzymes and creatine-phosphate kinase in "fast-twitch" and "slow-twitch" skeletal muscles of the chicken. Arch Biochem Biophys 214:642-656, 1982.

336. Petell, J.K. and Lebherz, H.G.: Regulation of fructose diphosphate aldolase concentrations in skeletal muscles of normal and dystrophic chickens. J Biol Chem 254: 7411-7414, 1979.

337. Shackelford, J.E. and Lebherz, H.G.: Effect of denervation on the levels and rates of synthesis of specific enzymes in "fast-twitch" (breast) muscle fibers of the chicken. J Biol Chem 256:6423-6429, 1981.

338. Markelonis, G., Oh, T.H. and Derr, D.: Stimulation of protein synthesis in cultured skeletal muscle by a trophic protein from sciatic nerves. Exp Neurol 70:598-612, 1980.

339. Markelonis, G., Oh, T.H., Eldefrawi, M.E. and Guth, L.: A myotrophic protein increases the number of acetylcholine receptors and receptor clusters in cultured skeletal muscle. Dev Biol 89:353-361, 1982.

340. Markelonis, G. and Oh, T.H.: A protein fraction from peripheral nerve having neurotrophic effects on skeletal muscle cells in culture. Exp Neurol 58:285-295, 1978.

341. Richler, C. and Yaffe, D.: The in vitro cultivation and differentiation capacities of myogenic cell lines. Develop Biol 23:1-22, 1970.

342. Karin, M. and Mintz, B.: Receptor-mediated endocytosis of transferrin in developmentally totipotent mouse teratocarcinoma stem cells. J Biol Chem 256:3245-3552, 1981.

343. Ward, J.H., Kushner, J.P. and Kaplan, J.: Regulation of HeLa cell transferrin receptors. J Biol Chem 257:10217-10323, 1982.

344. Hasegawa, T. and Ozawa, E.: Transferrin receptor on chick fibroblast cell surface and the binding affinity in relevance to the growth promoting activity of transferrin. Develop Growth and Differ 24:581-587, 1982.

345. Ozawa, E., Kimura, I., Hasegawa, T., Li, I., Saito, K., Hagiwara, Y. and Shimo-Oka, T.: Iron-bound transferrin as a myotrophic factor. In: Muscular Dystrophy: Bio-

medical Aspects. S. Ebashi and E. Ozawa, eds. Japan Sci. Soc. Press, Tokyo/Springer-Verlag, Berlin, pp. 53-60, 1983.

346. Ettienne, E.M., Swartz, K. and Singer, R.H.: Increased turnover of proteins from the sarcoplasmic reticulum of dystrophic chicken muscle cells in tissue culture. J Biol Chem 256:6408-6412, 1980.

347. Moxley, R.T., Livingston, J.R., Lockwood, D.H., Griggs, R.C. and Hill, R.L.: Abnormal regulation of monocyte insulin-binding affinity after glucose ingestion in patients with myotonic dystrophy. Proc Natl Acad Sci, USA, 78:2567-2571, 1981.

348. Smith, P.B., Grefrath, S.P. and Appel, S.H.: β-adrenergic receptor-adenylate cyclase of denervated sarcolemmal membrane. Exp Neurol 59:361-371, 1978.

349. Jeffry, P.L. and Appel, S.H.: Denervation alterations in surface membrane glycoprotein glycosyltransferases of mammalian skeletal muscle. Exp Neurol 61:432-441, 1978.

350. Trowbridge, I.S. and Lopez, F.: Monoclonal antibody to transferrin receptor blocks transferrin binding and inhibits human tumor cell growth in vitro. Proc Natl Acad Sci USA, 79:1175-1179, 1982.

351. Hamilton, T.A., Wada, H.G. and Sussman, H.H.: Identification of transferrin receptors on the surface of human cultured cells. Proc Natl Acad Sci USA, 76:6404-6410, 1979.

352. Wada, H.G., Hass, P.E. and Sussman, H.H.: Transferrin receptor in human placental brush border membranes. J Biol Chem 254:12629-12635, 1979.

353. Trowbridge, I.S. and Omary, M.B.: Human cell surface glycoprotein related to cell proliferation is the receptor for transferrin. Proc Natl Acad Sci USA, 78:3039-3043, 1981.

354. Octave, J.-N., Schneider, Y.-J., Crichton, R.R. and Trouet, A.: Transferrin uptake by cultured rat embryo fibroblasts. Eur J. Biochem 115:611-618, 1981.

355. Omary, M.B. and Trowbridge, I.S.: Biosynthesis of the human transferrin receptor in cultured cells. J Biol Chem 256:12888-12892, 1981.

356. Bleil, J.D. and Bretscher, M.S.: Transferrin receptor and its recycling in HeLa cells. EMBO J 1:351-355, 1982.

357. Racker, E. and Spector, M.: Warburg effect revisited: merger of biochemistry and molecular biology. Science 213: 303-307, 1981.

358. Matsuda, R., Spector, D.H. and Strohman, R.C.: Regenerating adult chicken skeletal muscle and satellite cell cultures express embryonic patterns of myosin and tropomyosin isoforms. Dev Biol 100:478-488, 1983.

359. Matsuda, R., Spector, D. and Strohman, R.C.: There is selective accumulation of a growth factor in chicken skeletal muscles. I. Transferrin accumulation in adult anterior latissimus dorsi. Dev Biol In press.

360. Matsuda, R., Spector, D. and Strohman, R.C.: There is selective accumulation of a growth factor in chicken skeletal muscle. II. Transferrin accumulation in dystrophic fast muscle. Dev Biol In press.

361. Ozawa, E. and Hagiwara, Y.: Avian and mammalian transferrins are required for chick and rat myogenic cell growth in vitro respectively. Proc Japan Acad Ser B 57:406-409, 1981.

362. Ozawa, E.: In: Gene Expression in Muscle. Plenum Press, New York, In press.

363. Gibson, M.C. and Schultz, E.: The distribution of satellite cells and their relationship to specific fiber types in soleus and extensor digitorum longus muscles. The Anatomical Record 202:329-337, 1983.

364. Campion, D.: The muscle satellite cell: A review. Internat Rev Cytol 87:225-251, 1984.

365. Lowey, S. and Risby, D.: Light chains from fast and slow muscle myosins. Nature 234:81-85, 1971.

366. Sarker, S., Streter, F. and Gergely, J.: Light chains of myosins from white, red, and cardiac muscle, Proc Natl Acad Sci 68:946-950, 1971.

367. Gauthier, G., and Lowey, S.: Polymorphism of myosin among skeletal muscle types. J Cell Biol 74:760-779, 1977.

368. Gauthier, G. and Lowey, S.: Distribution of myosin isoenzymes among skeletal muscle fiber types. J Cell Biol 81: 10-25, 1979.

369. Dalla Libera, L., Sartore, S., Pierobon-Bormioli, S. and Schiaffino, S.: Fast-white and fast-red isomyosins in guinea pig muscles. Biochem Biophys Res Commu 96: 1662-1670, 1980.

370. Mabuchi, K., Szvetko, D., Pinter, K. and Sreter, F.: Type IIB to IIA fiber transformation in intermittently stimulated rabbit muscles. Am J Physiol 11:C373-381, 1982.

371. Weeds, A., Trentham, D., Kean, C. and Buller, A.: Myosin from cross-innervated cat muscles. Nature 247:135-139, 1974.

372. Eccles, J., Eccles, R. and Lundberg, R.: The action potentials of the alpha motoneurons supplying fast and slow muscles. J Physiol 142:275-291, 1958.

373. Salmons, S. and Sreter, F.: Significance of impulse activity in the transformation of skeletal muscle type. Nature 262:30-34, 1976.

374. Salmons, S. and Vrbova, G.: The influence of activity on some contractile characteristics of mammalian fast and slow muscle. J Physiol 201:535-549, 1969.

375. Winder, W., Fitts, R., Holloszy, J., Kaiser, K. and Brooke, M.: Effects of thyroid hormone on different types of skeletal muscle. In: Plasticity of Muscle (Pette, D. ed.) pp. 581-591, Walter de Gruyter, Berlin, 1980.

376. Ianuzzo, C., Patel, P., Chen, V. and O'Brien, P.: A possible thyroidal trophic influence on fast and slow skeletal muscle myosin. In: Plasticity of Muscle (Pette, D., ed.) pp. 593-605, Walter de Gruyter, Berlin, 1980.

377. McKeran, R., Slavin, G., Andres, T., Ward, P. and Mair, W.: Muscle fiber changes in hypothyroid myopathy. J Clin Pathol 28:659-663, 1975.

378. Johnson, M., Mastaglia, F., Montgomery, A., Pope, B. and Weeds, A.: Changes in myosin light chains in the rat soleus after thyroidectomy. FEBS Lett 110:230-235, 1980.

379. Rubinstein, N. and Kelly, A.: Development of muscle fiber specialization in the rat hindlimb. J Cell Biol 90: 128-144, 1981.

380. Whalen, R., Schwartz, K., Sell, S., and Gros, F.: Contractile protein isozymes in development: Identification of an embryonic form of myosin heavy chain. Proc Natl Acad Sci 76:5197-5201, 1979.

381. Whalen, R., Sell, S., Butler-Browne, G., Schwartz, K., Bouveret, P. and Pinset-Harstrom, I.: Three myosin heavy chain isozymes appear sequentially in rat muscle development. Nature 292:805-809, 1981.

382. Lyons, G., Gambke, B., Kelly, A. and Rubinstein, N.: Myosin isozymes in the sexually dimorphic temporalis muscle in the guinea pig. Submitted for publication.

383. Lyons, G., Haselgrove, J., Kelly, A. and Rubinstein, N.: Myosin transitions in developing fast and slow muscles of the rat hindlimb. Different 25:168-175, 1983.

384. Bandman, E., Matsuda, R., and Strohman, R.: Developmental appearance of myosin heavy and light chain isoforms in vivo and in vitro in chicken skeletal muscle. Develop Biol 93:508-518, 1982.

385. Lowey, S., Benfield, P., LeBlanc, D., Waller, G., Winkelmann, D., and Gauthier, G.: Characterization of myosin from embryonic and developing chicken pectoralis muscle. In: Muscle Development (Pearson, H. and Epstein, H., eds.), pp. 15-24, Cold Spring Harbor Laboratory, 1982.

386. Bader, D., Masaki, T. and Fischman, D.: Immunochemical analysis of myosin heavy chain during avain myogenesis. J Cell Biol 95:763-770, 1982.

387. Rubinstein, N. and Kelly, A.: Myogenic and neurogenic contributions to the development of fast and slow twitch muscles in the rat. Develop Biol 62:252-261, 1978.

388. Agard, D., Steinberg, R. and Stroud, R.: Quantitative analysis of electropheretograms: A mathematical approach to super resolution. Analyt Biochem 111: 257-268, 1981.

389. Fitzsimmons, R. and Hoh, J.: Embryonic and foetal myosins in human skeletal muscle. J Neurol Sci 52:367-384, 1981.

390. Gambke, B., and Rubinstein, N.: A monoclonal antibody to the embryonic myosin heavy chain of the rat. Submitted for publication.

391. Gambke, B., Lyons, G., Haselgrove, J., Kelly, A., Rubinstein, N.: Thyroidal and neural control of myosin transitions during development of rat fast and slow muscles. FEBS Lett. 156:335-339, 1983.

392. Butler, J. and Cosmos, E.: Differentiation of the avian latissimus dorsi primordium: Analysis of fiber type expression using the myosin ATPase histochemical reaction. J Exper Zool 218:219-232, 1981.

393. Kelly, A., Lyons, G., Gambke, B. and Rubinstein, N.: Influences of testosterone in contractile proteins of the guinea pig temporalis muscle. In: Gene Expression in Muscle. Strohman, R. and Wolf, S. (eds.) Plenum Press, New York, In press.

394. Kockhakian, C.D., and Tillotson, C.: Influence of several C_{19} steroids on the growth of individual muscles of the guinea pig. Endocrin 60:607-618, 1957.

395. Gutmann, E. and Hanzlikova, V.: Effect of androgens on histochemical fiber type. Histochemie 24:287-291, 1970.

396. Rowlerson, A., Mascarello, F., Vegetti, A. and Carpene, E.: The fiber-type composition of the first branchial arch muscles in carnivora and primates. J Muscle Res & Cell Motil 4:443-472, 1983.

397. Resko, J.A.: Androgens in systemic plasma of male guinea pigs during development and after castration in adulthood. Endocrin 86:1444-1447, 1970.

398. Rigaudiere, N., Pelardy, G., Robert, A. and Delost, P.: Changes in the concentration of testosterone and androstenedione in the plasma and testis of the guinea pig from birth to death. J Reprod Fert 48: 291-300, 1976.

399. Bergamini, L.: Different mechanisms of testosterone action on glycogen metabolism in rat perianal and skeletal muscles. Endocrin 96:77-84, 1975.

400. Brooke, M.H., Williamson, E. and Kaiser, K.K.: The behavior of four fiber types in developing and reinnervated muscle. Arch Neurol 25:360-366, 1971.

401. Max, S.: Androgens enhance 2-deoxyglucose uptake by the rat levator ani muscle in vivo. J Cell Biol 95, 38a, 1982.

402. Hoh, J.F.Y., McGrath, P. and White, R.: Electrophoretic analysis of multiple forms of myosin in fast twitch and slow twitch muscles of the chick. Biochem J 157:87-95, 1976.

403. Lyons, G.E., Haselgrove, J., Kelly, A.M. and Rubinstein, N.A.: Myosin transitions in developing fast and slow muscles of the rat hind limb. Differentiation 25:168-175, 1983.

404. Salmons, S. and Vrbova, G.: J Physiol (Lond.) 201:535-549, 1969.

405. Pette, D., Smith, M.E., Staudte, H.W. and Vrbova, G.: Pflugers Arch 338:257-272, 1973.

406. Heilig, A. and Pette, D.: Plasticity of Muscle, Pette, D. ed. Walter de Gruyter, Berlin, New York, pp. 409-420, 1980.

407. Eisenberg, B.R., Salmons, S.: Cell Tissue Res 220:449-471, 1981.

408. Reichmann, H., Hoppeler, H. and Pette, D.: Pflugers Arch In preparation, 1984.

409. Pette, D., Ramirez, B., Muller, W., Simon, R., Exner, G.U. and Hildebrand, R.: Pflugers Arch 361:1-7, 1975.

410. Pette, D., Muller, W., Leisner, E. and Vrbova, G.: Pflugers Arch 364:103-112, 1976.

411. Pette, D. and Tyler, K.R.: J Physiol (Lond.) 338:1-9, 1983.

412. Buchegger, A., Nemeth, P.M., Pette, D. and Reichmann, H.: J Physiol (Lond.) In press.

413. Klug, G., Wiehrer, W., Reichmann, H., Leberer, E. and Pette, D.: Pflugers Arch In press.

414. Ramirez, B.U. and Pette, D.: FEBS Lett 49:188-190, 1974.

415. Heilmann, C. and Pette, D.: Eur J Biochem 93:437-446, 1979.

416. Heilmann, C., Muller, W. and Pette, D.: J Membr Biol 59:143-149, 1981.

417. Wiehrer, W. and Pette, D.: FEBS Lett 158:317-320, 1983.

418. Salmons, S. and Sreter, F.A.: Nature (Lond.) 263:30-34, 1976.

419. Sarzala, M.G., Szymanska, G., Wiehrer, W. and Pette, D.: Eur J Biochem 123:241-245, 1982.

420. Klug, G., Reichmann, H. and Pette, D.: FEBS Lett 152:180-182, 1983.

421. Blum, H.E., Lehky, P., Kohler, L., Stein, E.A. and Fisher, E.H.: J Biol Chem 252:2834-2838, 1977.

422. Celio, M.R. and Heizmann, C.W.: Nature (Lond.) 201:535-549, 1982.

423. Sreter, F.A., Gergely, J., Salmons, S. and Romanul, F.: Nature New Biol (Lond.) 241:17-19, 1973.

424. Pette, D. and Schnez, U.: FEBS Lett 83:128-130, 1977.

425. Seedorf, K., Seedorf, U. and Pette, D.: FEBS Lett 158:321-324, 1983.

426. Sreter, F.A., Elzinga, M., Mabuchi, K., Salmons, S. and Luff, A.R.: FEBS Lett 57:107-111, 1975.

427. Roy, R.K., Mabuchi, K., Sarkar, S., Mis, S. and Sreter, F.A.: Biochem Biophys Res Commun 89:181-187, 1979.

428. Heilig, A., Seedorf, K., Seedorf, U. and Pette, D.: Exp Biol Med Karger, Basel. In press.

429. Heilig, A. and Pette, D.: FEBS Lett 151:211-214, 1983.

430. Dolken, G. and Pette, D.: Hoppe-Seyler's Z Physiol Chem 355:289-299, 1974.

431. Rubinstein, N., Mabuchi, K., Pepe, F., Salmons, S., Gergely, J. and Sreter, F.: J Cell Biol 79:252-261, 1978.

432. Sreter, F.A., Mabuchi, K., Kover, A., Gesztelyi, I., Nagy, Z., and Furka, I.: In: Plasticity of Muscle D. Pette, ed., Walter de Gruyter, Berlin, New York, pp. 441-452, 1980.

433. Martonosi, A., Roufa, D., Boland, R., Reyes, E. and Tillack, T.W.: J Biol Chem 252:318-322, 1977.

434. Holtzer, H., Sanger, J., Ishikawa, H. and Strahs, K.: Selected topics in skeletal myogenesis. In: Cold Spring Harbor Symposium on Quantitative Biology, Vol. 37, 549-566, 1972.

435. Dienstman, S. and Holtzer, H.: Myogenesis: A Cell Lineage Interpretation. In: The Cell Cycle and Cell Differentiation. J. Reinert and H. Holtzer, eds., Results and Problems in Cell Differentiation, Vol. 7, 1-25, Springer-Verlag, Heidelberg, 1975.

436. Chi, J., Rubinstein, N., Fellini, S. and Holtzer, H.: Synthesis of myosin heavy and light chains in muscle cultures. J Cell Biol 67:523-537, 1975.

437. Holtzer, H., Croop, J.M., Toyama, Y., Bennett, G.S., Fellini, S.A. and West, C.: Differences in differentiation programs between presumptive myoblasts and their daughters, the definitive myoblasts and myotubes. In: Plasticity of Muscle. D. Pette, ed., pp. 133-146, Walter de Gruyter, Berlin, 1980.

438. Holtzer, H., Bennett, G.S., Tapscott, S.J., Croop, J.M., Toyama, Y.: Intermediate-sized filaments: Changes in synthesis and distribution in cells of myogenic and neurogenic lineages. Cold Spring Harbor Symposium on Quantitative Biology, Vol. 46, Organization of the Cytoplasm, pp. 317-329, Cold Spring Harbor Press, 1982.

439. Croop, J.M., Dubyak, G., Dlugosz, A., Scarpa, A. and Holtzer, H.: Effects of TPA on myofibril integrity and Ca^{+2} content in developing myotubes. Develop Biol 89: 460-474, 1982.

440. Toyama, Y., Forry-Schaudies, S., Hoffman, B. and Holtzer, H.: Effects of taxol and colcemid on myofibrillogenesis. Proc Natl Acad Sci USA, 79:6556-6566, 1982.

441. Antin, P. and Holtzer, H.: Reversible blocking of myogenesis by a chemical carcinogen. Anat Rec 202:8A, 1982.

442. Fallon, J. and Nachmias, V.: Localization of cytoplasmic and skeletal myosins in developing muscle cells by double-label immunofluorescence. J Cell Biol 87:237-247, 1980.

443. Fellini, S.A., Bennett, G.S. and Holtzer, H.: Selective binding of antibody against gizzard 10nm filaments to different cell types in myogenic cultures. Am J Anat 153:451-457, 1978.

444. Bennett, G.S., Fellini, S.A., Toyama, Y., and Holtzer, H.: Redistribution of intermediate filament subunits during skeletal myogenesis and maturation in vitro. J Cell Biol 82:577-584, 1979.

445. Ishikawa, H., Bischoff, R.E. and Holtzer, H.: The formation of arrowhead complexes with heavy meromyosin in a variety of cell types. J Cell Biol, 43:312-328, 1969.

446. Gard, D. and Lazarides, E.: The synthesis and distribution of desmin in vimentin during myogenesis in vitro. Cell 19:263-275, 1980.

447. Cohen, R., Pacifici, M., Rubinstein, N., Biehl, J. and Holtzer, H.,: Effects of a tumor promoter (PMA) on myogenesis. Nature 266:538-540, 1977.

448. Croop, J.M. and Holtzer, H.: Response of fibrogenic and myogenic cells to cytochalasin-B and to colcemid. I. Light microscopic observations. J Cell Biol 65:271-285, 1975.

449. Holtzer, H., Fellini, S., Rubinstein, N., Chi, J. and Strahs, K.: Cells, myosins, and 100 A filaments. In: Cell Motility, Cold Spring Harbor Symposium on Motile Systems, R. Goldman, T. Pollard and J. Rosenbaum, eds. pp. 823-829, Cold Spring Harbor Press, 1976.

450. Holtzer, H., Rubinstein, N., Fellini, S.A., Yeoh, G., Birnbaum, J., Chi, J. and Okayama, M.: Lineages, quantal cell cycles and the generation of cell diversity. Quart Rev Biophysics 8:524-557, 1974.

451. Holtzer, H., Sasse, J., Antin, P., Tokunaka, S., Pacifici, M., Horwitz, A. and Holtzer, S.: In: Developmental Processes in Normal and Diseased Muscle, Experimental Biology and Medicine, Vol. 9, H. Eppenberger and J-C Perriard, eds. pp. 126-134, S. Kargel, Basel, 1984.

452. Antin, P.B., Forry-Schaudies, S., Friedman, T.M., Tapscott, S.J. and Holtzer, H.: Taxol induces postmitotic myoblasts to assemble interdigitating microtubule-myosin arrays which exclude actin filaments. J Cell Biol 89:300-308, 1981.

453. Garrels, J.I.: Changes in protein synthesis during myogeneasis in a clonal cell line. Develop Biol 73:134-152, 1979.

454. Whalen, R.G., Butler-Browne, G.S. and Gros, F.: Identification of a novel form of myosin light chain present in embryonic muscle tissue and cultured muscle cells. J Mol Biol 126:415-431, 1978.

455. Whalen, R.G., Butler-Browne, G.S., Sell, S. and Gros, F.: Transitions in contractile protein isozymes during muscle cell differentiation. Biochimie 61:625-632, 1979a.

456. Bader, D., Masaki, T., Fischman, D.A.: Immunochemical analysis of myosin heavy chain during avian myogenesis in vivo and in vitro. J Cell Biol 95:763-770, 1982.

457. Butler-Browne, G.S. and Whalen, R.G.: Myosin isozyme transitions occurring during the postnatal development in the rat soleus muscle. Develop Biol 102: In press.

458. Brooke, M.H. and Kaiser, K.K.: Muscle fiber types: How many and what kind? Arch Neurol 23:369-379, 1970.

459. Whalen, R.G.: In: Gene Expression in Muscle. Strohman, R.C. and Wolf, S. editors, Plenum Press, New York, In press.

460. Harrison, R.G.: An experimental study of the relation of the nervous system to the developing musculature in the embryo of the frog. Am J Anat 3:197-220, 1904.

461. Le Douarin, N.: A biological cell labeling technique and its use in experimental embryology. Develop Biol 30:217-222, 1973.

462. Chevallier, A., Kieny, M. and Mauger, A.: Limb-somite relationship: origin of the limb musculature. J Embryol Exp Morph 41:245, 1977.

463. Christ, B., Jacob, H.J. and Jacob, M.: Experimental analysis of the origin of the wing musculature in avian embryos. Anat Embryol 150:171, 1977.

464. Wachtler, F., Christ, B. and Jacob, H.J.: On the determination of mesodermal tissues in the avian embryonic wing bird. Anat Embryol 161:283-289, 1982.

465. Holtzer, H., Biehl, J., Payette, R., Sasse, J., Pacifici, M. and Holtzer, S.: Cell diversification: Differing rules of cell lineages and cell-cell interactions. In: Limb Development and Regeneration. Part B. R.O. Kelly, P.F. Goetinck and J.A. MacCabe, editors, Alan R. Liss, Inc., New York, 271-280, 1983.

466. Newman, S.A. and Leonard, C.M.: Against programs: Limb development without developmental information. In: Limb Development and Regeneration. Part A. R.O. Kelly, P.I. Goetinck and J.A. MacCabe, editors. Alan R. Liss, Inc., New York, 251-256, 1983.

467. Hirose, G. and Jacobson, M.: Clonal organization of the central nervous system of the frog. I. Clones stemming from individual blastomeres of the 16-cell and earlier stages. Develop Biol 71:191-202, 1979.

468. Moody, S.A. and Jacobson, M.: Compartmental relationships between Anuran primary spinal motoneurons and somitic muscle fibers that they first innervate. J Neurosci 3:1670-1682, 1983.

469. Lance-Jones, C. and Landmesser, L.: Pathway selection by chick lumbosacral motoneurons during normal development. Proc R Soc Lond B 214:1-18, 1981.

470. Lance-Jones, C. and Landmesser, L.: Pathway selection by embryonic chick motoneurons in an experimentally altered environment. Proc R Soc Lond B 214:19-52, 1981.

471. Bonner, P.H. and Hauschka, S.D.: Clonal analysis of vertebrate myogenes. I. Early developmental events in the chick limb bud. Develop Biol 37:317-328, 1974.

472. Vrbova, G., Gordon, T. and Jones, R.: Nerve-muscle interaction. Chapman and Hall, 1978.

473. Stockdale, F.E., Baden, H. and Raman, N.: Slow muscle myoblasts differentiating in vitro synthesize both slow and fast myosin light chains. Develop Biol 82:168-171, 1981.

474. Blau, H.M., Chiu, C.-P. and Webster, C.: Cytoplasmic activation of human nuclear genes in stable heterokaryons. Cell 32:1171-1180, 1983.

475. Wright, E.W.: Induction of muscle genes in neural cells. J Cell Biol 98:427-435, 1984.

476. Fischman, D.A.: Introduction: Myofibrillar assembly. In: Muscle Development: Molecular and Cellular Control. M.L. Pearson and H.F. Epstein, editors. Cold Spring Laboratory, New York, 397-401, 1982.

477. Bader, D., Masaki, T. and Fischman, D.A.: Immunochemical analysis of myosin heavy chain during avian myogenesis in vivo and in vitro. J Cell Biol 95:763-770, 1982.

478. Reinach, F.C., Masaki, T., Shafiq, S., Obinata, T. and Fischman, D.A.: Isoforms of C-protein in adult chicken skeletal muscle: Detection with monoclonal antibodies. J Cell Biol 95:78-84, 1982.

479. Reinach, F.C., Masaki, T. and Fischman, D.A.: Characterization of the C-protein from posterior latissimus dorsi muscle of the adult chicken: Heterogeneity within a single sarcomere. J Cell Biol 96:297-300, 1983.

480. Obinata, T., Reinach, F.C., Bader, D.M., Masaki, T., Kitani, S. and Fischman, D.A.: Immunochemical analysis of C-protein isoform transitions during the development of chicken skeletal muscle. Develop Biol 101:116-124, 1984.

481. Offer, G.: C-protein and the periodicity of the thick filaments of vertebrate skeletal muscle. Cold Spring Harbor Symp Quant Biol 37:87-93, 1972.

482. Jeacocke, S.A. and England, P.: Phosphorylation of a myofibrillar protein, Mr 150,000 in perfused rat heart, and the tentative identification of this as C-protein. FEBS Lett 122:129-132, 1980.

483. Masaki, T. and Yoshisaki, C.: Differentiation of myosin in chick embryos. J Biochem 76:123-131, 1974.

484. Toyota, N. and Shimada, Y.: Isoform variants of troponin in skeletal and cardiac muscle cells cultured with and without nerves. Cell 33:297-304, 1983.

485. Sweeney, L.J., Clark, W.A., Zak, R. and Manasek, F.J.: Myosin heavy chain expression during cardiac embryogenesis in the chick. J Cell Biol 97:51a, 1983.

486. Cooper, T.A. and Ordahl, C.P. Submitted, 1984.

487. Minty, A.J., Alonso, S., Caravatti, M. and Buckingham, M.E.: Cell 30:185, 1982.

488. Sreter, F.A., Balint, M. and Gergely, J.: Structural and functional changes of myosin during development: Comparison of adult fast, slow and cardiac myosin. Develop Biol 46:317-325, 1975.

489. Huxley, H.E.: Introductory remarks: The relevance of studies on muscle to problems of cell motility. In "Cell Motility." Edited by R. Goldman, T. Pollard and J. Rosenbaum (Cold Spring Harbor Laboratory: Cold Spring Harbor), pp. 115-126.

490. McLachlan, A.D. and Karn, J.: Periodic charge distributions in the myosin rod amino acid sequence match cross-bridge spacings in muscle. Nature 299:226-231, 1982.

491. Korn, E.D.: Biochemistry of actomyosin-dependent cell motility (a review). Proc Natl Acad Sci USA, 75:588-599, 1978.

492. Straub, F.B.: Actin. Stud Inst Med Chem Univ Szeged III, 23-37, 1943.

493. Schachat, F., Garcea, R.L. and Epstein, H.F.: Myosins exist as homodimers of heavy chains: demonstration with specific antibody purified by nematode mutant myosin affinity chromatography. Cell 15:405-411, 1978.

494. Mackenzie, J.M., Jr., Schachat, F. and Epstein, H.F.: Immunocytochemical localization of two myosins within the same muscle cells in Caenorhabditis elegans. Cell 15:413-419, 1978.

495. Miller, D.M. III, Ortiz, I., Berliner, G.C. and Epstein, H.F.: Differential localization of two myosins within nematode thick filaments. Cell 34:477-490, 1983.

496. Epstein, H.F., Berman, S.A. and Miller, D.M., III: Myosin synthesis and assembly in normal and mutant nematode body-wall muscle. In: "Muscle Development: Molecular and Cellular Control." Edited by M.L. Pearson and H.F. Epstein (Cold Spring Harbor Laboratory: Cold Spring Harbor) pp. 419-427, 1982.

497. Garrels, J.I.: Quantitative two-dimensional gel electrophoresis of proteins. In Methods in Enzymology, Recombinant DNA Vol. 100, pp. 411-423, 1983.

498. Garrels, J.I., Farrar, J.T., and Burwell, C.B., IV.: The QUEST system of computer-analyzed two-dimensional electrophoresis of proteins. In Two-dimensional Gel Electrophoresis of Proteins: Methods and Applications J.E. Celis and R. Bravo (Eds.) pp. 37-91, Academic Press, New York, 1984.

499. Matsumura, F., Lin, J.J.-C., Yamashiro-Matsumura, S., Thomas, G.P. and Topp, W.C.: Differential expression of tropomyosin forms in the microfilaments isolated from normal and transformed rat cultured cells. J Biol Chem 258:13954-13964, 1984.

500. Matsumura, F., Yamashiro-Matsumura, S. and Lin, J.J.-C.: Isolation and characterization of tropomyosin-containing microfilaments from cultured cells. J Biol Chem 258: 6636-6644, 1983.

501. Miyachi, K., Fritzler, M.J., and Tan, E.M.: Autoantibody to a nuclear antigen in proliferating cells. J Immunol 121:2228-2234, 1978.

502. Bravo, R., Fey, S.J., Bellatin, J., Larsen, P.M., Arevalo, J., and Celis, J.E.: Identification of a nuclear and of a cytoplasmic polypeptide whose relative proportions are sensitive to changes in the rate of cell proliferation. Exp Cell Res 136:311-319, 1981.

503. Mathews, M.B., Bernstein, R.M., Franza, B.R., Jr., and Garrels, J.I.: The identity of the 'proliferating cell nuclear antigen' and 'cyclin.' Nature In press.

504. Burnette, W.N.: "Western Blotting": electrophoretic transfer of proteins from sodium dodecyl-sulfate-polyacrylamide gels to unmodified nitrocellulose and radiographic detection with antibody and radioiodinated protein A. Anal Biochem 112:195-203, 1981.

505. Chiu, C.-P. and Blau, H.M.: Reprogramming of cell differentiation in the absence of DNA synthesis. Cell In press.

506. Santi, D.V., Garret, C.E. and Barr, P.J.: On the mechanism of inhibition of DNA-cytosine methyltransferases by cytosine analogs. Cell 33:9-10, 1983.

507. Walsh, F.S. and Ritter, M.A.: Surface antigen differentiation during human myogenesis in culture. Nature 289:60-64, 1981.

508. Konigsberg, I.R., Sollman, P.A. and Mixter, L.O.: The duration of the terminal G_1 of fusing myoblasts. Dev Biol 63:11-26, 1978.

509. Brown, J.E. and Weiss, M.C.: Activation of production of mouse liver enzymes in rat hepatoma-mouse lymphoid cell hybrids. Cell 6:481-494, 1975.

510. Darlington, G.J., Rankin, J.K. and Schlanger, G.: Expression of human hepatic genes in somatic cell hybrids. Somatic Cell Genet 8:403-412, 1982.

511. Butler-Browne, G.S. and Whalen, R.G.: Myosin isozyme transitions occurring during the post-natal development of the rat soleus muscle. Develop Biol 102: In press.

512. d'Albis, A., Pantaloni, C. and Bechet, J.-J.: An electrophoretic study of native myosin isozymes and their subunit content. Eur J Biochem 99:261-272, 1979.

513. Starr, R. and Offer, G.: Polarity of the myosin molecule. J Mol Biol 81:17-31, 1973.

514. Zweig, S.E.: The muscle specificity and structure of two closely related fast-twitch white muscle myosin heavy chain isozymes. J Biol Chem 256:11847-11853, 1981.

515. Brown, W.E., Salmons, S. and Whalen, R.G.: The sequential replacement of myosin subunit isoforms during muscle type transformation induced by long term stimulation. J Biol Chem 258:14686-14692, 1983.

516. Butler-Browne, G.S., Herlicoviez, D. and Whalen, R.G.: Effects of hypothyroidism on myosin isozyme transitions in developing rat muscle. FEBS Lett 166:71-75, 1984.

517. Seo, H., Wunderlich, C., Vassart, G. and Refetoff, S.: Growth hormone responses to thyroid hormone in the neonatal rat. Resistance and anamnestic response. J Clin Invest 67:569-574, 1981.

518. Kugelberg, E.: Adaptive transformation of rat soleus motor units during growth. Histochemistry and contraction speed. J Neurol Sci 27:269-279, 1976.

519. Harris, J.B. and Johnson, M.A.: Further observations on the pathological responses of rat skeletal muscle to toxins isolated from the venom of the Australian tiger snake. Notechis scutatus. Clin Exp Pharmacol & Physiol 5:587-600, 1978.

520. Bischoff, R.: Tissue culture studies on the origin of myogenic cells during muscle regeneration in the rat. In: Muscle Regeneration. A. Mauro, editor, pp. 13-31, Raven Press, New York, 1979.

521. Roy, R.K., Sreter, F.A. and Sarkar, S.: Changes in tropomyosin subunits and myosin light chains during development of chicken and rabbit skeletal muscles. Dev Biol 69:15-30, 1979.

522. Hoh, J.F.Y.: Developmental changes in chicken skeletal myosin isozymes. FEBS Lett 98:267-270, 1979.

523. Amphlett, G., Perry, S.V., Suska, H., Brown, M. and Vrbova, G.: Cross innervation and the regulatory system of rabbit soleus muscle. Nature (Lond.) 257: 602-604, 1975.

524. Matsuda, R., Spector, D. and Strohman, R.C.: Denervated skeletal muscle displays discordinate regulation for the synthesis of several myofibrillar proteins. Proc Natl Acad Sci USA, 81:1122-1125, 1974.

525. Rowland, L.P.: Arch Neurol 33:315-321, 1976.

526. Schotland, D.L., Bonilla, E. and van Meter, M.: Science 196:1005-1007, 1977.

527. Bradley, W.G. and Fulthorpe, J.J.: Neurology 28:670-677, 1978.

528. Strickland, K.P., Hudson, A.J. and Thaker, J.H.: Ann NY Acad Sci 317:187-205, 1979.

529. Duncan, C.J.: Experientia 34:1531-1535, 1978.

530. Bodensteiner, J.B. and Engel, A.G.: Neurology (Minneap.) 28:439-446, 1978.

531. Beery, E., Klein, S., Nordenberg, J. and Beitner, R.: Biochem Int 1:526-531, 1980.

532. Wakelam, M.J.O. and Pette, D.: Biochem J 204:765-769, 1982.

533. Beitner, R.: Trends Biochem Sci 4:228-230, 1979.

534. Beitner, R., Haberman, S., Nordenberg, J. and Cohen, T.J.: Biochim Biophys Acta 542:537-541, 1978.

535. Beitner, R. and Nordenberg, J.: FEBS Lett 98:199-202, 1979.

536. Heizmann, C.W., Berchtold, M.W. and Rowlerson, A.M.: Proc Natl Acad Sci USA 79:7243-7247, 1982.

537. Blum, H.E., Lehky, P., Kohler, L., Stein, E.A. and Fischer, E.H.: J Biol Chem 252:2834-2838, 1977.

538. Klug, G., Reichman, H. and Pette, D.: FEBS Lett 152:180-182, 1983.

539. Nylen, E.G. and Wrogemann, K.: Exp Neurol 80:69-80, 1983.

540. Beitner, R., Nordenberg, J., Cohen, T.J. and Beery, E.: Int J Biochem 11:467-472, 1980.

541. Beitner, R. and Cohen, T.J.: IRCS Med Sci 7:24, 1979.

542. Wakelam, M.J.O., Emmerich, M. and Pette, D.: Biochem J 208:517-519, 1982.

543. Frucht, H., Kaplansky, M. and Beitner, R.: Biochem Med In press.

544. Klug, G., Wiehrer, W., Reichmann, H., Leberer, E. and Pette, D. Pflugers Arch In press.

545. Pette, D., Heilig, A., Klug, G., Reichmann, H., Seedorf, U., and Wiehrer, W.: In: Gene Expression in Muscle. Strohman, R. and Wolf, S. eds. In press

546. Green, H.J., Klug, G.A., Reichmann, H., Seedorf, U., Wiehrer, W. and Pette, D., Pflugers Arch In press.

547. Feit, H. and Domke, R.: Cell Motil 2:309-315, 1982.

548. Obinata, T., Takano-Ohmuro, H. and Matsuda, R.: FEBS Lett 120:195-198, 1980.

549. Stewart, P.A., Percy, M.E., Chang, L.W. and Thompson, M.W.: Muscle and Nerve 4:165-173, 1981.

550. Reichmann, H. and Pette, D.: Muscle and Nerve. In press.

551. Lowey, S., Benfield, P.A., LeBlanc, D.D., Waller, G.S., Winkelmann, D.A. and Gauthier, G.F. Characterization of myosins from embryonic and developing chicken pectoralis muscle. In: Muscle Development: Molecular and Cellular Control, Pearson, M.L. and Epstein, H.F., editors. Cold Spring Harbor Laboratory, New York, 15-24, 1982.

552. Umeda, P.K., Kavinsky, C.J., Sinha, A.M., Hsu, J.-J., Jakovcic, S. and Rabinowitz, M.: Cloned mRNA sequences for two types of embryonic myosin heavy chains from chick skeletal muscle. II. Expression during development using S1 nuclease mapping. J Biol Chem 258:5206, 1983.

553. Kavinsky, C.J., Umeda, P.K., Sinha, A.M., Elzinga, M., Tong, S.W., Zak, R., Jakovcic, S. and Rabinowitz, M.: Cloned mRNA sequences for two types of embryonic myosin heavy chains from chick skeletal muscle. I. DNA and derived amino acid sequence of light meromyosin. J Biol Chem 258:5196, 1983.

554, Barany, M.: ATPase activity of myosin correlated with speed of muscle shortening. J Gen Physiol 50:197, 1967.

555. Strzelecka-Golaszewska, H. and Piwowar, U.: Interaction of myosin filaments and minifilaments with actin: a comparative study. J Musc Res Cell Motility 4:25, 1984.

556. Reisler, E., Smith, C. and Seegan, G.: Myosin minifilaments. J Mol Biol 143:129, 1980.

557. Reisler, E.: Kinetic studies with synthetic myosin minifilaments show the equivalence of actomyosin and acto-HMM ATPases. J Biol Chem 225:9541, 1980.

558. Cheung, P. and Reisler, E.: The actomyosin ATPase of synthetic myosin minifilaments, filaments and heavy meromyosin. J Biol Chem 258:5040, 1983.

559. Lowey, S., Benfield, P.A., LeBlanc, D.D. and Waller, G.S.: Myosin isozymes in avian skeletal muscles. I. Sequential expression of myosin isozymes in developing chicken pectoralis muscles. J Musc Res Cell Motility 4:695, 1983.

560. Gordon, T. and Vrbova, G.: The influence of innervation on the differentiation of contractile speeds of developing chick muscles. Pflugers Arch Gesamte Physiol Menschen Tiere 360:199, 1975.

561. Rushbrook, J.I. and Stracher, A.: Comparison of adult, embryonic, and dystrophic myosin heavy chains from chicken muscle by sodium dodecyl sulfate/polyacrylamide gel electrophoresis and peptide mapping. Proc Natl Acad Sci USA 76:4331, 1979.

562. Winkelmann, D.A., Lowey, S. and Press, J.L.: Monoclonal antibodies localize changes on myosin heavy chain isozymes during avian myogenesis. Cell 34:295, 1983.

563. Lowey, S.: The structure of vertebrate muscle myosin. In: Myology, Banker, B.Q. and Engel, A.G., editors, In press.

564. Stockdale, F.E., Raman, N. and Baden, H.: Myosin light chains and the developmental origin of fast muscle. Proc Natl Acad Sci USA 75:931, 1981.

565. McLachlan, A. and Karn, J.: Periodic charge distributions in the myosin rod amino acid sequence match cross-bridge spacings in muscle. Nature (Lond.) 299:226, 1982.

566. Suzuki, H., Kamata, T., Onishi, H. and Watanabe, S.: Adenosine triphosphate-induced reversible change in the conformation of chicken gizzard myosin and heavy meromyosin. J Biochem 91:1699, 1982.

567. Onishi, H. and Wakabayashi, T.: Electron microscopic studies of myosin molecules from chicken gizzard muscle I. The formation of the intramolecular loop in the myosin tail. J Biochem (Tokyo) 92:871, 1982.

568. Trybus, K.M., Huiatt, T.W. and Lowey, S.: A bent monomeric conformation of myosin from smooth muscle. Proc Natl Acad Sci 79:6151, 1982.

569. Craig, R., Smith, R. and Kendrick-Jones, J.: Light-chain phosphorylation controls the conformation of vertebrate non-muscle and smooth muscle myosin molecules. Nature 302:436, 1983.

570. Trybus, K.M. and Lowey, S.: Conformational states of smooth muscle myosin. Effects of light chain phosphorylation and ionic strength. J Biol Chem In press, 1984a.

571. Trybus, K.M. and Lowey, S.: Smooth muscle myosin minifilaments. Biophys J 45:150a, 1984b.

572. Masaki, T. and Yoshizaki, C.: Differentiation of myosin in chick embryos. J Biochem (Tokyo) 76:123, 1974.

573. Benfield, P.A., Lowey, S., LeBlanc, D.D. and Waller, G.S.: Myosin isozymes in avian skeletal muscles. II. Fractionation of myosin isozymes from adult and embryonic chicken pectoralis muscle by immuno-affinity chromatography. J Musc Res Cell Motility 4:717, 1983.

574. Gauthier, G.F., Lowey, S., Benfield, P.A. and Hobbs, A.W.: Distribution and properties of myosin isozymes in developing avian and mammalian skeletal muscle fibers. J Cell Biol 92:471, 1982.

575. Sweeney, L.J., Clark, W.A., Jr., Umeda, P.K., Zak, R. and Manasek, F.J.: Immunofluorescence analysis of the primordial myosin detectable in embryonic striated muscle. Proc Natl Acad Sci 81:797, 1984.

576. Yguerībide, J., Epstein, H.F. and Stryer, L.: Segmental Flexibility in an Antibody Molecule. J Molec Biol 51:573-590, 1970.

577. Epstein, H.F., Miller, D.M. III, Gossett, L.A. and Hecht, R.M.: Myosin in Normal and Mutant Nematode Embryogenesis. Muscle Development: Molecular and Cellular Control. M.L. Pearson and H.F. Epstein, eds. pp. 7-14, Cold Spring Harbor, 1982.

578. Miller, D.M. III, Ortiz, I., Berliner, G.C. and Epstein, H.F.: Differential Localization of Two Myosins within Nematode Thick Filaments. Cell 34:477-490, 1983.

579. Botstein, D., White, R.L., Skolnick, M., and Davis, R.W.: Construction of a genetic linkage map in man using restriction fragment length polymorphisms. Am J Hum Genet 32:314, 1980.

580. Bender, W., Arkam, M., Karch, F., Beachy, P.A., Peifer, M., Spierer, P., Lewis, E.B., and Hogness, D.W.: Molecular genetics of the bithorax complex in Drosphilia melano gaster. Science 221:23-29, 1983.

581. Jacobs, P.A., Hunt, P.A., and Bart, R.D.: Duchenne muscular dystrophy (DMD) in a female with an X/autosome translocation: further evidence that the DMD locus is at Xp21. Am J Hum Genet 33:531, 1981.

582. Davies, K.E., Pearson, P.L., Harper, P.S., Murray, J.M. and O'Brien, T.: Linkage analysis of two cloned DNA sequences flanking the Duchenne muscular dystrophy locus on the short arm of the human X chromosome. Nucl Acids Res 1:2303-2312, 1983.

583. Kingston, H.M., Thomas, N.S., Pearson, P.L., Sarfarazi, M., and Harper, P.S.: Genetic linkage between Becker muscular dystrophy and a polymorphic DNA sequence on the short arm of the X chromosome. J Med Genet 20:255-258, 1983.

584. Davies, K.E., Young, B.B., Elles, R.G., Hill, M.E. and Williamson, R.: Cloning of a representative genomic library of the human X chromosome after sorting by flow cytometry. Nature 293:374-376, 1981.

585. Kunkel, L., Tantravahi, U., Eisenhard, M. and Latt, S.A.: Regional localization on the human X of DNA segments cloned from flow sorted chromosomes. Nucl Acids Res 10:1557, 1982.

586. Kunkel, L., Tantravahi, U., Kurnit, D., Bruns, G., Eisenhard, M. and Latt, S.A.: Identification and isolation of transcribed X chromosome DNA sequences. Nucl Acids Res 22:7961-7979, 1983.

587. Aldridge, J., Kunkel, L., Bruns, G., Tantravahi, U., Lalande, M., Brewster, T., Moreau, E., Wilson, M., Bromley, W., Roderick, T. and Latt, S.: A strategy to reveal high frequency RFLP's along the human X chromosome. Am J Hum Genet In press.

588. Whalen, R.G., Sell, S.M., Erikson, A., and Thornell, L.E.: Myosin subunit types in skeletal and cardiac tissues and their developmental distribution. Dev Biol 91: 478-484, 1982.

589. Chizzonite, R.E., Everett, W., Clark, W.A., Jaokovcic, S., Rabinowitz, M., and Zak, R.: Change in synthesis rates of α- and β-myosin heavy chains in rabbit heart after treatment with thyroid hormone. J Biol Chem 257:2056-2065, 1982.

590. Crow, M.T. and Stockdale, F.E.: Myosin isoforms and the cellular basis of skeletal muscle development. In: Experimental Biology and Medicine, 9, "Developmental Processes in Normal and Diseases Muscle," Edited by H.M. Eppenberger and J.C. Perriard, 165-174, Karger, Basel, 1984.

591. Heilig, A., Seedorf, K., Seedorf, U., and Pette, D.: Transcriptional and translational control of myosin light chain expression in adult muscle. In: Experimental Biology and Medicine, 9, "Developmental Processes in Normal and Diseased Muscle," Edited by H.M. Eppenberger and J.C. Perriard, 182-186, Karger, Basel, 1984.

592. Matsuda, R. and Strohman, R.: Changes in myofibrillar protein synthesis during regeneration in vivo and in vitro. Expl Biol Med 9:175-181, 1984.

593. Nudel, U., Mayer, Y., Zakut, R., Shani, M., Czosnek, H., Aloni, B. and Yaffe, D.: The structure and expression of rat actin genes. In: Experimental Biology and Medicine, 9, Edited by H.M. Eppenberger and J.C. Perriard. 219-227, Karger, Basel, 1984.

594. Mayer, Y., Czosnek, H., Zeelon, P.E., Yaffe, D. and Nudel, U.: Expression of the genes coding for the skeletal muscle and cardiac actins in the heart. Nucl Acids Res 12:1087-1100, 1984.

595. Hentschal, C.C. and Birnstiel, M.C.: The organization and expression of histone gene families. Cell 25:301-313, 1981.

596. Artavanis-Tsakonas, S., Schedle, P., Mirault, M.-E., Moran, L. and Lis, J.: Genes of the 70,000 dalton heat shock protein in two cloned D. melanogaster DNA segments. Cell 17:9-18, 1979.

597. Spradling, A.C.: The organization and amplification of two chromosomal domains containing Drosophila chorion genes. Cell 27:193-201, 1981.

598. Eickbush, T.H. and Kafatos, F.C.: A walk in the chorion locus of Bombix mori. Cell 29:633-643, 1982.

599. Czosnek, H., Nudel, U., Shani, M., Barker, P.E., Pravtcheva, D.D., Ruddle, F.H. and Yaffe, D.: The genes coding for the muscle contractile proteins, myosin heavy chain, myosin light chain 2, and skeletal muscle actin are located on three different mouse chromosomes. EMBO J 11:1299-1305, 1982.

600. Czosnek, H., Nudel, U., Mayer, Y., Barker, P.E., Pravtcheva, D.D., Ruddle, F.H. and Yaffe, D.: The genes coding for the cardiac muscle actin, the skeletal muscle actin and the cytoplasmic β-actin are located on three different mouse chromosomes. EMBO J 2:1977-1979, 1983.

601. Green, M.C. ed.: Genetic Variants and Strains of the Laboratory Mouse. Published by Gustav Fischer Verlag, Stuttgart/NY, 1981.

602. Michelson, A.M., Russel, E.S. and Harman, P.S.: Dystrophia muscularis: A hereditary primary myopathy in the house mouse. Proc Natl Acad Sci USA, 41:1079-1084, 1955.

603. Weintraub, H. and Groudine, M.: Chromosomal subunits in active genes have an altered conformation. 1976.

604. Garel, A. and Axel, R.: Selective digestion of transcriptionally active ovalbumin genes from oviduct nuclei. Proc Natl Acad Sci USA, 73:3966-3970, 1976.

605. Carmon, Y., Czosnek, H., Nudel, U., Shani, M. and Yaffe, D.: DNAase I sensitivity of genes expressed during myogenesis. Nucl Acids Res 10:3085-3098, 1982.

606. Shani, M., Zevin-Sonkin, D., Saxel, O., Carmon, Y., Katcoff, D., Nudel, U., and Yaffe, D.: The correlation between the synthesis of skeletal muscle actin, myosin heavy chain and myosin light chain and the accumulation of the corresponding mRNA sequences during myogenesis. Dev Biol 86:483-492, 1981.

607. Nudel, U., Katcoff, D., Carmon, Y., Zevin-Sonkin, D., Levi, Z., Shaul, Y., Shani, M., and Yaffe, D.: Identification of recombinant phages containing sequences from different rat myosin heavy chain genes. Nucl Acids Res 8:2133-2146, 1980.

608. Nudel, U., Zakut, r., Shani, M., Neuman, S., Levy, Z. and Yaffe, D.: The nucleotide sequence of the rat cytoplasmic β-actin gene. Nucl Acids Res 11:1759-1771, 1983.

609. Zakut, R., Shani, M., Givol, D., Neuman, S., Yaffe, D. and Nudel, U.: The nucleotide sequence of the rat skeletal muscle actin gene. Nature 298:857-859, 1982.

610. Graham, F.L. and Van der, E.B.: A new technique for the assay of human adenovirus 5 DNA. Virol 52:456-467, 1973.

611. Wigler, M., Pellicer, A., Silverstein, S. and Axel, R.: Biochemical transfer of single-copy eucaryotic genes using total cellular DNA as donor. Cell 14:725-731, 1978.

612. Melloul, D., Aloni, B., Calvo, J., Yaffe, D., and Nudel, U.: Developmentally regulated expression of chimeric genes containing muscle actin DNA sequences in transfected myogenic cells. EMBO J, In press.

613. Ordahl, C.P. and Cooper, T.A.: Strong homology in promoter and 3' untranslated regions of chick and rat α-actin genes. Nature 303:348-349, 1983.

614. Chao, M.V., Mellon, P., Charnay, F., Maniatis, T., Axel, R.: The regulated expression of β-globin genes introduced into mouse erythroleukemia cells. Cell 32:483-493, 1983.

615. Jahner, D., Stuhlmann, H., Stewart, C.L., Harbers, K., Lohler, J., Simon, I. and Jaenisch, R.: De novo methylation and expression of retroviral genomes during mouse embryogenesis. Nature 298:623-628, 1982.

616. Stewart, C.L., Stuhlman, C.L., Jahner, D. and Jaenisch, R.: De novo methylation, expression, and infectivity of retroviral genomes introduced into embryonal carcinoma cells. Proc Natl Acad Sci USA 79:4098-4102, 1982.

617. Jaenisch, R., Jahner, D., Nobis, P., Simon, I., Lohler, J., Harbers, K. and Grotkopp, D.: Chromosomal position and activation of retroviral genomes inserted into the germ line of mice. Cell 24:519-529, 1981.

618. Lacy, E., Roberts, S., Evans, E.P., Burtenshaw, M.D. and Costanini, F.D.: A foreign β-globin gene in transgenic mice: Integration at abnormal chromosomal positions and expression in appropriate tissue. Cell 34:343-358, 1983.

619. Davies, K.E., Pearson, P.L., Harper, P.S., Murray, J.M., O'Brien, T., Sarfarazi, M. and Williamson, R.: Linkage analysis of two cloned DNA sequences flanking the Duchenne muscular dystrophy locus on the short arm of the human X chromosome. Nucl Acids Res 11:2304-2312, 1983.

620. Cullen, M.J. and Fulthorpe, J.J.: Stages in fiber breakdown in Duchenne muscular dystrophy. J Neurol Sci 24:179-200, 1975.

621. Bugaisky, G. and Buckingham, M.E.: In preparation

622. Jakob, H., Buckingham, M.E., Cohen, A., Dupont, L., Fiszman, M., and Jacob, F.: A skeletal muscle cell line isolated from a mouse teratocarcinoma undergoes apparently normal terminal differentiation in vitro. Exp Cell Res 114: 403-412, 1978.

623. Whalen, R.G. and Sell, S.M.: Myosin from foetal hearts contains the skeletal embryonic light chain. Nature 286:731-733, 1980.

624. Barton, A. and Buckingham, M.E.: In preparation.

625. Robert, B., Weydert, A., Caravatti, M., Minty, A., Cohen, A., Daubas, P., Gros, F. and Buckingham, M.E.: cDNA recombinant plasmid complementary to mRNAs for light chains 1 and 3 of mouse skeletal muscle myosin. Proc Natl Acad Sci 79:2437-2441, 1982.

626. Rugh, R.: The Mouse; its Reproduction and Development. Burgers Publishing Co., USA, 1968.

627. Vandekerckhove, J., Couet, H.G. and Weber, K.: Molecular evolution of muscle specific actins: a protein chemical analysis. In: Actin - its structure and function in muscle and non-muscle cells, edited by dos Remedios. Sydney Academic Press, 1983.

628. Robert, B., Daubas, P., Akimenko, M.A., Cohen, A., Guenet, J.L. and Buckingham, M.E.: A single locus in the mouse encodes both myosin light chains 1 and 3, a second locus corresponds to a related pseudogene. Manuscript submitted for publication.

629. Weydert, A., Daubas, P., Caravatti, M., Minty, A., Bugaisky, G., Cohen, A., Robert, B. and Buckingham, M.E.: Sequential accumulation of mRNAs encoding different myosin heavy chain isoforms during skeletal muscle development in vivo detected with a recombinant plasmid identified as coding for an adult fast myosin heavy chain from mouse skeletal muscle. J Biol Chem 258:13867-13918.

630. Jenkins, N.A., Copeland, N.G., Taylor, B.A. and Lee, B.K.: Diluted coat colour mutation of DBA/2J mice is associated with the site of integration of an ecotropic Mu LV genome. Nature 293:370-374, 1981.

631. Bonhomme, F., Catalan, J., Britton-Davidian, J., Chapman, V.M., Moriwaki, K., Nevo, E. and Thaler, L.: Biochemical diversity and evolution in the genus mus. Biochem Genet 22:3-4. In press.

632. Minty, A.J., Caravatti, M., Robert, B., Cohen, A., Daubas, P., Weydert, A., Gros, F. and Buckingham, M.E.: Mouse actin mRNAs: Construction and characterization of a recombinant plasmid molecule containing a complementary DNA transcript of mouse α-actin mRNA. J Biol Chem 256:1008-1014, 1981.

633. Dubay, M. and Petes, T.D.: Recombination between genes located on non homologous chromosomes in Saccharomyces Cerevisiae. Genet 101:369-404, 1982.

634. Wydro, R.M., Nguyen, H.T., Gubits, R.M. and Nadal-Ginard, B.: Characterization of sarcomeric myosin heavy chain genes. J Biol Chem 258:670-678, 1983.

635. Flavell, R.A. and Grosveld, F.G.: Globin genes: their structure and expression. In: Eukaryotic Genes, edited by Maclean, N., Gregory, S.P. and Flavell, R.A. Chapter 17, pp 299-314, Butterworths Publications, 1983.

636. Nadal-Ginard, B., Medford, R.M., Nguyen, H.T., Periasamy, M., Wydro, R.M., Hornig, D., Gubits, R., Garfinkel, L.I., Wieczorek, D., Bekesi, E. and Mahdavi, V.: Structure and regulation of a mammalian sarcomeric myosin heavy-chain gene. Muscle Development: Molecular and Cellular Control. Pearson, M.L. and Epstein, H.F. eds. Cold Spring Harbor Laboratory, NY, pp. 143-168, 1982.

637. Medford, R.M., Wydro, R.M., Nguyen, H.T. and Nadal-Ginard, B.: Cytoplasmic processing of myosin heavy chain messenger RNA: Evidence provided by using a recombinant DNA plasmid. Proc Natl Acad Sci USA 77:5749-5753, 1980.

638. Periasamy, M., et al: Manuscript in preparation.

639. Mahdavi, V., Periasamy, M. and Nadal-Ginard, B.: Molecular characterization of two myosin heavy chain genes expressed in the adult heart. Nature 297:659-664, 1982.

640. Bois, D. and Nadal-Ginard, B.: Manuscript in preparation.

641. Mahdavi, V., Chambers, A.P. and Nadal-Ginard, B.: α-and β-cardiac myosin heavy chain genes are linked in the genome and organized according to their developmental expression. Proc Natl Acad Sci USA. In press.

642. Lompre, A.M., Nadal-Ginard, B. and Mahdavi, V.: Expression of the cardiac ventricular α-and β-myosin heavy chain genes is developmentally and hormonally regulated. Submitted for publication.

643. Leinwand, L.A., Fournier, R.E.K., Nadal-Ginard, B. and Shows, T.B.: Multigene family for sarcomeric myosin heavy chain in mouse and human DNA: Localization on a single chromosome. Science 221:766-769, 1983.

644. Periasamy, M. et al.: Myosin light chains 1 and 3 of rat fast skeletal muscle are encoded by a single gene. Submitted for publication.

645. Garfinkel, L.I., Periasamy, M. and Nadal-Ginard, B.: Cloning and characterization of cDNA sequences corresponding to myosin light chains 1, 2, and 3, troponin-C, troponin-T, α-tropomyosin and α-actin. J Biol Chem 257:11078-11086, 1982.

646. Medford, R.M., et al. Manuscript in preparation.

647. Putney, S.D., Herlihy, W.C. and Schimmel, P.: A new troponin T and cDNA clones for 13 different muscle proteins, found by shotgun sequencing. Nature 302:718-721, 1983.

648. Nguyen, H.T., et al. Manuscript in preparation.

PARTICIPANTS

Everett Bandman, Ph.D., Assistant Professor, Department of Food Science and Technology, University of California, Davis, California.

Helen M. Blau, Ph.D., Assistant Professor, Department of Pharmacology, Stanford University School of Medicine, Stanford, California.

Margaret Buckingham, Ph.D., Department de Biologie Moleculaire, Institut - PASTEUR, Paris, France.

Abe Eastwood, Ph.D., Associate Director of Research, Muscular Dystrophy Association, New York, New York.

Charles P. Emerson, Ph.D., Professor of Biology, Department of Biology, University of Virginia, Charlottesville, Virginia.

Henry F. Epstein, M.D., Professor of Neurology, Cell Biology and Biochemistry, Baylor College of Medicine, Houston, Texas.

Donald Fischman, M.D., Harvey Klein Professor of Biomedical Sciences, Chairman, Department of Cell Biology and Anatomy, Cornell University Medical College, New York, New York.

James Garrels, Ph.D., Senior Staff Investigator, Cold Spring Harbor Laboratories, Cold Spring Harbor, New York.

Stephen D. Hauschka, Ph.D., Professor of Biochemistry, University of Washington, Seattle, Washington.

Joseph Y.H. Hoh, Ph.D., Professor of Physiology, University of Sydney, New South Wales, Australia.

Howard Holtzer, M.D., Professor of Anatomy, University of Pennsylvania School of Medicine, Philadelphia, Pennsylvania

R. Rodney Howell, M.D., Professor and Chairman, Department of Pediatrics, University of Texas Medical Center, Houston, Texas.

Laurence H. Kedes, M.D., Professor of Medicine, VA Hospital, Stanford University School of Medicine, Palo Alto, California.

Alan Kelly, Ph.D., Professor of Pathology, School of Veterinary Medicine, University of Pennsylvania, Philadelphia, Pennsylvania.

Louis Kunkel, Ph.D., Assistant Professor of Pediatrics, Children's Hospital Medical Center, Boston, Massachusetts.

Samuel Latt, M.D., Professor of Pediatrics and Genetics, Children's Hospital Medical Center and Harvard Medical School, Boston, Massachusetts.

Susan Lowey, Ph.D., Professor of Biochemistry, Rosentiel Center, Brandeis University, Waltham, Massachusetts.

Ryoichi Matsuda, Ph.D., Assistant Professor, Department of Zoology, University of California, Berkeley, California.

Alexander Mauro, M.D., Professor of Biophysics, Rockefeller University, New York, New York.

Armand Miranda, Ph.D., Assistant Professor of Pathology, Research Center for Muscular Dystrophy, Columbia University, New York, New York.

T.H. Oh, Ph.D., Associate Professor of Anatomy, University of Maryland School of Medicine, Baltimore, Maryland.

Eijiro Ozawa, Ph.D., Division of Cell Biology, National Center for Nervous, Mental and Muscular Disorders, Kodaira, Tokyo, Japan.

Dirk Pette, M.D., Professor of Biochemistry, Universitat Konstanz, Fachbereich Biologie, Konstanz, West Germany.

Lewis P. Rowland, M.D., Henry & Lucy Moses Professor and Chairman, Department of Neurology, Director of Neurological Service, Columbia Presbyterian Medical Center, New York, New York.

Neil Rubinstein, Ph.D., Associate Professor of Anatomy, Department of Anatomy, University of Pennsylvania, Philadelphia, Pennsylvania.

Edward Schultz, Ph.D., Associate Professor of Anatomy, Department of Anatomy, University of Wisconsin, Madison, Wisconsin

Emanuel E. Strehler, Ph.D., Research Fellow, Children's Hospital Medical Center, Harvard Medical School, Boston, Massachusetts.

Richard C. Strohman, Ph.D., Professor of Zoology, Department of Zoology, University of California, Berkeley, California.

Robert Whalen, Ph.D., Department de Biologie Moleculaire, Institut - PASTEUR, Paris, France.

Stewart Wolf, M.D., Director, Totts Gap Medical Research Laboratories, Bangor, Pennsylvania; Professor of Medicine, Temple University, Philadelphia, Pennsylvania.

Donald Wood, Ph.D., Associate Director of Research, Muscular Dystrophy Association, New York, New York.

David Yaffe, M.D., Professor of Cell Biology, The Weizmann Institute of Science, Rehovot, Israel.

INDEX

www.ingramcontent.com/pod-product-compliance
Ingram Content Group UK Ltd.
Pitfield, Milton Keynes, MK11 3LW, UK
UKHW051131260726
13967UKWH00010B/2980

* 9 7 8 1 4 6 8 4 4 9 0 8 2 *